Diabetic Retinopathy - Advancement in Understanding the Pathophysiology and Management Strategies

Edited by Mohd Imtiaz Nawaz

Published in London, United Kingdom

Diabetic Retinopathy - Advancement in Understanding the Pathophysiology and Management Strategies
http://dx.doi.org/10.5772/intechopen.1001713
Edited by Mohd Imtiaz Nawaz

Contributors
Alaa M. Mansour, Ana Lisa Carauni, Babak Baban, Balkissou Adamou Dodo, Durgul Acan, Erick A. Quiroz-Gonzalez, Fabio Patelli, Godefroy Koki, Inna Hadja, Joobin Khadamy, Josiane Mare Njoya, Khaled Elmasry, Lily Chacra, Luca M. Rossetti, Maria Laura Scopelliti, Miguel A. Quiroz-Gonzalez, Miguel A. Quiroz-Reyes, Mohd Imtiaz Nawaz, Nikita Dash, Patrice Esame, Roberta Rissotto, Samar Habib

First published in London, United Kingdom, 2024 by IntechOpen
IntechOpen is the global imprint of INTECHOPEN LIMITED, registered in England and Wales, registration number: 11086078, 167-169 Great Portland Street, London, W1W 5PF, United Kingdom

For EU product safety concerns: IN TECH d.o.o., Prolaz Marije Krucifikse Kozulić 3, 51000 Rijeka, Croatia, info@intechopen.com or visit our website at intechopen.com.

British Library Cataloguing-in-Publication Data
A catalogue record for this book is available from the British Library

Diabetic Retinopathy - Advancement in Understanding the Pathophysiology and Management Strategies
Edited by Mohd Imtiaz Nawaz
p. cm.
Print ISBN 978-0-85466-680-5
Online ISBN 978-0-85466-679-9
eBook (PDF) ISBN 978-0-85466-681-2

Meet the editor

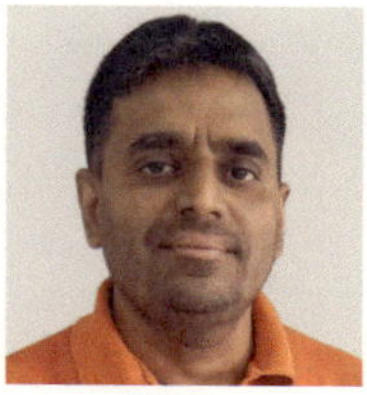

Mohd Imtiaz Nawaz, Ph.D., has 14 years of research experience in the pathophysiology of diabetic retinopathy (DR), a major vision-threatening eye complication in diabetic patients. He obtained his bachelor's and post-graduate degrees in biotechnology from premier universities in India. He was awarded a Ph.D. with "Doctor Europaeus" certification in Biomedical Sciences and Translational Medicine from the Department of Molecular and Translational Medicine, University of Brescia, Italy. He is currently an assistant professor in the Department of Ophthalmology, College of Medicine, King Saud University (KSU), KSA. His research areas include diabetes, diabetic retinopathy, cellular and molecular biology, angiogenesis, inflammation, oxidative stress, neurodegeneration, and biological activities of peptides. Dr. Nawaz has authored fifty-two peer-reviewed research articles and four book chapters and has edited several books. He has presented his research work at national and international conferences. He is the recipient of several fellowships, awards, and travel grants. He is also a journal reviewer, associate editor, and editorial board member of several international journals.

Contents

Preface

Diabetic retinopathy (DR) is a common neurovascular disease of the retina that causes serious vision loss in adults worldwide. Clinically, DR is classified as early-stage, non-proliferative diabetic retinopathy (NPDR) and advanced-stage proliferative diabetic retinopathy (PDR). PDR is the most advanced stage of the disease, characterized by retinal neovascularization, vitreous hemorrhage, traction retinal detachment, and formation of a fibrovascular epiretinal membrane.

Oxidative stress, inflammation, and angiogenesis are closely related processes that play a pivotal role in the initiation and progression of DR-associated pathogenesis. Prolonged and poorly managed hyperglycemia in diabetics leads to activation of neurovascular cells in the retina, causing the release of various locally acting factors, especially cytokines, into the retinal interstitium, vitreoretinal interface, and vitreous body. This creates a pathological signaling depot that, through systemic elevation of angio-inflammatory factors, triggers multiple biochemical pathways. These pathways, through secondary mediators and transcription factors, contribute to the biochemical derangements that advance DR.

Unfortunately, despite extensive laboratory and clinical investigations over the past several decades, the root cause of diabetes-associated vision loss remains uncertain. Moreover, the available treatment strategies, including laser photocoagulation, vitrectomy, excision of the epiretinal membranes, and pharmaceuticals, are either destructive or have limited successful implementation. Additionally, treatment interventions for PDR are also limited. Thus, there is a need for focused research to understand the mechanisms of initiation and progression of the disease and to explore new approaches for appropriate detection and cost-effective management of DR at its earliest stage, rather than waiting for the onset of non-manageable forms of vision-threatening lesions.

As such, this book, which is organized into three sections, provides a comprehensive overview of recent insights into DR. It covers cellular and molecular mechanisms, the role of angio-inflammatory mediators, and limitations of current treatment strategies. The final section explores potential future therapies, such as oral treatments, intravenous multi-target angiogenesis inhibitors, and gene therapy, aiming to enhance the management of DR.

Mohd Imtiaz Nawaz
Dr. Nasser Al-Rashid Research Chair in Ophthalmology,
Department of Ophthalmology,
College of Medicine,
King Saud University,
Riyadh, Saudi Arabia

Section 1

Understanding the Altered Pathophysiology and Pathological Pathways of Diabetic Retinopathy

Chapter 1

Perspective Chapter: Translational Implications of Proliferative Diabetic Retinopathy (PDR) Vitreous Fluid

Mohd Imtiaz Nawaz

Abstract

Proliferative diabetic retinopathy (PDR) is a neurovascular disease of the retina that causes severe vision loss in working adults worldwide. Hyperglycemia-induced dysregulated metabolic process activates neuro-vascular cells releasing numerous locally acting factors, particularly cytokines, into the vitreoretinal interface or vitreous body. In the pathological setting, vitreous forms an overwhelming "reservoir" by engaging an elevated level of various angiogenic and inflammatory mediators. Furthermore, an increase in the systemic level of angio-inflammatory factors in diabetic vitreous creates a depot of pathological signaling pathways by activating secondary mediators and transcriptional factors that propagate PDR pathogenesis. This chapter aims to discuss the relevance of the impaired vitreous microenvironment in sustaining and accelerating the pathogenesis of PDR. Additionally, we will discuss the PDR-vitreous fluid as helpful material for studying the patho-clinical events in the diabetic retina and obtaining pre-clinical, experimental evidence for developing new therapeutic drug candidates for PDR therapy.

Keywords: proliferative diabetic retinopathy (PDR), PDR-vitreous fluid, angiogenesis, inflammation, VEGF, translational implications

1. Introduction

Diabetes is a leading health problem of the twenty-first century. A chronic condition occurs when the body cannot produce enough insulin or respond appropriately to the insulin to metabolize the blood glucose. Globally, the World Health Organization (WHO) has ranked diabetes as the sixth leading cause of death, and every 6 seconds, a person dies from diabetes-related disorders. By 2040, the global prevalence of the diabetes epidemic has been projected to affect over 642 million people [1]. According to the International Diabetes Federation (IDF), alone in 2015, the estimated global economic burden to treat diabetes was around 700 billion USD (IDF Diabetes Atlas, 7th Ed., 2015). Clinically, diabetes and diabetes-associated complications are usually symptomless in their early stage.

Moreover, the incidents of undiagnosed diabetes and impaired glucose tolerance raise future concerns. There is not much success in the prevention or treatment of diabetes-associated complications. Thus, urgent measures are required to reduce the burden of diabetes which severely affects healthcare providers and people.

Clinically, diabetes is a metabolic disease and, in the long term, damages the macro- and microvessels of the heart, nerves, kidney, and retina. The pathogenesis of diabetes-associated complications is exceptionally complex. Several hyperglycemia-induced pathways have been proposed in the last few decades that subsequently initiate a cascade of pathological events via simultaneous involvement of oxidative stress, inflammation, and angiogenesis. Diabetes-associated complication includes nephropathy, neuropathy, and diabetic retinopathy (DR).

Diabetic retinopathy is a disease that damages the tiny blood vessels in the retina (the light-sensitive tissue that lines the back of the eye). It is the most common diabetic eye disease and is the leading cause of blindness among working adults worldwide. The risk of developing DR depends mainly on two factors, the type of diabetes and the duration of diabetes. Nearly, all patients with type 1 diabetes and about 77% of those with type 2 diabetes develop some form of retinopathy within the first 20 years of the disease (Report of WHO consultation in Geneva, Switzerland, 9–11 November 2005). The incidence of retinopathy usually increases with increasing duration. The correlation between the duration of diabetes and the development of retinopathy was first demonstrated in the Wisconsin Epidemiologic Study of Diabetic Retinopathy (WESDR), which showed that the prevalence of retinopathy was 8% at the first 3 years, 25% at 5 years, 60% at 10 years, and 80% at 15 years after the onset of diabetes. Among them, the prevalence of proliferative DR varied from 2.0% in persons who had diabetes for less than 5 years to 15.5% in persons who had diabetes for 15 or more years [2]. Extrapolating population-based studies to the global number of diabetic individuals, it is estimated that the number of people with DR will grow to 191.0 million by 2030 [3]. As the incidence of diabetes, moreover not adequately managed, is increasing exponentially, there is the possibility that, in the future, more individuals will suffer from severe forms of diabetic retinopathy.

The research in diabetic retinopathy has four main limiting factors.

1. Lack of proper animal models.

2. Unavailability of human retina samples at different degrees of pathology.

3. Lack of seriousness and or awareness of patients to understand the magnitude of diabetes complications

4. The success reports of most of the drugs in ameliorating diabetes-associated complications in the animal model are hardly translated into clinical practice.

Thus, there is an urgent need to develop a new approach for the detection, management, and cost-effective treatment of DR at its earliest stage, rather than wait for the onset of non-manageable forms of vision-threatening lesions.

Clinically, the vitreous fluid reflects events that are taking place in the retina during the pathogenesis of many eye disorders, including proliferative DR. Indeed, it is widely accepted that vitreous fluid acts as a surrogate or overwhelming reservoir to accelerate the events of DR. Studies demonstrate that the vitreoretinal surface act as a scaffold for the formation of retinal NV and vitreous hemorrhage in PDR [4]. Thus, vitreous fluid obtained from diabetic patients undergoing vitreoretinal surgery can be used to investigate the molecular events of disease and the intervention of potential therapeutic targets. Accordingly, the aim of this chapter is to study the changes occurring in the vitreous body during the onset of diabetes; to discuss the usefulness of PDR-vitreous fluid for studying the ongoing pathological events in the diabetic retina; and to obtain pre-clinical, experimental evidence for developing new therapeutic drug candidates for PDR therapy.

2. Clinical classification of DR

Diabetic retinopathy is regarded as microangiopathy, involving microvascular lesions that have been used as the criteria for evaluating and classifying the pathogenesis of DR [4]. Clinically, DR has been divided into an early, non-proliferative diabetic retinopathy (NPDR) and a later, advanced-stage proliferative diabetic retinopathy (PDR). NPDR is manifested by visible features, including microaneurysms, retinal hemorrhages, and intraretinal microvascular abnormalities (IRMA). Diabetic macular edema (DME), which occurs due to the breakdown of the blood-retinal barrier (BRB), is secondary to increased retinal vascular permeability and is the most common cause of vision loss in NPDR. PDR is the most advanced stage of DR, characterized by retinal neovascularization (NV), vitreous hemorrhage, traction retinal detachment, and the formation of a fibrovascular epiretinal membrane (ERM). Excessive neurovascular damage, retinal ischemia/hypoxia, and leukostasis are considered major players in the initiation and progression of PDR (Reviewed in [5, 6]).

3. Pathogenesis of proliferative DR (PDR)

Normal vision depends on intact cell-cell communication among the neuronal, glial, microglial, vascular, and pigmented epithelial cells of the retina. Diabetic retinopathy is a multifactorial condition arising from the complex interplay between biochemical and metabolic abnormalities, and it involves almost all cells of the retina.

3.1 Cellular causes

The retina consists of several cells, and the normal vision depends on intact cell-cell communication among them. The normal BRB is maintained by signaling between neurons, glia, pericytes, and endothelium to provide an ideal microenvironment. However, hyperglycemia-mediated activation of metabolic pathways dysregulates the normal functioning of most of the retinal cells, including blood capillaries and surrounding supporting cells. Diabetes damages vascular cells (endothelial cells and pericytes), neurons (photoreceptors, bipolar, and ganglions), glia (Muller cells and astrocytes), microglia, and pigmented epithelial cells.

Diabetic retinopathy is classically defined by its vascular lesions. However, several studies demonstrate that microangiopathy is only a single aspect of widespread retinal dysfunction. Indeed, the increase in apoptosis of most cells in the retina is observed in animal models of DR and post-mortem analysis of retinas from diabetic patients [7]. Moreover, collective evidence supports the hypothesis that neurodegeneration, together with functional changes in the microvasculature, has an essential role in the progression of diabetic retinopathy [8]. Before establishing visible histopathological changes due to neuro-vascular damage in the diabetic eye, cells are activated to produce several mediators such as growth factors, vasoactive agents, and adhesion molecules [5]. The factors released, primarily cytokines, are detrimental to surrounding cells and, through the feed-forward cycle (paracrine signaling), simultaneously activate another cell to release locally acting cytokines [9]. The increase in the systemic level of these factors induces several biochemical pathways that are implicated in the initiation and progression of DR.

3.2 Molecular causes

Pathogenesis associated with PDR is enormously complicated. During the past few decades, hyperglycemia has been considered the major contributor and upstream inducer in the initiation and progression of damage in the diabetic retina. Various interconnecting biochemical pathways have been suggested as potential links between hyperglycemia and DR (**Figure 1**). These include activation of protein kinase C (PKC) [10, 11], poly(ADP-ribose) polymerase (PARP) [12], stimulation of sorbitol-aldose reductase (polyol) [13], hexosamine pathway [14], activation of rennin-angiotensin system (RAS) [15], increased formation of advanced glycation end products (AGEs) [16], and production of excess reactive oxygen species (ROS) [17]. A growing body of evidence suggests that hypertension and dyslipidemia are also major risk factors in the development and progression of DR [18, 19]. After that, flux through all these pathways leads to a cascade of events to initiate angio-inflammation responses and promote neuro-vascular damage of the diabetic retina (**Figure 1**). Consequently, several randomized clinical data indicate that tight glycemic and blood pressure control,

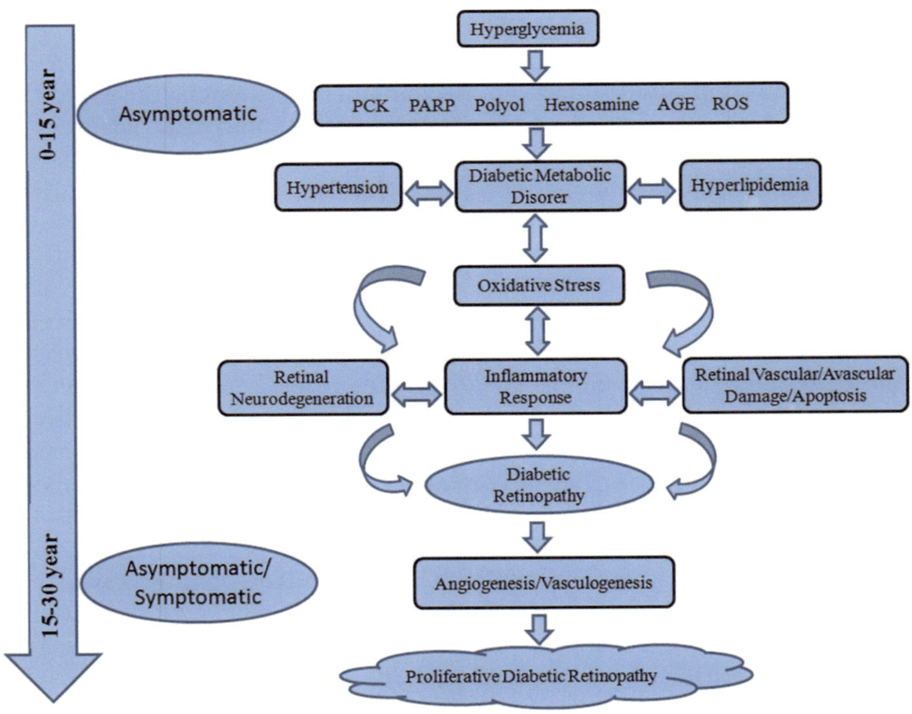

Figure 1.
A schematic presentation of hyperglycemia-induced complications in proliferative diabetic retinopathy.

including lipid-lowering agents, have beneficial effects in reducing the incidence and progression of DR (reviewed in [20, 21]). Despite these measures still, the number of DR patients is growing. Indeed, each therapeutic approach has its limitations. The concept of metabolic memory also remains a major hindrance to the effective management of diabetic complications [22]. The mechanisms for metabolic memory are not fully known, but vitreous may be highly relevant to the storage of this long-term signal. The resistance of DR to reverse could be attributed to the accumulation of metabolites such as AGEs and ROS, which are not easily removed even after good glycemic or blood pressure control is established [23]. Moreover, current pharmacological interventions are often non-selective, lack specificity, and in the long term, show side effects. For the last several decades, laser photocoagulation (a destructive technique) and vitrectomy remain the two conventional approaches for treating severe sight-threatening conditions such as macular edema, vitreous hemorrhage, the formation of the epiretinal membrane, and NV that are hallmark features of PDR [21]. Despite extensive laboratory and clinical investigations, the fundamental root cause of vision loss due to diabetes remains uncertain. The involvement and crosstalk of various molecular pathways in hyperglycemia-induced diabetic retinopathy are summarized schematically in **Figure 1**.

4. Anatomical/structural and molecular study of the vitreous body

4.1 Anatomical consideration

Anatomically, the eye's interior has two fluid-filled cavities: the anterior segment and the posterior segment, which play a vital role in maintaining ocular function. The anterior segment (space between the cornea and lens) is divided into two by the pupil (aperture of the iris), creating the anterior chamber and the posterior chamber that is filled with aqueous humor (**Figure 2**). Conversely, the posterior segment is filled with vitreous humor (commonly called vitreous). Usually, vitreous does not undergo

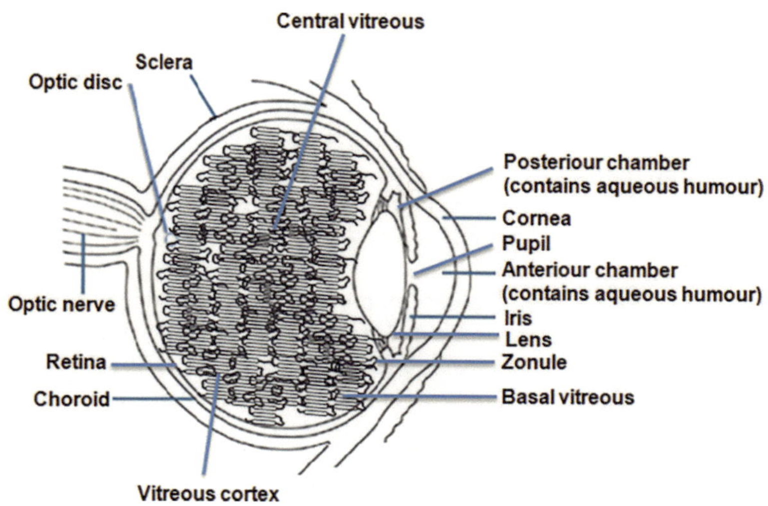

Figure 2.
A schematic illustration of vitreous distribution within a human eye. Depending on differing rheological properties, and fibrillar collagen concentration, vitreous is subdivided into different regions.

a regular formation and drainage process as does the aqueous humor. Vitreous is a spherical structure surrounded by the retina, lens, and, pars plana of the eye. The vitreous body can be divided into the central vitreous, the basal vitreous, the vitreous cortex, and the zonule [24]. Each vitreous region has different viscoelasticity due to the differences in collagen fibrillar concentration and orientation. The posterior vitreous cortex (vitreoretinal interface) is attached to the retina via intermediary macromolecules such as laminin, fibronectin, chondroitin sulfate, and other extracellular matrix components. Generally, the posterior vitreous cortex is considered a "metabolic center" of the vitreous. The vitreous is normally acellular; however, phagocytic mononuclear hyalocytes are found in the vitreous cortex and basal vitreous [24]. The diagram showing the human eye's general anatomy with the vitreous distribution and orientation is summarized in **Figure 2**.

4.2 Molecular constituents

Vitreous, permanently formed at birth, is a delicate transparent gel made up of water (99%), and salts (0.9%), and the remaining constituent includes a variety of proteins and polysaccharides. Structurally, the healthy adult human vitreous constitutes parallel collagen fibrils packed into bundles aggregate to form visible fibers. The collagen fibrils are at their lowest concentration within the central vitreous or higher in the basal vitreous. Vitreous collagen fibrils are morphologically distinct from collagen in other connective tissues. Indeed, they are almost similar to cartilage-collagen composed of $\alpha1$ type II chains [25, 26]. A study with a pepsinized form of collagen has demonstrated that vitreous fibril is made of a central core of collagen types V/XI molecule surrounded by type II collagen. The extensions of the N-propeptide form of type II collagen from the surface of the fibril mediate interaction with other extracellular components of the vitreous. Additionally, the presence of type IX collagen on the surface of vitreous collagen fibril probably plays a significant role in this regard [27, 28]. The human vitreous also contains a small amount of type VI collagen that forms separate microfibrils [29, 30]. Type VI collagen has been shown to link together the heterotypic collagen fibril and hyaluronic acid in the vitreous [31]. The study shows the presence of minor collagen protein endostatin, an inhibitor of angiogenesis and its progenitor collagen type XVIII in the vitreous [32]. The distribution of endostatin encompasses the internal limiting lamina of the retina, the anterior vitreous behind the lens, and the ciliary body. The distribution of endostatin provides inhibition of cell migration and proliferation within the vitreous body, thus preventing vessels from sprouting into the vitreous avascular compartments [33]. The loss-of-function mutation in collagen XVIII causes severe myopia, vitreoretinal degeneration, and retinal detachment in a patient with Knobloch syndrome, suggesting its critical role in the eye [34].

In mammalian vitreous, the glycosaminoglycans (GAGs) and water molecules fill the interfibrillar space. The predominant GAGs of mammalian vitreous is non-sulfated hyaluronan (HA), while sulfated GAGs, including chondroitin sulfate (CS) and heparan sulfate (HS), represent a minor component of the vitreous [35]. All GAGs, except HA, are usually covalently linked to a protein core, called proteoglycan, and post-synthesis undergo a varying degree of modifications by sulphation, epimerization, and acetylation/deacetylation. Polymeric HA is composed of the repeating disaccharide unit [β1-4glucuronic acid β1-3 N-acetylglucosamine]n, which forms a network through entanglement within the vitreous body. This initial biosynthetic product of HA is very long, and it is modified before being secreted into the extracellular environment. It is believed that collagen fibril is spaced apart by HA via interaction with the CS chains of type IX collagen. However, this shielding diminishes with aging, resulting in vitreous liquefaction and weakening of vitreoretinal adhesion [36].

Proteomic analysis using an in-depth mass spectrometric approach suggests that human vitreous microfibrils contain a few minor non-collagenous glycoproteins. Among them, fibrillin represents the major structural component of the zonules, whereas opticin is intense in the basal and cortical regions [37, 38]. Studies showed that vitreous has fibrillin-1 and fibrillin-2 isoforms. In patients with Marfan syndrome, a mutation in the gene encoding fibrillin-1 can cause ectopia lentis, vitreous liquefaction and an increased propensity toward rhegmatogenous retinal detachment [39, 40]. The presence of opticin, which belongs to the family of leucine-rich repeat protein/proteoglycans, plays a role in vitreoretinal adhesion and provides an anti-angiogenic environment in the vitreous. The study demonstrates that opticin binds to retinal growth hormone [41], type II collagen-containing fibrils, and GAGs, including HS and CS [42]. The murine oxygen-induced retinopathy (IOR) model concluded that opticin is an anti-angiogenic mediator that inhibits pre-retinal NV in a dose-dependent manner. Moreover, the opticin knockout mice produce significant pre-retinal NV compared to the wild-type mice [43]. This suggests that, among several molecules, opticin may be the most important one that contributes to vitreous anti-angiogenic properties.

The study also showed the presence of the sizeable versican-like proteoglycan [44]. The versican-like proteoglycan in the vitreous is bound to HA, which the link proteins stabilize to form a considerable supramolecular complex. The formation of this complex contributes to maintaining the integrity and viscoelasticity of the vitreous [45].

5. Aging of the vitreous body

The network of collagen fibrils is essential to maintain the gel state of the vitreous. Human adult vitreous consists of a combination of gel and liquid. The gel is composed of a fragile, fibrous collagen network, and the liquid is viscoelastic HA. The vitreous viscoelasticity is dependent on a combination of the concentration and molecular size of the HA molecules. After birth, no new collagen fibrils, but only HA molecules, are produced to keep pace with and fill the globe as it develops. Up to 4 years, no liquid vitreous is found in human eyes [46]. However, as the eye grows, up to the age of 20 years, the fluid volume slowly increases and fills about 20% of the total vitreous volume. With age, the volume of the liquid vitreous increases, and, consequentially, the volume of the gel vitreous steadily decreases. The remodeling of the vitreous matrix starts at a very early age and continues the old age, albeit at a slower pace. The phenomenon of liquefaction of the vitreous body, known as "synchisis," is the most common degenerative change occurring in a geriatric condition causing mild to severe vision loss. It is not known what initiates synchisis, but some invoke metabolic dysfunction or/and light-induced production of ROSs may cause conformational changes in vitreous macromolecules [47, 48]. The ultrastructural study shows that, in aging vitreous, the collagen fibrils aggregate into macroscopic strands that result in their distribution within the vitreous gel [49]. The collagen microfibrils are connected and spaced apart by the CS chains of type IX collagen. However, with aging, there is also a loss of type IX collagen from the fibril surface, combined with increased surface exposure of type II collagen, leading to collagen fibrillar aggregation [36]. Hyaluronidase digestion of HA results in deflation and relaxation of the collagen network in the vitreous body [50]. Usually, in aging vitreous, the HA level significantly decreases [51]. Like any other tissue in the body, the vitreous is also vulnerable to aging. With aging, vitreous liquefaction occurs due to the localized breakdown of the gel structure and aggregation of the fibrils [52]. Moreover, the phenomenon of vitreous liquefaction is a frequent precursor for "vitreochisis" (a split in the posterior vitreous) and posterior vitreous detachment (PVD), which indeed can cause a precocious retinal break and detachment [53].

During PVD, the posterior vitreous cortex separates from the retina's internal limiting membrane (ILM). In aging vitreous, the frequency of occurrence of partial or complete PVD increases [54]. An individual who experiences synchisis without concurrent dehiscence at the vitreoretinal interface may experience anomalous PVD [55]. Usually, PVD is not a serious threat to vision, but the patient notes a spider-like floater in front of the eye, which moves in the gaze direction. In acute PVD, there is a strong vitreoretinal adhesion at the peripheral retina, thus causing a retinal tear. Scanning electron micrographs of the retinal surface after PVD showed remnants of an outermost layer of cortical vitreous collagen remaining on the ILM [56, 57]. This split in the posterior vitreous cortex (vitreoschisis) induces a different set of vitreomacular pathologies [58] and is prevalent in modulating the events in proliferative diabetic retinopathy.

6. Vitreous state during diabetes

At first glance, the vitreous appears to be a redundant tissue; however, the vitreous body and the vitreoretinal interface have a crucial influence on the pathophysiology of the eye. Firstly, the vitreous fluid acts as a biochemical depot to mitigate the biochemical derangements of diabetes-associated complications. Secondly, diabetic vitreous plays a significant role in accelerating the events of visual loss. Most of the effects in the vitreous are due to intrinsic changes that occur in response to diabetes. With the progression of diabetes, the set of pathologic changes in the vitreous, concurrent with events at the retina, is known as "diabetic vitreopathy" [59]. Thus, the study of vitreous alteration in diabetes at the molecular and structural level is needed to understand their role in the progression of DR and the development of possible therapeutic interventions.

6.1 Structural alteration

HA interacts with collagen fibrils to form a three-dimensional supramolecular complex by separating collagen fibrils in a normal vitreous. HA stabilizes and maintains the vitreous transparency to minimize light scattering and maximize photon transmission to the retina. However, not unlike aging, the diabetic vitreous undergoes metabolic derangement. It causes collagen's cross-linking primarily by glycation and depolymerization of HA, resulting in premature vitreous liquefaction and PVD. Non-invasive dynamic light scattering (DLS) measurement found macroscopic fibers of greater heterogeneity and larger particle sizes in vitreous subjects with diabetes as compared to age-matched controls [60]. The collagenous nature of macroscopic fibers was investigated and confirmed using electron microscopy and Raman spectroscopy [61, 62]. DLS spectroscopy was employed for in vivo analysis of the abnormal molecular behavior of vitreous molecules in patients with diabetes afflicted with a varied degree of diabetic retinopathy [63].

The duration and severity of diabetes affect the structure of the vitreous body and the posterior vitreoretinal interface. The vitreoretinal interface is a site of normal physiology. It has three components: the inner limiting membrane (ILM), the posterior vitreous cortex, and an intervening extracellular matrix (ECM) responsible for vitreoretinal adhesion. Diabetes causes changes in each of these three components and contributes to a variety of vitreoretinal disorders. Changes in the posterior vitreous cortex and ILM increase vitreoretinal adhesion and may contribute to the tendency to initiate DR-associated vitreoschisis, PVD, vitreous hemorrhage, and retinal NV. The ILM is the basement for retinal Müller cells and is composed of collagen type IV fibers, glycosaminoglycans, laminin, and fibronectin. ILM provides a support surface to inner neuro-vascular cells. However, prolonged diabetes is considered to be deleterious, affecting the vitreoretinal interface, and might be one of the reasons for the uncontrolled vasculogenesis in the eyes [64]. On histological examination, due to the invasion of macrophages, the thickness of the ILM in the DR group is significantly increased compared with that in the control group [65]. It is hypothesized that this thick and disrupted ILM is less conductive, that is, preventing egress of fluid or inversely causing accumulation of fluid in the macula (small area at the center of the retina). The source of the fluid is due to leakage in the retinal blood vessels. Both in normal and chronic diabetic conditions, the phenomenon of cell proliferation, migration, differentiation, and adhesion of cells and other cellular functions are influenced by components of surrounding ECM (mainly fibronectin and laminin). The events of cross-linking due to non-enzymatic glycation and the formation of AGEs may occur between proteins of cortical vitreous (primarily type II collagen) and the proteins of ILM (primarily type IV collagen). The study demonstrated that the formation of AGEs in the ILM activates pathological AGE/RAGE signaling pathways in underlying Müller cells [66]. Indeed, the accommodation of AGEs within the ILM can disrupt normal interactions between Müller cells and the component of ECM such as integrin signaling [67]. Added, changes at the vitreoretinal interface result in the generation of proliferating cellular vitreous, determined by the proliferation of different types of cells to form fibro-cellular ERMs. The formation of ERMs on the ILM surface of the retina consists of cellular components and ECM proteins such as fibronectin and collagen [68, 69]. In turn, cells of ERM are themselves a source of locally acting cytokines that exaggerate the events of PDR. A study of pre-retinal membranes as removed during vitrectomy in PDR suggests that multilayer membrane expresses ECM proteins, including type II collagen (vitreal collagen), that could in turn act as scaffolding in the formation of ERMs [68, 70]. Additionally, abnormalities at the vitreoretinal interface include retinal traction that lay serious complications in PDR. The possible consequence can be summarized as follows:

- If there is an insufficient weakening of vitreoretinal adhesion, there could be vitreoschisis that may provide a scaffold for the formation of cellular ERM.

- If there is sufficient weakening of vitreoretinal adhesion, an innocuous PVD may occur.

- If there is strong adhesion at the vitreoretinal interface, the traction may cause the rupture of abnormal new vessels and vitreous hemorrhage.

- There can be tractional retinal detachment if strong adhesion over a broad area at the vitreoretinal interface.

- If there is traction upon the macula, diabetic macular edema can be observed.

The firmly attached vitreous also represents a paracrine depot for pathological signals that may contribute to the progression of diabetic retinopathy.

6.2 Molecular alteration

As discussed, hyperglycemia causes activation of several metabolic stress pathways. An important outcome is the oxidation of sugars and the formation of AGEs. Studies demonstrate the localization of AGEs in retinal blood vessels, which correlates with the degree of retinopathy in diabetes patients [71, 72]. The study was supported by the accumulation of AGEs in the serum and the vitreous cavity of patients with DR [73, 74]. Systemically, AGE precursors target the receptor of AGE (RAGE) on endothelial cells, glia, mesangial cells, and macrophages. The activation of the AGE/RAGE axis causes the activation of numerous kinases, activating the pleiotropic transcription factor and ROS production. However, the most intriguing aspect is the formation of AGEs on the structural proteins of the vitreous, in particular, on the collagen, resulting in a crosslinking of collagen fibril and other proteins. This observation was supported by the fact that the elevated glucose level in diabetic vitreous increases the probability of collagen glycation [75]. Indeed, vitreous collagen derived from diabetic patients was found to have significantly higher levels of the crosslink dihydroxylysinonorleucine than that of control subjects [76]. Levels of AGEs were almost 20 times higher in diabetic vitreous compared with the vitreous of controls. The role of hyperglycemia-induced accommodation of AGEs in collagen cross-linking was characterized using Fourier transform Raman spectroscopy [62, 77].

The second mechanism suggests that AGEs in the diabetic vitreous may accelerate the depolymerization of HA, the second major macromolecule of vitreous. In the presence of riboflavin (a photosensitizer), the use of photo-induced vitreous liquefaction demonstrated that irradiation with white light causes oxidative damage and depolymerization of HA in vitreous [47, 78]. AGEs, which are usually higher in the diabetic vitreous, were explicitly shown to accelerate the associated depolymerization of HA and cause vitreous liquefaction [79, 80]. Thus, together, both cross-linking of vitreous collagen and degradation of HA may contribute to diabetes-related synchysis, vitreoschisis, and an early PVD [81].

7. Role of vitreous in accelerating the pathological events of PDR

The present prevalent concept of the pathology of proliferative diabetic retinopathy is mostly emphasized as a neuro-vascular disorder, without much consideration for the role of vitreous. In chronic diabetic conditions, the vitreous undergoes metabolic derangements to exacerbate the event of PDR. Indeed, the impact and involvement of vitreous in the initiation and progression of PDR could be termed "proliferative diabetic vitreoretinopathy" (PDVR) [4]. Clinically, PDR develops only if the vitreoretinal interface is partially or entirely attached to the retinal surface, which acts as a scaffold for the proliferation of new vessels. The process of retinal NV, an essential outcome of later stages of PDR, usually tends to occur at the site of the vitreoretinal junction. The newly formed vessels grow away from the retinal surface to breach into the cortex vitreous and entangle with vitreous microfibrils [82, 83]. Inversely, the study suggests that, in areas of PVD, the new vessels could also breach into the ILM and grow along the retinal surface to form abortive clumps [82, 84]. The clinical investigation confirmed that a partial PVD is more common than a complete

PVD in PDR diabetes [85]. Complete PVD was uncommon among those diabetic patients with PDR [86] and, conversely, vitrectomy prevented recurrence of retinal NV [87]. Thus, the occurrence of complete PVD is a protection against the formation of florid neovascularization and to development of aggressive PDR. It is likely that vitrectomy or vitreous detachment allows clearance of angiogenic factors away from the retinal surface and enhances oxygen circulation around the retinal surface [88] or oxygenation from the ciliary body. Together these observations support the concept of the involvement of vitreous, and especially of the vitreoretinal interface, in the progression of PDR.

Hyperglycemia causes activation of neurovascular cells by releasing numerous locally acting factors, particularly cytokines, into the retinal interstitium, or at the vitreoretinal interface, or into the vitreous body, creating a depot of pathological signaling. An increase in the systemic level of factors in diabetic patients induces several biochemical pathways through the activation of secondary mediators and transcriptional factors that mitigate biochemical derangements in the progression of PDR. Vitreous can thus form an overwhelming "reservoir" of pathological paracrine signals, such as AGE, angio-inflammatory mediators, and others [5]. The relative circulation of these cytokines into and out of lacunae within the vitreous is unknown. Still, a stagnant pocket of liquid within a vitreoschisis cavity could concentrate cytokines and produce a depot effect. The presence of a vitreoschisis cavity, especially around the macula, may increase the duration and potency of the cytokines within the diabetic retina [89]. The modern proteomic technique can simultaneously quantify the protein level in the human vitreous with or without diabetes [90]. Proteomic analysis from the diabetic vitreous sample demonstrates hundreds of locally produced mediators of the angio-inflammatory signaling pathway taking part in the progression of PDR. However, it is difficult to interpret the aggressive "paracrine depot effect" of diabetic vitreous for several reasons:

- Different experiments and technical approaches have different sensitivity. This could give variation in estimating the level of the analytes.

- Quantification of signaling proteins, like vascular endothelial growth factor (VEGF), does not relate to their potency in mediating signaling pathways.

- Due to technical limitations, sometimes cytokines with low concentrations are not detected. It could be because cytokines are bound tightly to vitreous components or, inversely, are prevented from acting locally by their sequestration.

- BRB breakdown or vitreous hemorrhage, which often occurs in PDR, produces an influx of serum proteins, such as growth factors, into the vitreous fluid. This could give an overestimation of the vitreous level of mediators in diabetic patients compared to control.

- The vitreous sample reflects the level of degree of diabetes-related pathology. However, individual patients or patients from different regions and ethnic groups often respond differently to disease.

Thus, a generalization of the involvement of the estimated level of mediators in PDR vitreous fluid cannot be compared with the degree of the pathogenesis of the disease. This cautions about the interpretation of data.

8. Therapies in the management of PDR

The management of modifiable risk factors, including hyperglycemia, hypertension, and dyslipidemia, is the first step to minimizing the risk of proliferative diabetic retinopathy. The Diabetes Control and Complications Trial (DCCT) and the United Kingdom Prospective Diabetes Study (UKPDS) demonstrated that the tight control of both blood glucose levels and hypertension is associated with a lower risk of retinopathy compared to conventional therapy in type 1 and type 2 diabetes [91, 92]. Treatment with lipid-lowering drugs reduces the level of serum cholesterol, low-density lipoprotein, triglycerides, and retinal hard exudates, including the risk of developing PDR [93]. However, there is no firm evidence supporting the concept of tight glucose and blood pressure treatment goals, especially in patients with advanced stages of DR. The data from several randomized controlled trials studies are not conclusive due to wide variation in age, disease progression, macrovascular risks, as well as the patient's lifestyle and disease management capabilities [94, 95]. Indeed, tight glycemic control has clinically two acute adverse effects: (a) there is a risk of early worsening of DR [91, 96] and (b) frequent severe hypoglycemic episodes [91]. Moreover, recommended goals from the clinical trials are most often difficult to achieve in many patients. Still, DR remains the leading cause of blindness in working adults worldwide, thereby further highlighting the need to develop effective treatment strategies.

The early treatment diabetic retinopathy study (ETDRS) and diabetic retinopathy study (DRS) have demonstrated current laser photocoagulation treatment for DR has changed little since its inception; albeit it is applied only after the onset of NV to reduce peripheral and night vision, it is uncomfortable, destructive, and expensive [21]. Moreover, despite repeated laser photocoagulation, it is established that, in about 50% of patients, retinopathy progresses, with scars continuously enlarging over time, leading to a decrease in night vision, color vision, and peripheral vision, as well as loss of 1–2 lines of visual acuity in some patients [97]. In the diabetic retinopathy vitrectomy study (DRVS), a microsurgical procedure in the eye is also employed to remove any scar tissue or blood leaks in the vitreous after vitreous hemorrhages, to protect the macula and to improve vision [98].

Although laser photocoagulation treatment and vitrectomy remain the standard care for treating severe complications of PDR, these treatments are either destructive or their successful implementation approaches are limited. Further, the treatment strategies, especially for advanced PDR, also rely chiefly on the conventional surgical removal of the epiretinal membranes from the retina's surface, allowing the retina to remodel and reattach. Despite dramatic developments, vitreoretinal surgery for epiretinal membranes is often dissatisfying anatomically and functionally [99, 100]. Thus, current treatment interventions for advanced PDR are limited. Novel pharmaceutical approaches are thus urgently needed for the management to reduce the incidence of the pathogenesis of diabetic retinopathy significantly.

9. Vascular endothelial growth factor (VEGF): a significant player in the pathogenesis of PDR

In the progression of PDR, recent evidence indicated that tissue hypoxia leads to an upregulation of various vasoactive effectors and angiogenic growth factors to initiate the process of retinal neovascularization. The presence of an increased level of a variety of growth factors in the vitreous and epiretinal membranes supports its role in the pathogenesis of PDR. Both pro- and anti-angiogenic proteins are detected in the vitreous throughout disease stages, with the balance moving toward the pro-angiogenic environment. Each angiogenic factor may likely operate in coordination or a cascade with other growth factors.

The vitreous gel structure promotes the persistence of angiogenic factors and aids in its eventual dispersion throughout the vitreous body. Among several growth factors, VEGF level is increased many folds in the diabetic eye is considered as a primary angiogenesis factor for vascular endothelial cells and increases vascular permeability. It is produced by multiple cell types in the retina in diabetes, including Mueller cells, ganglion cells, and pericytes. There are six members of the VEGF family: VEGF-A, VEGF-B, VEGF-C, VEGF-D, VEGF-E, and placental-derived growth factor (PlGF) [101]. VEGF-A is the most widely studied member about the pathogenesis of diabetic retinopathy. The complexity of the VEGF-A family is increased by alternative splicing or processing by matrix metalloproteinases to generate isoforms VEGF-A_{121}, VEGF-A_{145}, VEGF-A_{165}, and VEGF-A_{189} (the numbers indicating amino acid residues in the human polypeptides) [102]. Compared with VEGF-A_{121}, VEGF-A_{165} is more potent, and data from animal and clinical studies have demonstrated that it is a significant player in the development and progression of diabetic retinopathy [103, 104]. Decreased levels of the dominant-negative splice variant VEGF-A_{165b} were found in vitreous samples from patients with diabetic retinopathy, suggesting that a molecular switch between the VEGF-A_{165} (hereafter referred to as VEGF) and VEGF-A_{165b} could be involved in the development of diabetic retinopathy [105]. Presently, the role of VEGF-B in PDR remains unclear, and data indicate that they are either not involved or play a minor role in the pathogenesis of PDR [106]. However, a recent study reported that vitreous level VEGF-B was found to significantly increase in PDR patients. This increase is substantially higher as the disease is at a more advanced stage [107].

Studies with clinical specimens have shown a strong correlation between increased intraocular VEGF levels and PDR development. In the diabetic retina, many factors can contribute to the over-expression of VEGF, including tissue hypoxia, inflammatory cytokines, growth factors, and ROS [108]. VEGF increases vascular permeability in the ischemic retina and promotes angiogenesis via stimulation of endothelial cell growth, causing neovascularisation and breakdown of the BRB. To exaggerate the event of pathogenesis, the elevated level of VEGF enhances the adhesion of leukocytes to vascular walls. It increases the up-regulation of inflammatory mediators, including the leukocyte adhesion molecules like intercellular adhesion molecule-1 (ICAM-1) and vascular cell adhesion molecule-1 (VCAM-1) in the diabetic retina [109]. The elevated level of adhesion molecules promotes cytokine productions that, in turn, mediate the inflammatory response and stimulate the further release of VEGF.

10. Anti-VEGF therapies

The discovery of the role of VEGF in diabetic retinopathy has led to the development of anti-VEGF agents as therapies, and currently, four anti-VEGF agents have been used in the management of diabetic retinopathy: pegaptanib (Macugen; Pfizer, Inc., New York, USA), bevacizumab (Avastin; Genentech, Inc.), ranibizumab (Lucentis; Genentech, Inc., South San Francisco, California, USA), and aflibercept/VEGF Trap-Eye (Eylea; Pharmaceuticals, Inc., Tarrytown, New York, USA). Pegaptanib is a pegylated RNA aptamer directed against the VEGF-A_{165} isoform. It was the first FDA-approved ophthalmologic anti-VEGF agent for the treatment of retinal NV in DME [110]. In phases I, II, and III prospective clinical trials, pegaptanib appeared to improve visual acuity outcomes and regress neovascularization [111, 112]. Bevacizumab is a full-length recombinant humanized antibody active against all isoforms of VEGF-A. Case reports and small nonrandomized pilot studies have reported using the off-label intravitreal bevacizumab (IVB) to treat DME, vitreous hemorrhage, retinal or iris NV, and various complications of PDR [113–115]. However, to date, all studies regarding IVB (1.25 mg) for DME therapy have demonstrated transient beneficial effects with a requirement for repeated injections. Short-term results, according to the ETDRS criteria, suggest that combined IVB and pan-retinal photocoagulation achieved rapid clearance of VH, regression of retinal NV, and visual improvement in the treatment of high-risk PDR [116]. Ranibizumab is a recombinant humanized monoclonal antibody fragment that lacks the Fc domain and is specific to bind all isoforms of human VEGF-A. Few pilot studies of intravitreal ranibizumab injection demonstrated an improved visual acuity in patients with DME (reviewed in [117]. Aflibercept/VEGF Trap-Eye is a 115 kDa recombinant fusion protein consisting of the VEGF-binding domains of human VEGF receptors 1 (VEGFR1) and VEGFR2 fused to the Fc domain of human IgG1. Aflibercept is used against VEGF-A, and PlGF, and early clinical results suggest efficacy for the treatment of DR [118].

11. Limitation of anti-VEGF therapies

Withstanding all efforts, the results of several studies have not yielded promising results for the use of anti-VEGF treatments in DR-associated pathogenesis. The long-term effects of VEGF inhibition in the eye require close monitoring. Limitations to anti-VEGF interventions may exist and include short duration of action, the presence of adverse side effects, and poor response in a significant percentage of patients [119, 120]. As well, the constitutive expression of VEGF and its receptors in normal adult choriocapillaris and neuroretina suggests that it plays a neuroprotective role in the survival of vascular as well as neuronal elements [121], and there appears a link between the use of anti-VEGF drugs and the death of neuroretinal cells involved in visual function [122]. Furthermore, various pro-inflammatory and angiogenic factors other than VEGF may play a role in PDR (reviewed in [5, 123]), causing resistance to anti-VEGF interventions. This observation, therefore, indicates that the pathogenesis of PDR is multifactorial, and many other factors beyond VEGF may play a role in this process. Thus, novel approaches targeting additional pathways, increasing target affinity, and lengthening treatment durability are eagerly required for an efficacious therapy of PDR.

12. Implications of PDR vitreous fluid

The recent publication demonstrates that vitreous fluid obtained from vitreoretinal surgery can be widely used in exploring the pathological events taking place in the diabetic retina (reviewed in [124]). The most relevant applications are as follows:

a. Vitreous fluid as a tool in identifying biomarkers for early detection of diabetic retinopathy:

Diabetic retinopathy research has several limiting factors. Indeed, experimental data implicate that increased oxidative stress induced-angio-inflammatory response damages neurovascular components early in the diabetic retina and may further accelerate the DR-associated clinical pathology [125, 126]. Thus, vitreous fluid obtained from patients with early signs of DR, having a different pathological setting, could serve as a tool in identifying biomarkers for early detection of diabetic retinopathy. This could help to study cost-effective therapeutic intervention for the management of DR at its earliest stage, rather than waiting for the onset of non-manageable forms of the disease.

b. Angiogenic and inflammatory activity of PDR vitreous fluid

The capacity of PDR vitreous fluid to elicit a potent angiogenic and inflammatory activity in various preclinical *in vitro*, *ex vivo,* and *in vivo* experimental models has been recently described [124, 127, 128]. This capacity may represent a useful tool to study the involvement of dysregulated angio-inflammatory mediators in the pathogenesis of diabetic retinopathy.

c. PDR vitreous fluid for translational research

The use of PDR vitreous fluid as a stimulus in angiogenesis assays can provide preclinical experimental evidence for the discovery of new pharmacologic treatment strategies in the management of diabetic retinopathy [127–129].

As detailed, the clinical and experimental investigations point toward the fact that the vitreous plays a crucial role in developing PDR. Other than conventional methods, therapeutic aims must also be directed to prevent diabetic vitreopathy or eliminate vitreoretinal-adhesion, the events necessary for the development of retinal neovascularization PDR. The evidence that vitreous fluid is a sort of repository where inflammatory/angiogenic factors and metabolites accumulate [5], representing a surrogate of the events taking place in the diabetic retina, makes its use a valuable tool for a preclinical evaluation of therapeutic drugs. Accordingly, recent observations have shown that vitreous fluid samples obtained from PDR patients after *pars plana* vitrectomy can induce a series of angiogenic/inflammatory responses in endothelial cells in vitro and in vivo [129–134]. These activities have been exploited for the characterization of novel anti-angiogenic molecules with different mechanisms of action [129–131].

Keeping together this observation, the human vitreous fluid obtained from PDR patients after *pars plana* vitrectomy could be exploited as a novel tool to evaluate potential drug candidates for the treatment of PDR. Thus, in this context, a work by Sara Rezzola et al. developed a novel 3D-endothelial cell spheroid/human vitreous assay for a rapid and cost-effective experimental procedure suitable for the evaluation of the anti-angiogenic activity of novel extracellular and intracellular drug candidates using PDR vitreous fluid as a pro-angiogenic stimulus [127].

13. Concluding remarks

Diabetic retinopathy is a common neurovascular disease of the retina that causes serious vision loss in working adults worldwide. Angiogenesis and inflammation are closely related processes that play a pivotal role in the initiation and progression of proliferative diabetic retinopathy pathogenesis. Indeed, hyperglycemia causes activation of neurovascular cells through the release of numerous locally acting factors, particularly cytokines, into the retinal interstitium or at the vitreoretinal interface or into the vitreous body creating a depot of pathological signaling [124]. An increase in the systemic level of factors in diabetic vitreous in turn induces various biochemical pathways through the activation of secondary mediators and transcriptional factors that mitigate biochemical derangements in the progression of PDR [5, 127]. In the pathological setting, the vitreous can thus form an overwhelming "reservoir" through engaging an elevated level of a variety of angiogenic and inflammatory mediators. The relevance of impaired vitreous microenvironment, thus, plays a role both in sustaining and accelerating the angio-inflammatory responses during the pathogenesis of proliferative diabetic retinopathy. Additionally, vitreous fluid is a helpful material to study the ongoing pathological pathways in the diabetic retina and to demonstrate experimental evidence for developing new therapeutic drugs for the management of PDR.

Author details

Mohd Imtiaz Nawaz[1,2]

1 Department of Ophthalmology, College of Medicine, King Saud University, Riyadh, Saudi Arabia

2 Dr. Nasser Al-Rashid Research Chair in Ophthalmology, King Abdulaziz University Hospital, Riyadh, Saudi Arabia

*Address all correspondence to: mnawaz@ksu.edu.sa

References

[1] Ogurtsova K et al. IDF diabetes atlas: Global estimates for the prevalence of diabetes for 2015 and 2040. Diabetes Research and Clinical Practice. 2017;**128**:40-50

[2] Klein R et al. The Wisconsin epidemiologic study of diabetic retinopathy. III. Prevalence and risk of diabetic retinopathy when age at diagnosis is 30 or more years. Archives of Ophthalmology. 1984;**102**(4):527-532

[3] Zheng YF, He MG, Congdon N. The worldwide epidemic of diabetic retinopathy. Indian Journal of Ophthalmology. 2012;**60**(5):428-431

[4] Kroll P, Rodrigues EB, Hoerle S. Pathogenesis and classification of proliferative diabetic vitreoretinopathy. Ophthalmologica. 2007;**221**(2):78-94

[5] Semeraro F et al. Diabetic retinopathy: Vascular and inflammatory disease. Journal Diabetes Research. 2015;**2015**:582060

[6] Ola MS et al. Recent advances in understanding the biochemical and molecular mechanism of diabetic retinopathy. Journal of Diabetes and its Complications. 2012;**26**(1):56-64

[7] Barber AJ et al. Neural apoptosis in the retina during experimental and human diabetes—Early onset and effect of insulin. Journal of Clinical Investigation. 1998;**102**(4):783-791

[8] Ola MS et al. Neurodegeneration and neuroprotection in diabetic retinopathy. International Journal of Molecular Sciences. 2013;**14**(2):2559-2572

[9] Antonetti DA et al. Diabetic retinopathy—Seeing beyond glucose-induced microvascular disease. Diabetes. 2006;**55**(9):2401-2411

[10] Koya D, King GL. Protein kinase C activation and the development of diabetic complications. Diabetes. 1998;**47**(6):859-866

[11] Geraldes P, King GL. Activation of protein kinase C isoforms and its impact on diabetic complications. Circulation Research. 2010;**106**(8):1319-1331

[12] Zheng L, Szabo C, Kern TS. Poly(ADP-ribose) polymerase is involved in the development of diabetic retinopathy via regulation of nuclear factor-kappa B. Diabetes. 2004;**53**(11):2960-2967

[13] Lorenzi M. The polyol pathway as a mechanism for diabetic retinopathy: Attractive, elusive, and resilient. Experimental Diabetes Research. 2007;**2007**:61038

[14] Du XL et al. Hyperglycemia-induced mitochondrial superoxide overproduction activates the hexosamine pathway and induces plasminogen activator inhibitor-1 expression by increasing Sp1 glycosylation. Proceedings of the National Academy of Sciences of the United States of America. 2000;**97**(22):12222-12226

[15] Satofuka S et al. (pro)renin receptor-mediated signal transduction and tissue renin-angiotensin system contribute to diabetes-induced retinal inflammation. Diabetes. 2009;**58**(7):1625-1633

[16] Schleicher ED, Wagner E, Nerlich AG. Increased accumulation of the glycoxidation product N-epsilon(carboxymethyl)lysine in human tissues in diabetes and aging.

Journal of Clinical Investigation. 1997;**99**(3):457-468

[17] Ido Y, Kilo C, Williamson JR. Cytosolic NADH/NAD(+), free radicals, and vascular dysfunction in early diabetes mellitus. Diabetologia. 1997;**40**:S115-S117

[18] Cardoso CRL et al. Predictors of development and progression of retinopathy in patients with type 2 diabetes: Importance of blood pressure parameters. Scientific Reports. 2017;**7**(1):4867

[19] van Leiden HA et al. Blood pressure, lipids, and obesity are associated with reteinopathy—The Hoorn study. Diabetes Care. 2002;**25**(8):1320-1325

[20] Nawaz MI et al. Novel drugs and their targets in the potential treatment of diabetic retinopathy. Medical Science Monitor. 2013;**19**:300-308

[21] El-Asrar AM, Al-Mezaine HS, Ola MS. Changing paradigms in the treatment of diabetic retinopathy. Current Opinion in Ophthalmology. 2009;**20**(6):532-538

[22] Reddy MA, Zhang EL, Natarajan R. Epigenetic mechanisms in diabetic complications and metabolic memory. Diabetologia. 2015;**58**(3):443-455

[23] Kowluru RA. Diabetic retinopathy, metabolic memory and epigenetic modifications. Vision Research. 2017;**139**:30-38

[24] Bishop PN. Structural macromolecules and supramolecular organisation of the vitreous gel. Progress in Retinal and Eye Research. 2000;**19**(3):323-344

[25] Swann DA, Constable IJ, Harper E. Vitreous structure. 3. Composition of bovine vitreous collagen. Investigative Ophthalmology. 1972;**11**(9):735-738

[26] Swann DA, Caulfield JB, Broadhurst JB. The altered fibrous form of vitreous collagen following solubilization with pepsin. Biochimica et Biophysica Acta. 1976;**427**(1):365-370

[27] Seery CM, Davison PF. Collagens of the bovine vitreous. Investigative Ophthalmology and Visual Science. 1991;**32**(5):1540-1550

[28] Bishop PN et al. Extraction and characterization of the tissue forms of collagen types II and IX from bovine vitreous. The Biochemical Journal. 1994;**299**(Pt 2):497-505

[29] Bishop P et al. Type VI collagen is present in human and bovine vitreous. Graefe's Archive for Clinical and Experimental Ophthalmology. 1996;**234**(11):710-713

[30] Bu SC et al. The ultrastructural localization of type II, IV, and VI collagens at the vitreoretinal Interface. PLoS One. 2015;**10**(7):e0134325

[31] Kielty CM et al. Type VI collagen microfibrils: Evidence for a structural association with hyaluronan. The Journal of Cell Biology. 1992;**118**(4):979-990

[32] Maatta M et al. Collagen XVIII/endostatin shows a ubiquitous distribution in human ocular tissues and endostatin-containing fragments accumulate in ocular fluid samples. Graefe's Archive for Clinical and Experimental Ophthalmology. 2007;**245**(1):74-81

[33] Ohlmann AV et al. Localization of collagen XVIII and endostatin in the human eye. Current Eye Research. 2005;**30**(1):27-34

[34] Fukai N et al. Lack of collagen XVIII/endostatin results in eye abnormalities. The EMBO Journal. 2002;**21**(7):1535-1544

[35] Noulas AV et al. Variations in content and structure of glycosaminoglycans of the vitreous gel from different mammalian species. Biomedical Chromatography. 2004;**18**(7):457-461

[36] Bishop PN et al. Age-related changes on the surface of vitreous collagen fibrils. Investigative Ophthalmology and Visual Science. 2004;**45**(4):1041-1046

[37] Cain SA et al. Proteomic analysis of fibrillin-rich microfibrils. Proteomics. 2006;**6**(1):111-122

[38] Reich M et al. Proteomic analysis of vitreous humor in retinal vein occlusion. PLoS One. 2016;**11**(6):e0158001

[39] Yamanouchi K et al. Fibrillin-1 and fibrillin-2 are essential for formation of thick oxytalan fibers in human nonpigmented ciliary epithelial cells in vitro. Connective Tissue Research. 2012;**53**(1):14-20

[40] Milla E et al. Novel FBN1 mutation causes Marfan syndrome with bilateral ectopia lentis and refractory glaucoma. European Journal of Ophthalmology. 2012;**22**(4):667-669

[41] Sanders EJ et al. Opticin binds retinal growth hormone in the embryonic vitreous. Investigative Ophthalmology and Visual Science. 2003;**44**(12):5404-5409

[42] Hindson VJ et al. Opticin binds to heparan and chondroitin sulfate proteoglycans. Investigative Ophthalmology and Visual Science. 2005;**46**(12):4417-4423

[43] Le Goff MM et al. The vitreous glycoprotein opticin inhibits preretinal neovascularization. Investigative Ophthalmology and Visual Science. 2012;**53**(1):228-234

[44] Reardon A et al. The large chondroitin sulphate proteoglycan versican in mammalian vitreous. Matrix Biology. 1998;**17**(5):325-333

[45] Theocharis AD et al. Occurrence and structural characterization of versican-like proteoglycan in human vitreous. Biochimie. 2002;**84**(12):1237-1243

[46] Sebag J. Aging of the vitreous. Eye-Transactions of the Ophthalmological Societies of the United Kingdom. 1987;**1**:254-262

[47] Ueno N et al. Effects of visible-light irradiation on vitreous structure in the presence of a photosensitizer. Experimental Eye Research. 1987;**44**(6): 863-870

[48] Kakehashi A, Ueno N, Chakrabarti B. Molecular mechanisms of photochemically induced posterior vitreous detachment. Ophthalmic Research. 1994;**26**(1):51-59

[49] Sebag J. Age-related-changes in human vitreous structure. Graefes Archive for Clinical and Experimental Ophthalmology. 1987;**225**(2):89-93

[50] Bishop PN, McLeod D, Reardon A. Effects of hyaluronan lyase, hyaluronidase, and chondroitin ABC lyase on mammalian vitreous gel. Investigative Ophthalmology and Visual Science. 1999;**40**(10):2173-2178

[51] Itakura H et al. Decreased vitreal hyaluronan levels with aging. Ophthalmologica. 2009;**223**(1):32-35

[52] Los LI et al. Age-related liquefaction of the human vitreous body: LM and TEM evaluation of the role of

proteoglycans and collagen. Investigative Ophthalmology and Visual Science. 2003;**44**(7):2828-2833

[53] Hikichi T. Time course of posterior vitreous detachment in the second eye. Current Opinion in Ophthalmology. 2007;**18**(3):224-227

[54] Wang J et al. Age-dependent changes in the basal retinovitreous adhesion. Investigative Ophthalmology and Visual Science. 2003;**44**(5):1793-1800

[55] Sebag J. Anomalous posterior vitreous detachment: A unifying concept in vitreo-retinal disease. Graefe's Archive for Clinical and Experimental Ophthalmology. 2004;**242**(8):690-698

[56] Kishi S, Demaria C, Shimizu K. Vitreous cortex remnants at the fovea after spontaneous vitreous detachment. International Ophthalmology. 1986;**9**(4):253-260

[57] Sebag J. Vitreoschisis. Graefes Archive for Clinical and Experimental Ophthalmology. 2008;**246**(3):329-332

[58] Gupta P et al. Vitreoschisis in macular diseases. British Journal of Ophthalmology. 2011;**95**(3):376-380

[59] Sebag J. Diabetic vitreopathy. Ophthalmology. 1996;**103**(2):205-206

[60] Sebag J et al. Dynamic light scattering of diabetic vitreopathy. Diabetes Technology and Therapeutics. 1999;**1**(2):169-176

[61] Faulborn J, Dunker S, Bowald S. Diabetic vitreopathy—Findings using the celloidin embedding technique. Ophthalmologica. 1998;**212**(6):369-376

[62] Sebag J et al. Raman spectroscopy of human vitreous in proliferative diabetic retinopathy. Investigative Ophthalmology and Visual Science. 1994;**35**(7):2976-2980

[63] Fankhauser F. Analysis of diabetic vitreopathy with dynamic light scattering spectroscopy—Problems and solutions related to photon correlation. Acta Ophthalmologica. 2012;**90**(3):e173-e178

[64] Ljubimov AV et al. Basement membrane abnormalities in human eyes with diabetic retinopathy. The Journal of Histochemistry and Cytochemistry. 1996;**44**(12):1469-1479

[65] Matsunaga N et al. Histopathologic evaluation of the internal limiting membrane surgically excised from eyes with diabetic maculopathy. Retina. 2005;**25**(3):311-316

[66] Barile GR et al. The RAGE axis in early diabetic retinopathy. Investigative Ophthalmology and Visual Science. 2005;**46**(8):2916-2924

[67] Stitt AW. AGEs and diabetic retinopathy. Investigative Ophthalmology and Visual Science. 2010;**51**(10):4867-4874

[68] Hosoda Y et al. Epiretinal membrane of proliferative diabetic retinopathy: An immunohistochemical study. Ophthalmic Research. 1993;**25**(5):289-294

[69] Ioachim E et al. Immunohistochemical study of extracellular matrix components in epiretinal membranes of vitreoproliferative retinopathy and proliferative diabetic retinopathy. European Journal of Ophthalmology. 2005;**15**(3):384-391

[70] George B et al. Extracellular matrix proteins in epiretinal membranes and in diabetic retinopathy. Current Eye Research. 2009;**34**(2):134-144

[71] Murata T et al. The relationship between accumulation of advanced

glycation end products and expression of vascular endothelial growth factor in human diabetic retinas. Diabetologia. 1997;**40**(7):764-769

[72] Stitt AW. Advanced glycation: An important pathological event in diabetic and age related ocular disease. British Journal of Ophthalmology. 2001;**85**(6):746-753

[73] Ono Y et al. Increased serum levels of advanced glycation end-products and diabetic complications. Diabetes Research and Clinical Practice. 1998;**41**(2):131-137

[74] Katagiri M et al. Evaluation of vitreous levels of advanced glycation end products and angiogenic factors as biomarkers for severity of diabetic retinopathy. International Ophthalmology. 2018;**38**(2):607-615

[75] Lundquist O, Osterlin S. Glucose concentration in the vitreous of nondiabetic and diabetic human eyes. Graefe's Archive for Clinical and Experimental Ophthalmology. 1994;**232**(2):71-74

[76] Sebag J et al. Biochemical abnormalities in vitreous of humans with proliferative diabetic retinopathy. Archives of Ophthalmology. 1992;**110**(10):1472-1476

[77] Avery NC, Bailey AJ. The effects of the maillard reaction on the physical properties and cell interactions of collagen. Pathologie Biologie (Paris). 2006;**54**(7):387-395

[78] Akiba J, Ueno N, Chakrabarti B. Mechanisms of photo-induced vitreous liquefaction. Current Eye Research. 1994;**13**(7):505-512

[79] Deguine V et al. Free radical depolymerization of hyaluronan by maillard reaction products: Role in liquefaction of aging vitreous. International Journal of Biological Macromolecules. 1998;**22**(1):17-22

[80] Katsumura C et al. Effects of advanced glycation end products on hyaluronan photolysis: A new mechanism of diabetic vitreopathy. Ophthalmic Research. 2004;**36**(6):327-331

[81] Foos RY et al. Posterior vitreous detachment in diabetic subjects. Ophthalmology. 1980;**87**(2):122-128

[82] Faulborn J, Bowald S. Microproliferations in proliferative diabetic retinopathy and their relationship to the vitreous: Corresponding light and electron microscopic studies. Graefe's Archive for Clinical and Experimental Ophthalmology. 1985;**223**(3):130-138

[83] Muqit MM, Stanga PE. Swept-source optical coherence tomography imaging of the cortical vitreous and the vitreoretinal interface in proliferative diabetic retinopathy: Assessment of vitreoschisis, neovascularisation and the internal limiting membrane. The British Journal of Ophthalmology. 2014;**98**(7):994-997

[84] Wong HC, Sehmi KS, McLeod D. Abortive neovascular outgrowths discovered during vitrectomy for diabetic vitreous haemorrhage. Graefe's Archive for Clinical and Experimental Ophthalmology. 1989;**227**(3):237-240

[85] Tagawa H, McMeel JW, Trempe CL. Role of the vitreous in diabetic retinopathy. II. Active and inactive vitreous changes. Ophthalmology. 1986;**93**(9):1188-1192

[86] Akiba J, Arzabe CW, Trempe CL. Posterior vitreous detachment and neovascularization in diabetic

retinopathy. Ophthalmology. 1990;**97**(7):889-891

[87] Blankenship GW, Machemer R. Long-term diabetic vitrectomy results. Report of 10 year follow-up. Ophthalmology. 1985;**92**(4):503-506

[88] Stefansson E. Physiology of vitreous surgery. Graefe's Archive for Clinical and Experimental Ophthalmology. 2009;**247**(2):147-163

[89] Agarwal D et al. The vitreomacular Interface in diabetic retinopathy. Journal of Ophthalmology. 2015;**2015**:392983

[90] Wang H et al. Characterisation of the vitreous proteome in proliferative diabetic retinopathy. Proteome Science. 2012;**10**(1):15

[91] Nathan DM et al. The effect of intensive treatment of diabetes on the development and progression of long-term complications in insulin-dependent diabetes mellitus. The New England Journal of Medicine. 1993;**329**(14):977-986

[92] UK Prospective Diabetes Study Group. Tight blood pressure control and risk of macrovascular and microvascular complications in type 2 diabetes: UKPDS 38. UK Prospective Diabetes Study Group. BMJ. 1998;**317**(7160):703-713

[93] Chew EY et al. Association of elevated serum lipid levels with retinal hard exudate in diabetic retinopathy. Early treatment diabetic retinopathy study (ETDRS) report 22. Archives of Ophthalmology. 1996;**114**(9):1079-1084

[94] Fullerton B et al. Intensive glucose control versus conventional glucose control for type 1 diabetes mellitus. Cochrane Database of Systematic Reviews. 2014;**2**:CD009122

[95] Do DV et al. Blood pressure control for diabetic retinopathy. Cochrane Database of Systematic Reviews. 2015;**1**:CD006127

[96] Early worsening of diabetic retinopathy in the diabetes control and complications trial. Archives of Ophthalmology. 1998;**116**(7):874-886

[97] Maeshima K et al. Progressive enlargement of scattered photocoagulation scars in diabetic retinopathy. Retina. 2004;**24**(4):507-511

[98] Flynn HW Jr et al. Pars plana vitrectomy in the early treatment diabetic retinopathy study. ETDRS report number 17. The early treatment diabetic retinopathy study research group. Ophthalmology. 1992;**99**(9):1351-1357

[99] Charteris DG et al. Proliferative vitreoretinopathy-developments in adjunctive treatment and retinal pathology. Eye (London, England). 2002;**16**(4):369-374

[100] Pastor JC, de la Rua ER, Martin F. Proliferative vitreoretinopathy: Risk factors and pathobiology. Progress in Retinal and Eye Research. 2002;**21**(1):127-144

[101] Koch S, Claesson-Welsh L. Signal transduction by vascular endothelial growth factor receptors. Cold Spring Harbor Perspectives in Medicine. 2012;**2**(7):a006502

[102] Koch S et al. Signal transduction by vascular endothelial growth factor receptors. The Biochemical Journal. 2011;**437**(2):169-183

[103] Ishida S et al. VEGF164 is proinflammatory in the diabetic retina. Investigative Ophthalmology and Visual Science. 2003;**44**(5):2155-2162

[104] Wirostko B, Wong TY, Simo R. Vascular endothelial growth factor and diabetic complications. Progress in Retinal and Eye Research. 2008;**27**(6):608-621

[105] Perrin RM et al. Diabetic retinopathy is associated with a switch in splicing from anti- to pro-angiogenic isoforms of vascular endothelial growth factor. Diabetologia. 2005;**48**(11):2422-2427

[106] Kinoshita S et al. Vitreous levels of vascular endothelial growth factor-B in proliferative diabetic retinopathy. Acta Ophthalmologica. 2016;**94**(6):e521-e523

[107] Mesquita J et al. VEGF-B levels in the vitreous of diabetic and non-diabetic patients with ocular diseases and its correlation with structural parameters. Medicinal Sciences (Basel). 2017;**5**(3):17

[108] Penn JS et al. Vascular endothelial growth factor in eye disease. Progress in Retinal and Eye Research. 2008;**27**(4):331-371

[109] Joussen AM et al. Retinal vascular endothelial growth factor induces intercellular adhesion molecule-1 and endothelial nitric oxide synthase expression and initiates early diabetic retinal leukocyte adhesion in vivo. American Journal of Pathology. 2002;**160**(2):501-509

[110] Cunningham ET et al. A phase II randomized double-masked trial of pegaptanib, an anti-vascular endothelial growth factor aptamer, for diabetic macular edema. Ophthalmology. 2005;**112**(10):1747-1757

[111] Adamis AP et al. Changes in retinal neovascularization after pegaptanib (macugen) therapy in diabetic individuals. Ophthalmology. 2006;**113**(1):23-28

[112] Starita C et al. Vascular endothelial growth factor and the potential therapeutic use of pegaptanib (macugen) in diabetic retinopathy. Developments in Ophthalmology. 2007;**39**:122-148

[113] Castillo J et al. Preoperative bevacizumab administration in proliferative diabetic retinopathy patients undergoing vitrectomy: A randomized and controlled trial comparing interval variation. American Journal of Ophthalmology. 2017;**183**:1-10

[114] Parikh RN et al. Intravitreal bevacizumab for the treatment of vitreous Hemorrhage due to proliferative diabetic retinopathy. American Journal of Ophthalmology. 2017;**176**:194-202

[115] Avery RL et al. Intravitreal bevacizumab (avastin) in the treatment of proliferative diabetic retinopathy. Ophthalmology. 2006;**113**(10):1695 e1-1695 15

[116] Yang CS et al. Intravitreal bevacizumab (avastin) and panretinal photocoagulation in the treatment of high-risk proliferative diabetic retinopathy. Journal of Ocular Pharmacology and Therapeutics. 2013;**29**(6):550-555

[117] Dervenis N et al. Ranibizumab in the treatment of diabetic macular edema: A review of the current status, unmet needs, and emerging challenges. Advances in Therapy. 2017;**34**(6):1270-1282

[118] Do DV et al. One-year outcomes of the da Vinci study of VEGF trap-eye in eyes with diabetic macular edema. Ophthalmology. 2012;**119**(8):1658-1665

[119] Kieran MW, Kalluri R, Cho YJ. The VEGF pathway in cancer and disease: Responses, resistance, and the path forward. Cold Spring

Harbor Perspectives in Medicine. 2012;**2**(12):a006593

[120] van Wijngaarden P, Qureshi SH. Inhibitors of vascular endothelial growth factor (VEGF) in the management of neovascular age-related macular degeneration: A review of current practice. Clinical and Experimental Optometry. 2008;**91**(5):427-437

[121] Sun FY, Guo X. Molecular and cellular mechanisms of neuroprotection by vascular endothelial growth factor. Journal of Neuroscience Research. 2005;**79**(1-2):180-184

[122] Latzer P, Schlegel U, Theiss C. Morphological changes of cortical and hippocampal neurons after treatment with VEGF and bevacizumab. CNS Neuroscience and Therapeutics. 2016;**22**(6):440-450

[123] Urias EA et al. Novel therapeutic targets in diabetic macular edema: Beyond VEGF. Vision Research. 2017;**139**:221-227

[124] Nawaz IM et al. Human vitreous in proliferative diabetic retinopathy: Characterization and translational implications. Progress in Retinal and Eye Research. 2019;**72**:100756

[125] Kowluru RA, Mishra M. Oxidative stress, mitochondrial damage and diabetic retinopathy. Biochimica et Biophysica Acta. 2015;**1852**(11):2474-2483

[126] Simó R, Stitt AW, Gardner TW. Neurodegeneration in diabetic retinopathy: Does it really matter? Diabetologia. 2018;**61**(9):1902-1912

[127] Rezzola S et al. 3D endothelial cell spheroid/human vitreous humor assay for the characterization of anti-angiogenic inhibitors for the treatment of proliferative diabetic retinopathy. Angiogenesis. 2017;**20**(4):629-640

[128] Sara Rezzola et al. Inflammation and N-formyl peptide receptors mediate the angiogenic activity of human vitreous humour in proliferative diabetic retinopathy. 2017;**60**(4):719-728

[129] Rezzola S et al. Therapeutic potential of anti-angiogenic multitarget N,O-sulfated E. Coli K5 polysaccharide in diabetic retinopathy. Diabetes. 2015;**64**(7):2581-2592

[130] Dal Monte M et al. Antiangiogenic effectiveness of the urokinase receptor-derived peptide UPARANT in a model of oxygen-induced retinopathy. Investigative Ophthalmology and Visual Science. 2015;**56**(4):2392-2407

[131] Rezzola S et al. Inflammation and N-formyl peptide receptors mediate the angiogenic activity of human vitreous humour in proliferative diabetic retinopathy. Diabetologia. 2017;**60**(4):719-728

[132] Watanabe D et al. Erythropoietin as a retinal angiogenic factor in proliferative diabetic retinopathy. The New England Journal of Medicine. 2005;**353**(8):782-792

[133] Yang J et al. Vitreous humor and albumin augment the proliferation of cultured retinal precursor cells. Journal of Neuroscience Research. 2009;**87**(2):495-502

[134] Murugeswari P et al. Angiogenic potential of vitreous from proliferative diabetic retinopathy and Eales' disease patients. PLoS One. 2014;**9**(10):e107551

Chapter 2

Diabetic Macular Edema

Fabio Patelli, Ana Lisa Carauni, Roberta Rissotto, Lily Chacra, Maria Laura Scopelliti and Luca M. Rossetti

Abstract

Diabetic macular edema (DME) is defined as the buildup of fluid within the retina in the extracellular space, specifically at the level of the macula in the inner nuclear, outer plexiform, Henle's fiber layer, and subretinal space. Diabetes mellitus is one of the leading causes of visual impairment in industrialized countries and DME is the main reason for vision drop in diabetic patients. Several diagnostic methods are available for the characterization and staging of diabetic retinopathy (DR) and DME; the principal one for DME is optical coherence tomography (OCT), a quick and non-invasive technique that helps in decision-making for therapeutic choices based on biomarkers. Various classifications have been suggested over the years to aid in treatment management for DME. Current therapeutic options include laser photocoagulation, anti-VEGF (vascular endothelial growth factor) intravitreal injections or corticosteroids, and surgery. Recently, a surgical approach has been proposed with pars plana vitrectomy (PPV) in case vitreomacular traction is present together with DME. Refractory DME is a challenging scenario, and it may be managed by switching to a different class of intravitreal medications or with surgical intervention or micropulse laser. Future perspectives include artificial intelligence algorithms based on OCT and OCT-angiography images which may improve diagnosis and treatment of DME with better preservation of visual acuity in diabetic patients.

Keywords: macular edema, optical coherence tomography (OCT), fluorescein angiography, anti-VEGF, corticosteroids, laser photocoagulation, biomarkers, vitreoretinal surgery, artificial intelligence

1. Introduction

Diabetes mellitus (DM) is not just a health problem, but a global pandemic, with alarming projections indicating an increase in the number of people affected in the coming years. It is estimated that by 2040, the number of people affected by diabetes will soar to 642 million, an increase of 62% over 2015 [1]. This escalation is mainly attributed to the parallel rise in obesity rates and the lengthening life expectancy of the world's population, underscoring the urgency of addressing this burgeoning health crisis.

Within the broad spectrum of complications arising from this disease, diabetic retinopathy (DR) emerges as one of the leading causes of vision loss in individuals affected by this disease. Specifically, within the DR landscape, diabetic macular edema (DME) emerges as the main culprit responsible for the decrease in visual acuity (VA) in patients suffering from this complication.

The severity of DR, including proliferative DR (PDR), affects vision and is a critical prognostic indicator for overall life expectancy. It underscores the urgency of effective therapeutic interventions to prevent visual impairment and blindness [2].

Given the serious implications of DR and DME for both individual well-being and public health, it is imperative to explore and develop effective therapeutic strategies to mitigate its impact. This chapter aims to delve into the current landscape of therapeutic interventions for DR and DME, highlighting advances, challenges, and future directions in the field.

1.1 Materials and methods

All images used in this chapter belong to patients followed up in our retinal outpatient clinic at ASST Santi Paolo e Carlo Hospital in Milan, Italy, where the privacy and confidentiality of patients' identities are guaranteed.

Optical coherence tomography (OCT), infrared (IR), autofluorescence, and fluorescein angiography (FA) pictures were taken with Spectralis spectral-domain optical coherence tomography (SD-OCT) (Heidelberg Engineering, Heidelberg, Germany).

2. Pathophysiology

The gold standard for preventing DR and DME is good glycemic control, along with control of other DM parameters such as arterial tension and lipids. The most important factor in the pathogenesis of DR is hyperglycemia, which acts on different molecular pathways and damages the blood-retinal barrier (BRB). The pathological process leading to DME is highly complex, including a sequence of events such as angiogenesis, inflammation, and an overexpression of vascular endothelial growth factor (VEGF). It remains unclear whether angiogenesis following VEGF overexpression is a cause or a consequence of inflammation [3].

Diabetic retinopathy (DR) stems from three main factors: vascular wall lesions, alterations in blood flow, and platelet dysfunction. These factors, along with others, combine to form the underlying lesions of DR: exudation and ischemia.

Exudation and the resulting macular edema appear as a consequence of an imbalance between the liquid passing from retinal vessels to the extracellular space and the reabsorption of the liquid from the extracellular space into the vessels.

There are two types of macular edema: cytotoxic edema, where the liquid is intracellular, and vasogenic edema, where the liquid is extracellular. In DME, we have both forms of edema: cytotoxic edema at the earlier stages and vasogenic edema at the later stages [3].

Ischemia is induced by platelet dysfunction and arteriolar changes leading to vascular occlusion and diminished perfusion. Changes in blood flow, such as erythrocyte hyperaggregability, also contribute to this ischemic state. The obstruction and loss of retinal capillaries eventually lead to retinal hypoxia and ischemia. In an attempt to revascularize the ischemic areas, the retina produces VEGF.

Vascular endothelial growth factor, which is higher in the vitreous of DR patients, is involved in the genesis of PDR and DME by inducing changes in the vascular bed, the rupturing of the blood-retinal barrier, and the induction of angiogenesis [4].

3. Diagnostic methods in DME

Timely diagnosis of DME is crucial for the prevention of irreversible complications in individuals with diabetes. Tools such as OCT and fluorescein angiography (FA) help us to perform thorough assessments and targeted management strategies that aid in preserving visual health.

3.1 Fluorescein angiography

Fluorescein angiography (FA) allows the visualization of leakage from microaneurysms or capillaries and areas of retinal ischemia. Focal leakage from microaneurysms leads to focal DME, in contrast with diffuse DME when scarcely demarcated areas of capillary leakage are present. FA is a more invasive and time-consuming procedure than OCT, yet it is still the only imaging technique to detect vascular leakage (**Figures 1** and **2**). Moreover, it is crucial when planning a retinal laser treatment

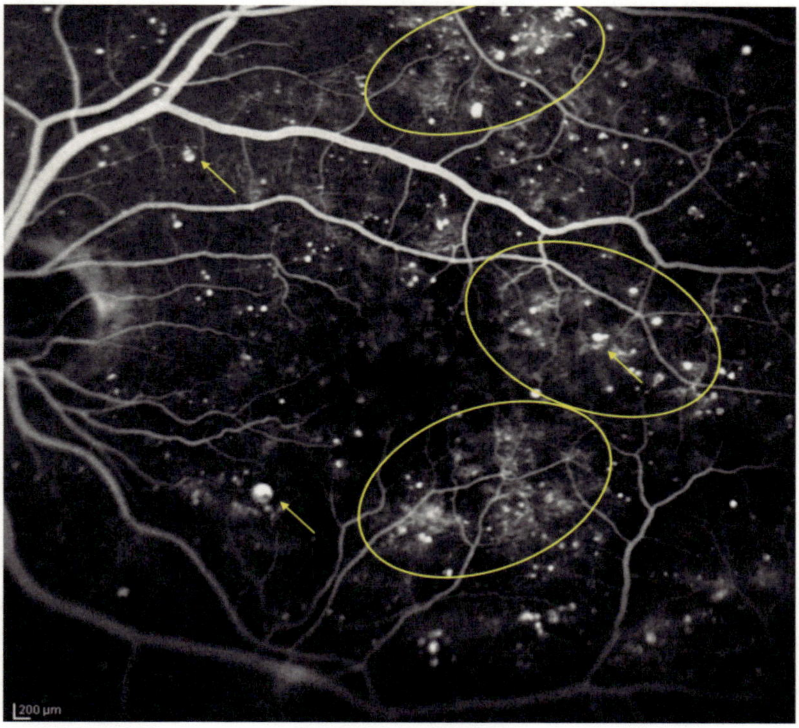

Figure 1.
Fluorescein angiography, SPECTRALIS® scanning laser angiography, intermediate phase, showing multiple microaneurysms in the context of diabetic retinopathy (arrows indicate some of the dozens of microaneurysms). Microaneurysms are visible as variably sized hyperfluorescent dots. Areas of multifocal leakage are visible as poorly demarcated hyperfluorescence (as seen in the circles) from incompetent retinal capillaries, microaneurysms, and microvascular abnormalities.

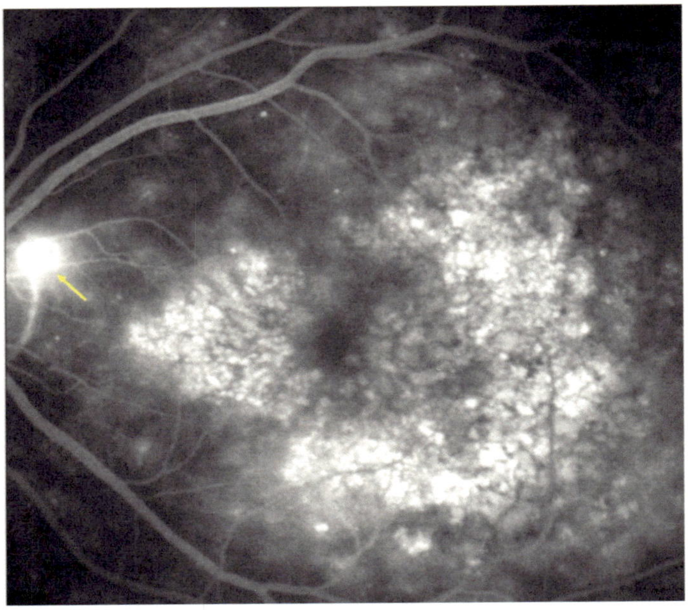

Figure 2.
Fluorescein angiography, SPECTRALIS® scanning laser angiography, late phase. Perifoveal cystoid macular edema is visible as areas of late pooling of the dye, and peripapillary neovessels are seen as bright spots of enhanced leakage (arrow).

since only FA enables the detection of peripheral ischemic areas. It is contraindicated during pregnancy and in case of allergy to fluorescein dye [5].

3.2 Fundus autofluorescence

Fundus autofluorescence (FAF) not only allows anatomical evaluation of the retina but also provides functional information concerning the metabolic activity of the retinal pigment epithelium (RPE). Therefore, it may be useful in assessing the visual potential of patients with long-standing DME. Abnormalities on FAF in patients with center-involving DME may display two different patterns: a "mosaic" pattern with alternating patchy hyper- and hypo-autofluorescence spots at the fovea and a "cystoid" pattern where the cystoid spaces are defined [5].

3.3 Optical coherence tomography (OCT)

Outdated time-domain OCT (TD-OCT) has been replaced by the faster and more detailed spectral- domain (SD-OCT) and swept-source (SS-OCT) machines.

The primary morphological changes of DME can be visualized with OCT (**Figure 3**), namely subretinal fluid (between RPE and neurosensory retina) and cystoid macular edema (within the neurosensory retina). Additional features include disorganization of inner retinal layers (DRIL), alterations of the external limiting membrane, exudates and hyperreflective foci, changes in choroidal thickness, and vitreomacular interface abnormalities (VMIA) including vitreomacular adhesion, vitreomacular traction, and epiretinal membrane (ERM). Identifying VMIA is essential for differentiating between primary DME and secondary causes

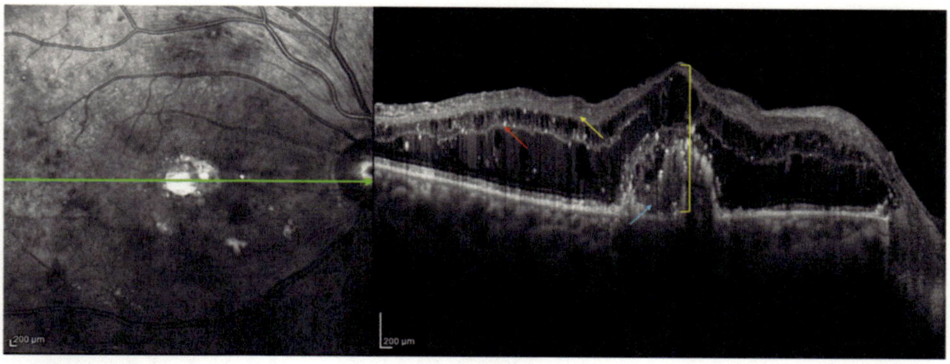

Figure 3.
Spectral-domain optical coherence tomography SD-OCT image (Spectralis, Heidelberg) of diabetic macular edema showing retinal thickening (yellow bracket), intraretinal cysts, disorganization of inner retinal layers (DRIL) (yellow arrow), hyperreflective foci (red arrow), and subfoveal exudates (blue arrow) with disruption of the external retinal layers.

of VMIA, or a combined mechanism. Moreover, OCT is the most useful imaging technique in clinical practice for monitoring intravitreal treatment response in patients. In particular, intraretinal cysts located in the inner nuclear layer tend to be more responsive to either anti-VEGF or corticosteroids than fluid accumulation in the outer nuclear layer [6].

The International Council of Ophthalmology (ICO) guidelines for diabetic eye care have considered center-involved DME versus non-center-involved DME in 2018, depending on retinal thickness involvement or not of the central subfield zone (1 mm in diameter) [7].

In addition to the location of the edema, the Diabetic Retinopathy Clinical Research Network (DRCR.net) has given recommendations on central subfield treatment thresholds based on sex-matched standards. These thresholds are different for each OCT device, considering that thickness measurements cannot be compared between different machines, thus each device must have its own normative database and algorithms [8].

Regarding SD-OCT Staging of diabetic maculopathy, four different stages of the disease may be identified based on foveal thickness, intraretinal cysts' size, ellipsoid zone (EZ) and/or external limiting membrane (ELM) status, and DRIL. Namely, early DM, advanced DM, severe DM, and atrophic maculopathy.

The characteristics of intraretinal cysts may also give hints on DME severity, based on the size of cystoid spaces, up to retinal cystoid degeneration where large coalescent macrocysts characterize severe, long-standing disease with Müller cell dysfunction [9].

3.4 Biomarkers of diabetic macular edema

3.4.1 OCT

Optical coherence tomography is a non-invasive and fast tool that provides *in vivo* retinal images. OCT technology is the most used modality for the screening, classification, monitoring, and treatment assessment of DME in our modern day. The management and treatment of DME is based on the evaluation of various biomarkers (**Figures 4–6**).

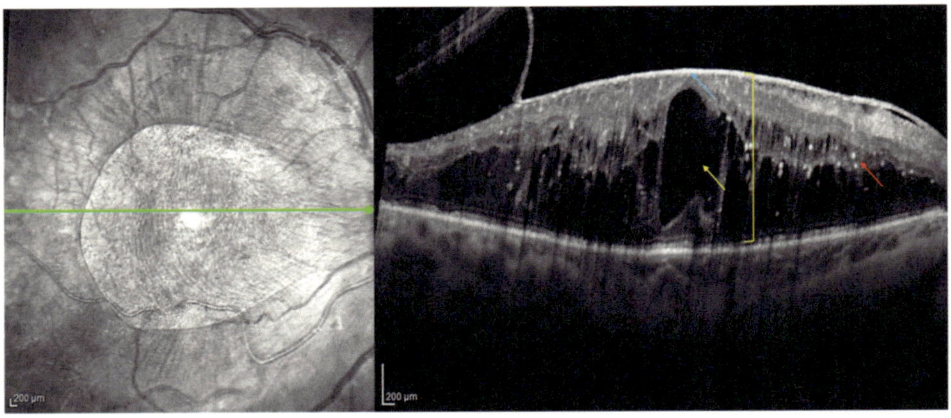

Figure 4.
Spectral-domain optical coherence tomography (SD-OCT) image (Spectralis, Heidelberg) showing diffuse retinal thickening (yellow bracket), macular edema with an elevated foveal contour, and significant intraretinal cystic spaces (yellow arrow), a dense epiretinal membrane overlying the macular surface (blue arrow), hyperreflective foci (red arrow), disorganization of the inner retinal layers and the external limiting membrane and photoreceptor layers.

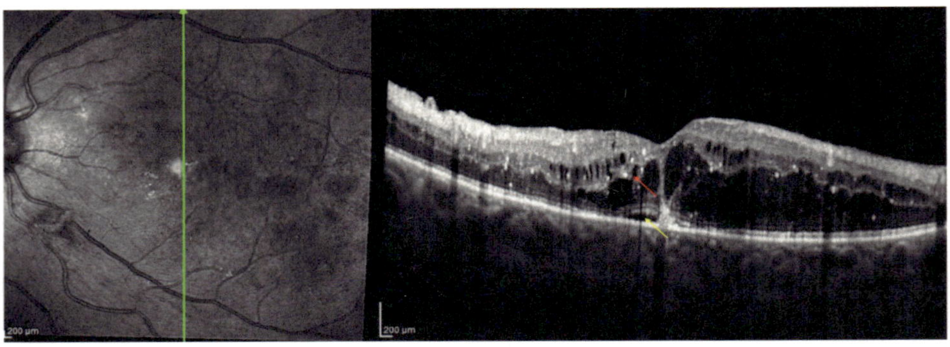

Figure 5.
Spectral-domain optical coherence tomography (SD-OCT) image (Spectralis, Heidelberg) showing intraretinal fluid with a small neuroretinal detachment (yellow arrow), hyperreflective foci (red arrow), large cystic spaces, and exudates.

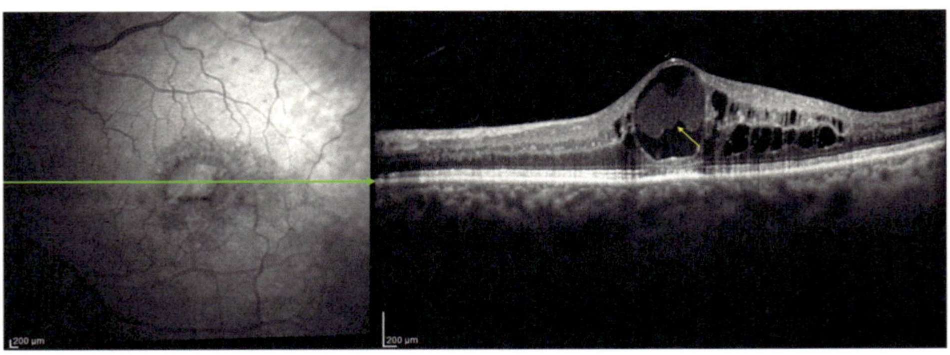

Figure 6.
Spectral-domain optical coherence tomography (SD-OCT) image (Spectralis, Heidelberg) at the fovea showing cystic macular edema, foveal macrocyst with mixed internal reflectivity (yellow arrow).

Biomarkers of DME on OCT include

- intraretinal fluid (IRF) [10]
- disorganization of inner retinal layers (DRIL) [7]
- subretinal fluid (SRF) [10]
- alterations in the inner and outer photoreceptor layers [11]
- alterations in the external limiting membrane (ELM)
- hyperreflective foci
- changes in choroidal thickness

Optical coherence tomography also provides a quantitative measure, the central retinal thickness (CRT), which may be due to diffuse retinal thickening and/or SRF and IRF. The evaluation of CRT and its variation between follow-ups is commonly used in clinical practice to obtain an overview of the DME status. However, it is not enough to determine the decision of treating or retreating a patient with DME.

The SAVE protocol classifies DME based on SRF, the area of the affected retina by IRC, and vitreoretinal interface abnormalities [12]. It uses both OCT and FA to better understand the source of leakage and the prognosis of visual outcomes with different therapeutic approaches [6, 12].

The optimal recommendation is to monitor disease activity every month with OCT, even if no treatment is needed or intended to identify morphological changes as early as possible [13].

3.4.1.1 Angio OCT

Optical coherence tomography angiography (OCT-A) is a non-invasive technology that provides retinal and choroidal microvasculature assessment using motion contrast imaging [14].

While conventional FA permits us to visualize the superficial plexus, OCT-A identifies vascular changes in the deep retinal plexi caused by various retinal diseases, including diabetic retinopathy [15–17]. OCT-A does not require the use of fluorescein, which eliminates fluorescein leakage and allows for better visualization of capillaries (**Figure** 7).

Several studies have shown that OCT-A is less effective at detecting microaneurysms compared to FA. This might be due to the relatively low blood flow in capillaries, which renders the detection of blood flow using motion contrast imaging more challenging [5].

Despite these findings, OCT-A has the advantage of localizing these lesions in their exact intraretinal location [18].

Other DR clinical findings, such as arteriolar wall staining, neovascularization, and intraretinal microvascular abnormalities (IRMA), have different appearances on OCT angiography and fluorescein angiography. On OCT-A, wall staining and arteriolar narrowing are seen as intense attenuation of microcirculation caliber. IRMA are seen as dilated terminal vessels surrounded by capillary loss [15].

Retinal neovessels are detected by observing the flow signal above the internal limiting membrane.

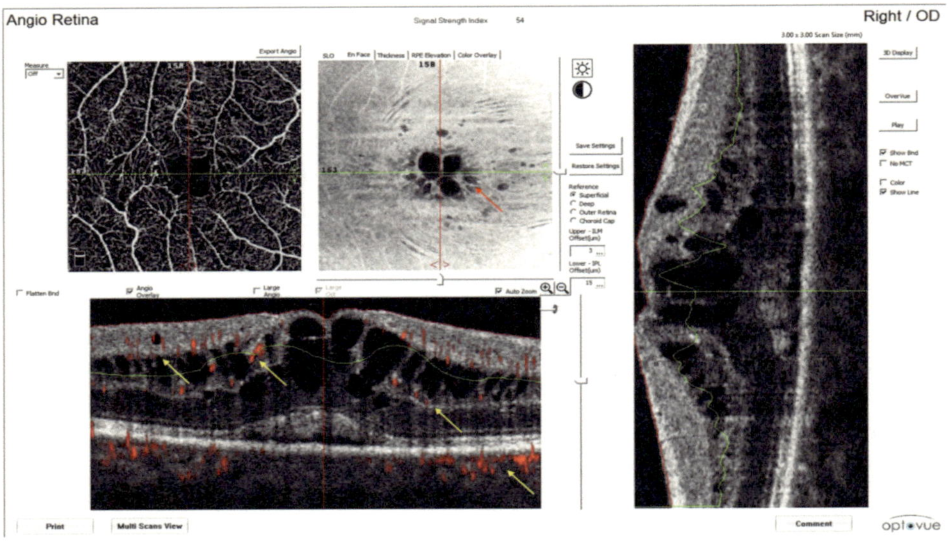

Figure 7.
Optical coherence tomography (OCT) angiography illustrating intraretinal cysts (red arrow) in DME and blood flow (yellow arrows) in the retina and choroid in the macular region that corresponds to 3–3 mm en face flow images from RTVue-100 Optovue OCT.

Hyperfluorescent lesions on fluorescein angiography that appeared indistinguishable from a microaneurysm (MA) were identified as near vision (NV) using OCT-A. This might explain why some patients with vitreous hemorrhage do not have definitive signs of NV on FA [15].

4. DME classification

The Early Treatment Diabetic Retinopathy Study Research Group (ETDRS) defined clinically significant diabetic macular edema (CSDME) as any one of the following:

- retinal edema located at or within 500 μm of the center of the macula
- hard exudates at or within 500 μm of the center associated with thickening of the adjacent retina
- a zone of thickening larger than one disk area located within 1 disk diameter of the center of the macula

The Diabetic Macular Edema Diseases Severity Scales (DMDSSE) defined:

- Edema *absent* as any of the following:
  - Retinal thickness apparently regular to the posterior pole
  - Absence of hard exudates to the back pole
- Edema *present* as any of the following:

- Retinal areas with an apparent increase in the thickness to the back pole
- Presence of hard exudates to the back pole

- Edema *Mild*
    - Increase of the retinal thickness or hard exudates not involving the macula
- Edema *Moderate*
    - Increase of the retinal thickness or hard exudates next to the macula
- Edema *Severe*
    - Increase of the retinal thickness or hard exudates involving the macula

Various attempts have been made to classify DME based on its location (center- and non-center-involved), extent (focal and diffuse), and nature (vasogenic and non-vasogenic). Nevertheless, a classification involving all these features obtained with SD-OCT is still missing [2, 19–21].

Optical coherence tomography has also been shown to be effective for both the qualitative and quantitative description of DME. The widely accepted classification is proposed by Kim et al.

They described and classified five patterns of DME according to OCT [22]:

- Diffuse retinal Thickening (DRT)
- Cystoid macular edema (CME) (**Figure 8**)
- Serous retinal detachment (SRD) without Posterior hyaloid traction (PHT) (**Figure 9**)
- PHT without Traction retinal detachment (TRD) (**Figures 10** and **11**)
- PHT with TRD (**Figure 12**)

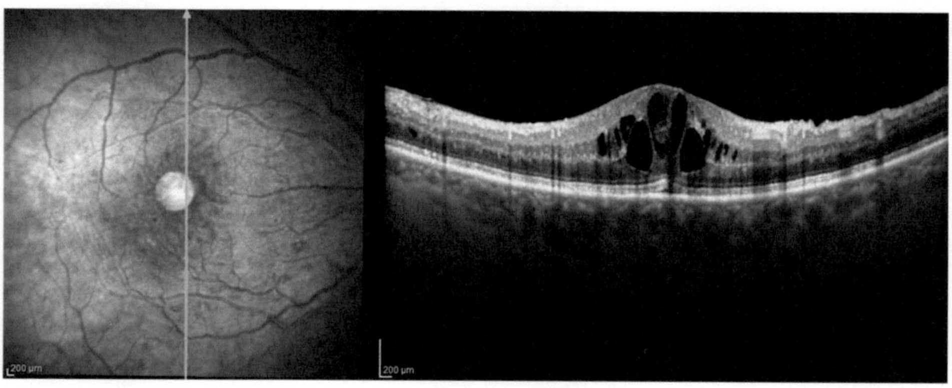

Figure 8.
Spectral-domain optical coherence tomography (OCT-SD) image (Spectralis, Heidelberg) shows irregularities in the outer retinal layers due to cystoid macular edema with intraretinal cysts disrupting the retinal layers.

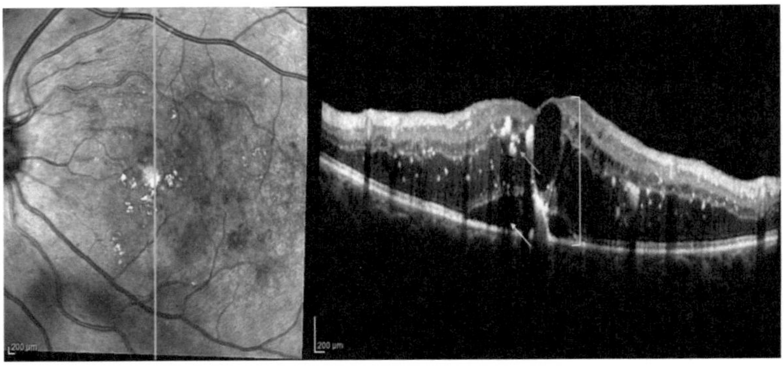

Figure 9.
Spectral-domain optical coherence tomography (OCT-SD) image (Spectralis, Heidelberg) shows serous retinal detachment (SRD) (yellow arrow) without Posterior hyaloid traction (PHT), diffuse retinal thickening (yellow bracket), and dense foveal exudates (blue arrow).

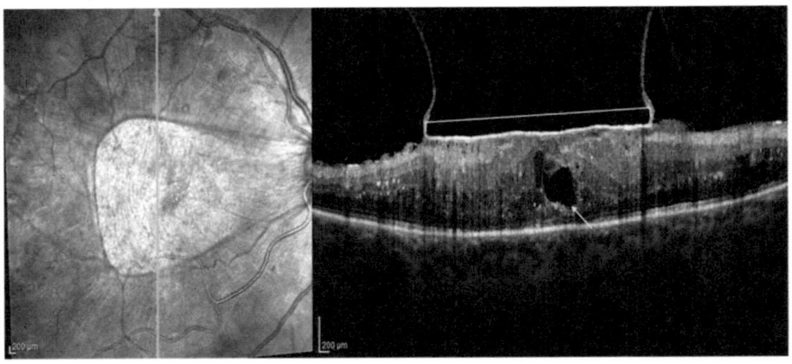

Figure 10.
Spectral-domain optical coherence tomography (OCT-SD) image (Spectralis, Heidelberg) shows Posterior hyaloid traction (bracket) without Traction retinal detachment, intraretinal cysts (arrow), and disturbance of the normal organization of retinal layers.

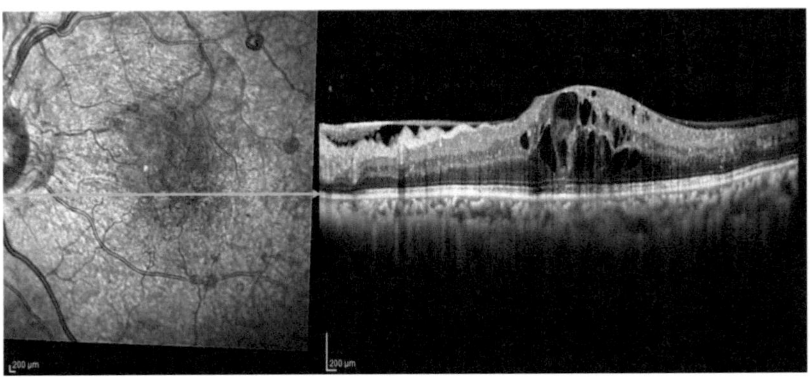

Figure 11.
Posterior hyaloid traction without Traction retinal detachment. Conservation of the outer layers is evident, along with the presence of cystoid macular edema and traction of the posterior hyaloid (Spectralis, Heidelberg).

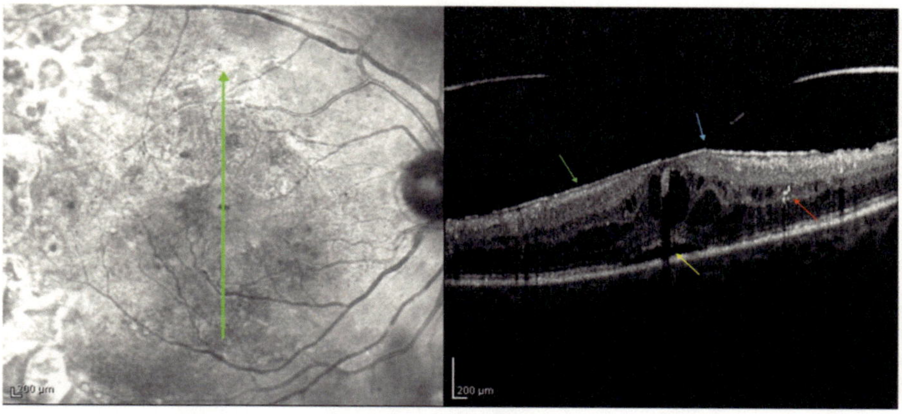

Figure 12.
Posterior hyaloid traction with Traction retinal detachment. A small retinal detachment can be observed with overlying intraretinal fluid (yellow arrow), hyperreflective foci and exudates (red arrow), epiretinal membrane (green arrow), and traction of the hyaloid (blue arrow) (Spectralis, Heidelberg).

5. Therapeutic options

Tighter control of systemic factors, such as hypertension, hyperglycemia, and hyperlipidemia, is generally beneficial in reducing retinopathy in patients with both type 1 and type 2 diabetes mellitus [23].

5.1 Laser photocoagulation

Laser photocoagulation has been a cornerstone in the management of diabetic macular edema. It reduces edema and prevents further vision loss by destroying the ischemic retina to increase oxygen perfusion to the viable retina and reduce the release of cytokines, angiogenic factors, and VEGF [24].

Subtypes of laser photocoagulation include Focal/grid, which is used for well-defined areas of edema, and Panretinal, which is more extensive. The type of approach used depends on the type of macular edema.

Despite its importance in the treatment of DME, laser photocoagulation has limited use in the case of macular DME due to the expansion of retinal atrophy over time and the consequent risk of vision loss from central scars.

Focal laser energy should be applied to leaking MA in combination with grid laser treatment of areas of diffuse macular leakage and non-perfusion in thickened retinas. Complications associated with laser treatment include color vision, night vision, and contrast sensitivity impairment, along with enlargement of laser scars, secondary choroidal neovascularization, subretinal fibrosis, and visual-field sensitivity deterioration. Vision loss, along with other listed complications, has led to the investigation of pharmacological therapies for DME. The two main categories are anti-VEGF agents and corticosteroids.

The ETDRS demonstrated that patients with clinically significant macular edema who were treated with focal photocoagulation experienced a 50% decrease in the risk of moderate visual loss compared to the control group [25]. However, only 3% experienced an improvement in visual acuity of 3 or more lines.

The DRCR.net Protocol I evaluated the role of prompt or deferred laser treatment in addition to ranibizumab therapy in improving best corrected visual acuity (BCVA) after five years of treatment. This study showed that the number of patients achieving a > 15-letter BCVA gain was higher in patients with deferred laser therapy.

In the presence of DME and high-risk non-PDR or PDR, DRCR.net Protocol S data revealed the superiority of anti-VEGF (ranibizumab) therapy as the sole intervention that improves BCVA and additionally induces regression of PDR (**Figures 13** and **14**) [26].

5.2 Anti-VEGF

Before the introduction of anti-VEGF agents in the twenty-first century, the treatment of DME was limited to laser photocoagulation. It was not until 1994 that a

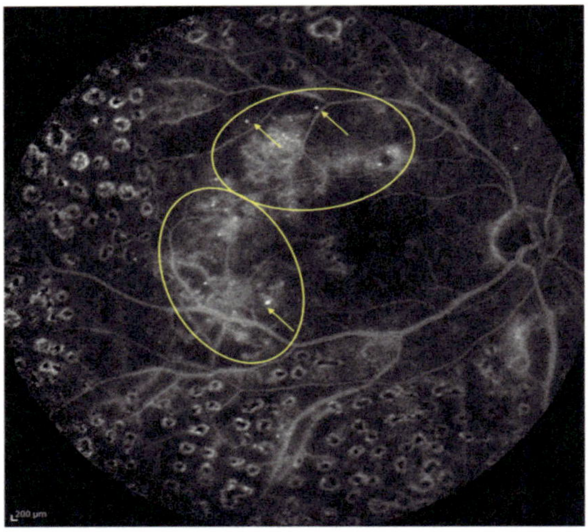

Figure 13.
Fluorescein angiography, SPECTRALIS® scanning laser angiography, intermediate phase, showing signs of previous retinal laser treatment for ischemic areas. Multiple microaneurysms (arrows) and areas of leakage (circles) from microaneurysms and microvascular abnormalities are also evident.

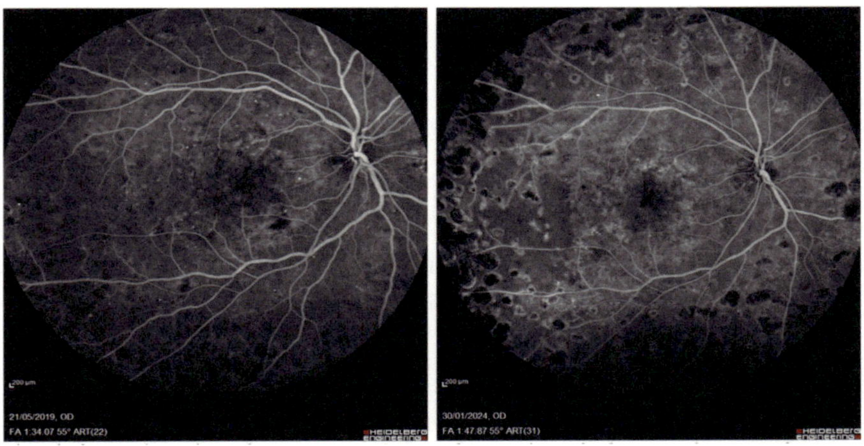

Figure 14.
Fluorescein angiography, SPECTRALIS® scanning laser angiography demonstrating pre- and postphotocoagulation laser treatment for ischemic areas in diabetic retinopathy with residual ischemic areas temporal to the fovea.

study published in the American Journal of Pathology demonstrated that the hypoxic retina produces vascular endothelial growth factor (VEGF), changing definitively the understanding of this pathology [27]. In this study, primate retinas were subjected to laser photocoagulation to induce ischemia and the result was iris neovascularization along with elevated levels of messenger VEGF-mRNA and VEGF protein, demonstrating a role for VEGF in angiogenesis. Along with this significant finding, in 1997 Bevacizumab began to be used for the adjuvant treatment of metastatic colon cancer, prompting the development of the first ocular antiangiogenic, pegylated anti-VEGF aptamer pegaptanib, whose trade name was Macugen. In 2004, pegaptanib was the world's first antiangiogenic approved for ocular neovascularization in humans, thus beginning the era of anti-VEGF.

Vascular endothelial growth factor levels in the vitreous and retina are increased in patients with diabetic retinopathy and have been shown to increase vascular permeability through activation of the protein kinase C pathway, a protein located at the tight junctions between endothelial cells [28, 29]. Treatment with vascular endothelial growth factor inhibitors (anti-VEGF) reduces this process and the abnormal angiogenesis that leads to edema formation in diabetic retinopathy and improves visual acuity in patients with DME [28].

Four intravitreal anti-VEGF agents dominate the global DME market at the time of writing this chapter: Bevacizumab, Ranibizumab, Aflibercept, and Faricimab. Numerous studies have been performed comparing the safety and efficacy of various anti-VEGFs and between the use of corticosteroids and laser treatment. **Table 1** describes some of the main studies and their results [30–33].

Virgili G. et al. in a meta-analysis considered 6007 patients with DME. The result showed that approximately 10% of people improved their vision by 3 or more ETDRS lines with laser after one year, while the ranibizumab group as well as the bevacizumab group improved vision after one year in 30% of patients. Aflibercept achieved this gain in 40% of patients [34]. Also, the RISE and RIDE trials comparing ranibizumab with laser and the VISTA and VIVID trials comparing aflibercept with laser were unable to demonstrate any benefit in the treatment of this pathology with laser.

Considering a single study, we can assume that e.g. in Protocol T it was demonstrated that the use of antiangiogenics under study (bevacizumab, ranibizumab, and aflibercept) improves VA with less need for injections in the second year. Furthermore, it was observed that there is no difference in visual outcomes if the patient has a visual acuity >20/50, but if it is less than 20/50 the visual outcomes were better with the use of aflibercept and ranibizumab. This was also demonstrated in a meta-analysis conducted in 2021, where 45,032 eyes with DME were analyzed and the authors noted that the visual outcome was significantly higher by +3.01 ETDRS letters for aflibercept compared to bevacizumab [35].

In 2022, Faricimab was approved by the US Food and Drug Administration (FDA) and it is the first bispecific antibody approved for the eye, as it is designed to block the angiopoietin-2 (Ang-2) and vascular endothelial growth factor A (VEGF-A) pathways.

The YOSEMITE and RHINE studies showed that administering Faricimab at intervals of up to four months resulted in visual gains that were not inferior to those of aflibercept administered every two months. In the RHINE study, the mean increase in vision at one year was +10.8 and + 11.8 letters in the Faricimab and 2-month extension treatment arms, respectively, and + 10.3 letters in the aflibercept group. This increase in application interval brought great advantages to the use of anti-VEGF, as many patients did not adhere to monthly anti-VEGF treatment. Greater reductions in central subfield thickness (CST) and intraretinal fluid were also demonstrated with Faricimab [30].

Study	Study desing	Primary endpoint	Results
Rise & ride	randomized, parallel, multi-centre clinical trials	To compare the effectiveness of different doses of Ranibizumab versus SHAM with laser rescue in DME. Patients received monthly injections of • 0.3 mg ranibizumab • 0.5 mg ranibizumab • sham	Ranibizumab is effective in treating DME. The average number of injections was 24. More patients in the sham group received macular laser or panphotocoagulation.
Restore	Phase IIIb, multicenter, 12-month, randomized core study and 24-month open-label extension study.	To demonstrate the superiority of ranibizumab 0.5 mg with or without laser vs. laser treatment alone in improving VA over 1 year in patient with DME: • 0.5 mg ranibizumab • 0.5 mg ranibizumab + Laser • sham & Laser	Ranibizumab alone or combined with laser resulted in a higher number of patients with a gain of >15 ETDRS letters.
Resolve	A 12-month, randomized, controlled, double-masked, multicenter phase II study	Efficacy and safety of ranibizumab in diabetic macular oedema: • 0.3 mg ranibizumab • 0.5 mg ranibizumab • sham	At one year, there was a statistically superior increase in VA in the ranibizumab group, with an increase of 10.3 letters. Foveolar thickness decreased by 194.2 versus 48.4 µm in the ranibizumab and sham groups, respectively.
DRCR protocolo I	multicenter randomized clinical trial	To assess the efficacy and safety of: • Sham + focal laser • Ranibizumab with focal laser • Ranibizumab • triamcinolone + focal laser	• The ranibizumab group with laser and delayed laser had better visual acuity and macular thickness on macular OCT, however in pseudophakic patients final VA was achieved. • Lower VA is obtained if focal laser is performed at baseline with ranibizumab instead of delayed laser. Results at 5 years: The visual acuity gained in the first year has been maintained up to 5 years with progressive decrease in the number of applications, the delayed laser was associated with better visual acuity.
DRCR protocolo T	multicentre randomized clinical trial	Comparison of the three antiangiogenic agents in 660 patients with central DME using monthly use: • ranibizumab 0.3 mg • aflibercept 2.0 mg • bevacizumab 1.25 mg	All 3 anti-VEGFs demonstrated improvement in VA with less need for injections in the second year. In patients with good baseline visual acuity there is no difference between antiangiogenics, however, in patients with visual acuity <20/50 aflibercept and ranibizumab was better than bevacizumab More thromboembolic events with ranibizumab.

Study	Study desing	Primary endpoint	Results
DRCR protocolo TX	Single-visit 5-year follow-up study of patients who were enrolled in Protocol T	A Comparative Effectiveness Study of Intravitreal Aflibercept, Bevacizumab, and Ranibizumab for Diabetic Macular Edema, 5-year extension of Protocol T.	The mean change in VA at 5 years was +8 letters aflibercept, +7.6 letters ranibizumab, +6.6 letters bevacizumab. In terms of OCT CRT changes was −154 μm in all 3 groups.
Bolt	Prospective, randomized, masked, single-center, 2-year, 2-arm clinical trial.	Report 2-year outcome comparing bevacizumab versus macular laser therapy.	At two years the average best-corrected VA was 20/50 with Bevacizumab and 20/80 with laser.
VIVID/ VISTA	Two similarly designed phase 3 trials: VISTADME and VIVIDDM	To compare the safety and efficacy of aflibercept with macular laser photocoagulation for diabetic macular edema (DME) over 3 years. • 2 mg every 4 weeks • 2 mg every 8 weeks after 5 monthly doses • laser control	Both studies demonstrate superiority of aflibercept. The proportion of patients who gained more than 15 letters was 38.3%, 33.1% and 13% in VISTA and 38.2%, 31.1% and 12.1% in VIVID respectively. The most frequent adverse event was cataract 2.4%, 1% and 0.3%.
Kestrel and kite	Double-masked, 100-week, multicenter, active-controlled, randomized trials.	To compare the efficacy and safety of brolucizumab with aflibercept in patients with diabetic macular edema. Kestrel • 3 mg/ 6 mg brolocizumab • Aflibercept 2 mg Kite • 6 mg brolocizumab • Aflibercept 2 mg	Brolucizumab 6 mg showed robust visual gains and anatomical improvements. The incidence of ocular serious adverse events was 3.7% (brolucizumab 3 mg), 1.1% (brolucizumab 6 mg), and 2.1% (aflibercept) in KESTREL; and 2.2% (brolucizumab 6 mg) and 1.7% (aflibercept) in KITE.
Yosemite and rhine	Randomized, double-masked, non-inferiority trials across 353 sites worldwide up to the week 100	To reduce treatment burden and optimize patient outcomes in diabetic macular oedema, • 6.0 mg faricimab every 8 weeks • 6.0 mg faricimab per personalized treatment interval (PTI) • aflibercept 2.0 mg every 8 weeks (PTI dosing intervals were extended, maintained, or reduced (every 4 weeks up to every 16 weeks) based on disease activity at active dosing visits.)	Robust vision gains and anatomical improvements with faricimab were achieved with adjustable dosing up to every 16 weeks, demonstrating the potential for faricimab to extend the durability of treatment for patients with diabetic macular oedema.

Table 1.
A summary of various studies conducted over the years, with emphasis on their design, main objective, and salient results. Table columns: Study: Name of the clinical study. Study Design: Description of the methodological design of the study and the duration of the study. Primary endpoint: The main objective or research question the study sought to answer. Results: Main findings or results of the study that summarize its most important conclusions.

Comparing the different agents on the market and analyzing the studies mentioned in **Table 1**, it can be concluded that neither these nor the following studies and meta-analyses demonstrated any additional benefit of macular laser when administered together with anti-VEGF treatment, so that laser is no longer routinely recommended in diffuse DME (**Figures 15** and **16**).

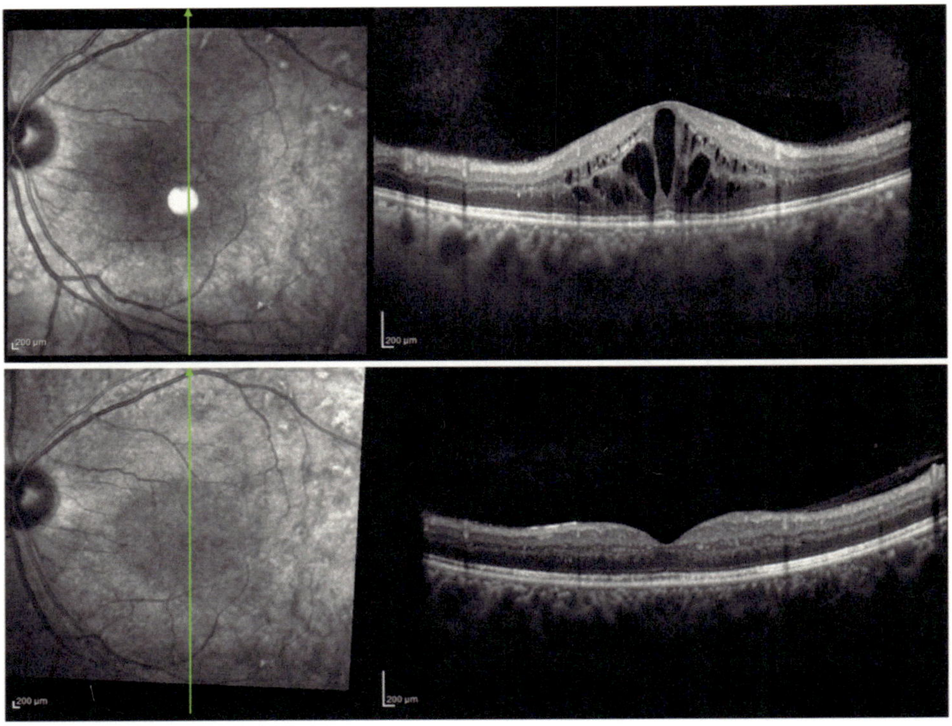

Figure 15.
Spectral-domain optical coherence tomography (SD-OCT) images demonstrating cystoid macular edema in diabetic retinopathy (picture above) and its resolution (picture below) at one month after intravitreal anti-VEGF injection.

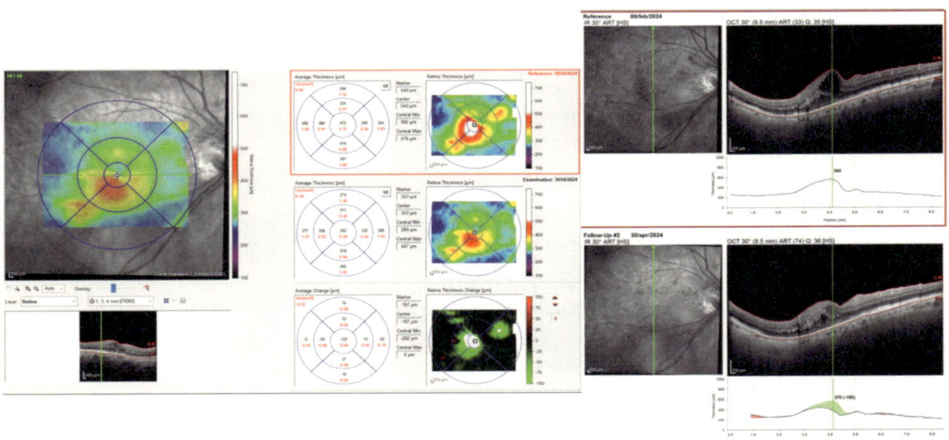

Figure 16.
Spectral-domain optical coherence tomography (SD-OCT) macular map and single-line images demonstrating changes in macular thickness due to reduction of intraretinal cystic spaces in DME after intravitreal anti-VEGF injection.

5.3 Corticosteroids

Recent evidence highlights the role of inflammation in the development of DME; therefore, one of the options for the treatment of this pathology is corticosteroids. Corticosteroids have an anti-inflammatory effect that decreases the

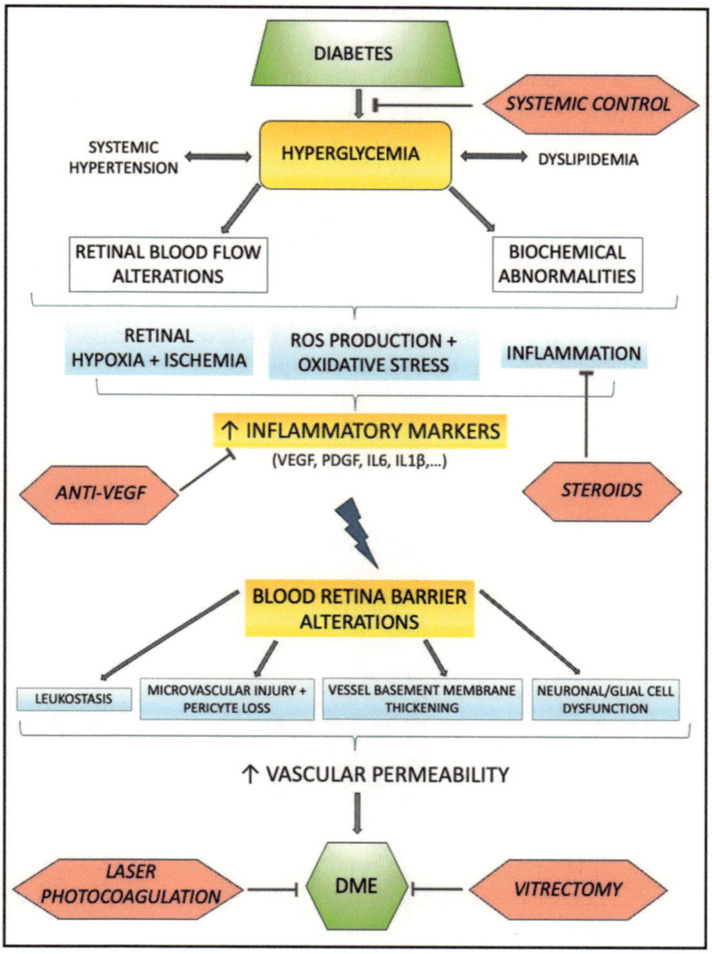

Figure 17.
The figure describes the main pathological pathways involved in diabetic macular edema and the principal therapeutic interventions (highlighted in red) aimed at ameliorating these changes or at interrupting the pathological mechanisms.

synthesis of VEGF and inflammatory mediators, which has been shown to improve the BRB function. It was also seen to downregulate intracellular adhesion molecule (ICAM)-1, which is implicated in increased retinal leukostasis, vascular permeability, and BRB breakdown in diabetes. However, its common adverse effects are the development of ocular hypertension and cataracts in phakic patients, which limits its therapeutic indication (**Figure 17**) [36].

Currently, the corticosteroids for intravitreal use on the market are triamcinolone acetonide, fluocinolone (Iluvien), and the posterior segment dexamethasone delivery system (Ozurdex). The use of corticosteroids has been studied in large protocols such as B and I which are published by the DRCR for the management of diabetic macular edema. The latter is an independent, multicenter, randomized, controlled clinical trial of 5-year duration, in which the use of sham injection + immediate laser, 0.5 mg ranibizumab + immediate laser, 0.5 mg ranibizumab + delayed laser (≥24 weeks), or 4 mg triamcinolone acetonide + immediate laser was compared in patients with DME. After one year, triamcinolone and laser treatment resulted in a 4-letter gain from baseline, compared with a

9-letter gain obtained by the ranibizumab group. In addition to having a lower visual gain, he had 50% intraocular pressure (IOP) elevation ≥10 mm Hg compared to the ranibizumab group (9%) or the laser group (11%), during two years of follow-up [37, 38].

Fluocinolone acetonide-Iluvien was approved by the FDA in 2014. The approved dose for fluocinolone acetonide (FLA) is 0.19 mg, with sustained release for at least one year [39]. In a randomized controlled study conducted over one year, the efficacy of FLA was compared with that of photocoagulation in diabetic macular edema. After this period, it was observed that 57% of patients treated with FLA had resolved DME, compared to 20% treated with photocoagulation alone [40]. However, after a 3-year follow-up, it was found that 95% of patients developed cataracts [41].

The dexamethasone drug delivery system (DDS) (Ozurdex, Allergan Inc., Irvine, California) is a biodegradable, sustained-release device approved by the FDA for the treatment of DME in patients who have not shown any response to anti-VEGF treatment, or patients with significant cardiovascular disease.

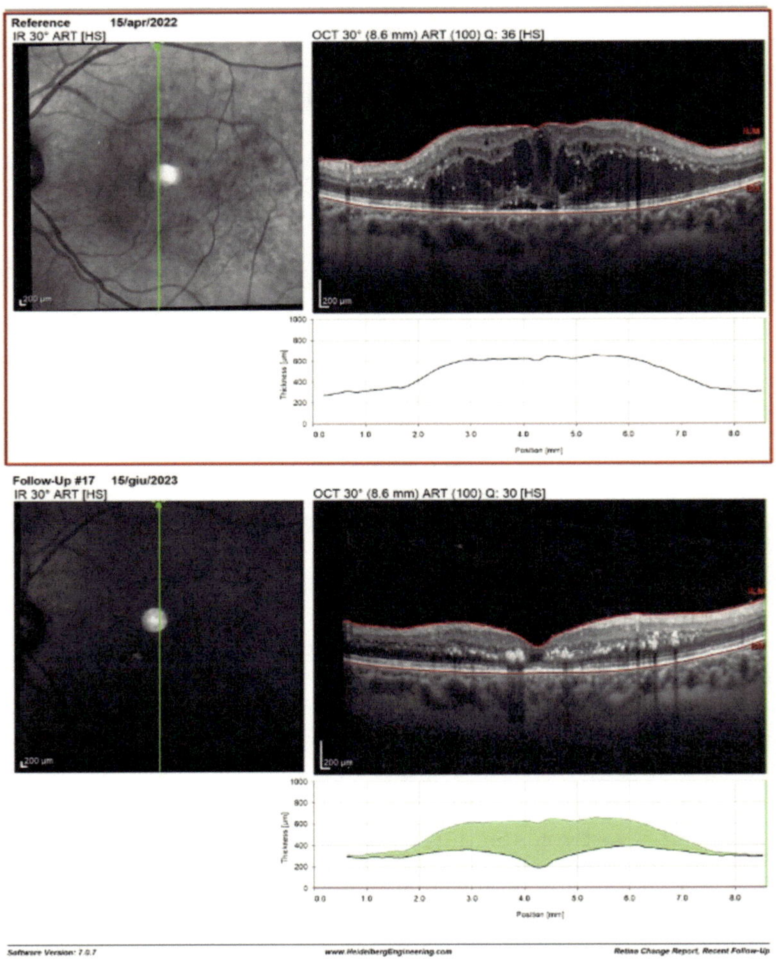

Figure 18.
The spectral-domain optical coherence tomography (SD-OCT) images demonstrating cystoid macular edema with subfoveal neuroretinal detachment, intraretinal hyper-reflective dots, intraretinal exudates in diabetic retinopathy (picture above), and the resolution of intraretinal edema and neuroretinal detachment with persistence of exudates (picture below) at two months after intravitreal corticosteroid implant.

Time	Antiangiogenic Limitations	Corticosteroid Limitations
Immediately	• Requires frequent injections • Second option in patients with a severe cardiovascular history • Subconjunctival hemorrhage	• Risk of increased intraocular pressure • Slightly more difficult application technique • Subconjunctival hemorrhage • Caution in patients with a history of viral infections such as herpes simplex. Should not be used in case of active ocular herpes simplex
0–3 months	• Variable response in different patients • Risk of ocular complications due to more frequent applications such as endophthalmitis	• Possible development of cataracts
3–12 months	• Need for continuous monitoring • Some patients may develop resistance • Costly ongoing treatment	• Need for repeated dosing • Potential for increased intraocular pressure
>12 months	• Risk of recurrence of macular oedema • risks of scloramalacia at injection sites • No adequate data on use in pregnant women	• Risk of eye infection • May not be effective in all patients • No adequate data on use in pregnant women

Table 2.
Limitations of antiangiogenic and corticosteroid treatments in patients with diabetic macular edema over time. It is important to note that these limitations may vary depending on the specific type of antiangiogenic or corticosteroid used, as well as individual patient characteristics. In addition, advances in research and the development of new treatments may change these limitations over time.

The implant releases the corticosteroid into the vitreous for a period of ≤6 months [42]. Therefore, retreatment is recommended after this period has elapsed and simultaneous administration in both eyes is not recommended. A phase 2 randomized controlled trial (RCT) in patients with persistent macular edema secondary to DME showed that over six months of dexamethasone DDS produced improvements in visual acuity, macular thickness, and fluorescein leakage (**Figure 18**) [43].

Similar results have been reached in the study by Boyer DS et al., where dexamethasone DDS was reported to improve final visual acuity and macular thickness in previously vitrectomized patients with diffuse DME [44].

Up to now, corticosteroids have proven to be a valuable tool in treating patients with DME, albeit often as a secondary option. This is particularly the case for patients who have not responded well to anti-VEGF treatment. Conversely, they might be preferred as a first-line option for patients with a significant cardiovascular history. Studies suggest that after continuous monthly anti-VEGF treatment over a 2-year period, these patients may face heightened risks of mortality and potential stroke [45]. Further limitations of both anti-VEGF agents and corticosteroids are outlined in **Table 2**.

5.4 Surgical management of diabetic macular edema

5.4.1 The role of the vitreous and vitrectomy in DME

The vitreous has been implicated as a cause of macular edema in people with diabetes via several mechanical and physiological mechanisms, all of which are postulated to lead to an increase in vascular permeability [46]. Suggested mechanisms include the following [47]:

1. destabilization of the vitreous by abnormal glycation and crosslinking of vitreous collagen, leading to traction on the macula

2. accumulation and concentration of factors causing vasal permeability in the premacular vitreous gel

3. accumulation of chemoattractant factors in the vitreous, leading to cellular migration to the posterior hyaloid, contraction, and macular traction

The reduction in DME followed by improved oxygenation and the release of mechanical traction on the macula, either by spontaneous posterior vitreous detachment or by vitrectomy, supports the suggested mechanisms and highlights the potential advantage of vitrectomy in these cases [48].

Vitrectomy improves oxygenation at the inner retinal surface by increasing the flow of oxygen-rich aqueous from the highly vascularized iris and ciliary body to the posterior pole. Increased oxygen tension counteracts the diabetes-induced retinal hypoxia responsible for VEGF upregulation and blood-retinal barrier breakdown, decreasing exudation from the retinal capillaries and resolving DME.

Kim et al. [22] noticed a significant association between decreased visual acuity and the presence of Posterior hyaloid traction (PHT) without tractional retinal detachment (TRD). The traction produced by the vitreomacular interface alone has been postulated to play a role in the development of DME. This vitreomacular interface has been thought to cause tangential traction, which could lead to macular edema. Hence, identifying the structural changes in patients with DME using OCT may allow more effective management of these patients.

5.4.2 Vitrectomy: when?

Vitrectomy should be taken into consideration as the primary therapeutic option if vitreo-macular traction is present and identified with biomicroscopy or OCT, to mechanically remove the traction itself (**Figures 10–12**) [49–53].

In the Diabetic Retinopathy Clinical Research Network (DRCR.net) trial, 241 eyes were enrolled [54], and a decrease in the mean subfield thickness from 412 microns to 278 microns was demonstrated six months after vitrectomy. Visual acuity significantly improved in eyes with worse VA at baseline ($P < 0.001$) and in eyes requiring ERM peeling ($P = 0.006$), even though the entire cohort's average VA (20/80) remained the same.

Moreover, eyes with a worse baseline VA were more likely to have a greater improvement in VA and a larger reduction in macular thickness. Although the most relevant decrease in macular thickness was shown in eyes with the greatest preoperative thickness, the trial could not clearly demonstrate that the final visual acuity is independently associated with baseline macular thickness. This is probably explained by the slight possible improvement when either or both macular thickness and visual acuity are relatively small.

A better outcome in VA was present when ERM was removed during vitrectomy, while the amount of macular thickness reduction was not affected, possibly indicating a resolution in metamorphopsias rather than an improvement in DME. Instead, a relevant decrease in retinal thickness was observed with internal limiting membrane (ILM) peeling, with no improvement in VA.

Factors associated with changes in anatomic outcomes or VA after pars plana vitrectomy (PPV) for DME were evaluated only in a few studies in the literature. Kumagai et al. [55] conducted a retrospective study demonstrating that VA at 1-year examination was better after ILM removal as compared to ILM preservation, after evaluating 486 eyes that underwent lensectomy and PPV for diffuse non-tractional DME.

Tamura et al. [56] carried out a histopathologic analysis of the ILM after vitrectomy and peeling from eyes with diffuse diabetic macular edema. ILM examined by light microscopy revealed the presence of five cell types on the vitreous side of the specimens, namely glial cells, fibroblast-like cells, macrophages, neutrophils, and lymphocytes, while immunohistochemistry corroborated the presence of glial cells and macrophages.

The advantages of ILM removal in eyes with DME are underlined in several papers; nevertheless, the major issue is the difficulty in preoperative DME characteristics standardization, given that previous laser treatments or intravitreal steroid/anti-VEGF are likely to interfere.

Randomized clinical trials (RCTs) with an appropriate follow-up have not been conducted yet concerning vitrectomy compared with other methods in DME management; therefore, its application and role remain unclear, with regard to its potential risks and benefits.

Diffuse DME without evident traction may not benefit from vitrectomy; moreover, low visual acuity after complete resolution of DME may be explained by macular ischemia [57, 58], photoreceptor dysfunction [51, 59], or accumulated subfoveal hard exudates [60]. The poor visual outcome may be predicted with a better photoreceptor layer visualization, as assessed by SD-OCT, especially for what concerns the integrity of the external limiting membrane (ELM) and inner and outer segments (IS/OS) of the photoreceptor junction.

In conclusion, a surgical approach in patients with DME should aim at rapidly drying the retina as much as possible. It is clear that the posterior hyaloid should be completely removed, whereas ILM peeling remains controversial. Postoperative VA may be predicted with detailed SD-OCT evaluation of the ELM and IS/OS layer done before and after surgery; furthermore, a quick and long-lasting improvement in VA may be achieved with early vitrectomy to significantly reduce macular thickness. However, a randomized trial comparing vitrectomy with the current standard of care should be carried on.

As medical budgets become tighter, and alternative therapies, including anti-VEGF injections, become more expensive, vitrectomy may emerge as the preferred low-cost, longer-duration therapy.

6. Refractory or persistent DME

Medications used for vascular endothelial growth factor inhibition (anti-VEGF) have significantly changed visual and anatomical outcomes in people with diabetic macular edema (DME). However, success is not always assured, and some patients continue to experience persistent diabetic macular edema (PDME), despite intensive treatment. Approximately 30–65% of patients are thought to be refractory [61]. "Refractory or persistent macular edema" is defined as a < 10% or 20% decrease in central retinal thickness (CRT) compared to baseline data or when visual gain is suboptimal, i.e. patients achieve <5-letter increase in best corrected visual acuity (BCVA) on the ETDRS or less than one line of sight on the Snellen poster [62].

In daily practice, there is no standardized treatment for this pathology that supports the superiority of one strategy over another. Consequently, it is the treating professional who decides on the therapy, taking into account various clinical factors, complementary examinations, and the particular characteristics of each patient.

Several treatment options are currently being proposed. One is to switch to a drug with a different affinity for VEGF and which can block cytokines via other pathways, maximizing the therapeutic potential. This is generally used after an inadequate response after three to six injections, at the discretion of the treating ophthalmologist. Another option is to change the therapeutic agent to corticosteroids. Intravitreal corticosteroids such as dexamethasone or fluocinolone have been shown to achieve remarkable improvements in visual and anatomical outcomes in people who do not respond to anti-VEGF treatment, due to their anti-inflammatory and antiangiogenic effects. Finally, in cases where the origin of the lack of therapeutic response is an epiretinal membrane, vitreous traction, or macular ischemia, pars plana vitrectomy can be the option.

6.1 Analysis of the evidence

One of the hypotheses for the treatment of this type of pathology is "replacement of one antiangiogenic molecule by another," but the timing of switching anti-VEGF agents remains a matter of debate, as there are so far insufficient well-designed, prospective, randomized clinical trials assessing the efficacy of switching. Some advocate switching early, before permanent structural damage is observed due to persistent chronic macular edema, arguing for a more favorable long-term visual outcome. This idea is supported by findings obtained in Protocol I, where it is stated that if visual gain is poor after the first three applications of anti-VEGF, continuing with the same therapeutic agent will likely result in suboptimal visual gain.

A marked difference in efficacy in favor of aflibercept compared to bevacizumab was also observed in Protocol T. Therefore if the decision is made to switch from anti-VEGF after only three monthly applications, the most effective switch would be from bevacizumab to aflibercept or ranibizumab. Several investigations have supported this hypothesis, demonstrating similar results of a gain of 3–5 lines of sight in favor of switching [63, 64].

On the other hand, also in Protocol T, it is suggested that caution should be exercised when considering changing treatment for DME if there is a limited response in the first few months of treatment. This is because it was observed that in some cases, there is continued resolution of edema on OCT, especially with monthly and continuous use of aflibercept and ranibizumab, from week 12 to week 24. Similar results were observed in the Protocol I study, in which 30% of the treated patients, who did not achieve a BCVA of >5 letters in the first three anti-VEGF applications, achieved a BCVA > or equal to 10 letters at the end of the 3-year follow-up.

With the recent emergence of Faricimab, some studies have found benefits in its use in patients who are non-responders to aflibercept, especially in terms of treatment interval in patients with PDME. Visual and anatomical improvements were also demonstrated, but further long-term studies are required for confirmation [65, 66]. Rush et al. found that patients who switched from aflibercept to Faricimab showed significant improvements in both visual acuity and central macular thickness (CMT) compared to those who continued aflibercept treatment for persistent DME [65]. In their study, 37.5% of patients achieved a CMT < 300 μm, and 41.7% of patients showed an improvement of >0.2 logMAR (Logarithm of the Minimum Angle of Resolution) four months after switching to Faricimab. This could reduce the financial burden, the need for multiple visits and injections, the likelihood of infection, and systemic complications associated with treatment.

Another alternative frequently used in daily practice is the use of corticosteroids, either as an adjunct or as a single therapeutic agent. Considering that there is evidence suggesting that the late phase of DME may be due to inflammatory activities rather than angiogenic factors. Another reason is that not all patients respond to anti-VEGF. Up to 40% of participants in pivotal clinical trials did not reach a VA threshold of 20/40 [67]. In addition, dexamethasone intravitreal implants (DEX DDS) may extend the therapeutic interval in those who cannot cope with the intensive regimen required for anti-VEGF therapy.

6.2 Future developments

Given the high incidence of this disease and the challenge of treating it, new studies with innovative therapeutic approaches are underway, some of which include:

- RGX-314 (Regenxbio): is a virus-mediated gene therapy that enables the production of a Fab Anti-VEGF fragment. The study, called ALTITUDE (Aliskieren Trial in Type 2 Diabetes Using Cardio-Renal Endpoints), is in phase 2 and evaluates the efficacy, safety, and tolerability of RGX-314E gene therapy for diabetic retinopathy.

- OPT-302 (Opthea): is an anti-VEGF combination therapy against vascular endothelial growth factor-C and -D (VEGF-C and -D) and with available anti-VEGF agents. Phase 2 data from patients with refractory DME treated with combination therapy showed a 52% improvement in VA $\geq$ 5 letters at 12 weeks compared to baseline

- APX3330 (Ocuphire Pharma): is a Phase 2 oral therapy for the treatment of diabetic retinopathy. So far, it was demonstrated that up to 24 weeks, no treated patient showed a binocular worsening $\geq$3 steps of the Diabetic Retinopathy Severity Rating System (DRSS) from baseline, compared to 16% of placebo-treated patients.

In conclusion, the treatment of persistent diabetic macular edema is a major challenge for the treating ophthalmologist. The lack of consensus and the diversity of available therapeutic options reflect its complexity. Therefore, the choice of treatment requires a careful assessment of the patient's medical history, socioeconomic situation, and individual response to treatment.

Continued research and interdisciplinary collaboration are essential to advance the understanding and management of persistent diabetic macular edema.

7. Artificial intelligence and future perspectives

The complementary use of artificial intelligence (AI) in medicine, particularly in ophthalmology, has increased in recent years and this trend is expected to continue. This tool has proven useful in different pathologies, particularly in diabetic macular edema (DME), thanks to AI's great capacity to analyze a large amount of data quickly and accurately. This has allowed it to be used as a means of screening, diagnosis, and treatment, marking a significant milestone in ophthalmology and changing the approach to the disease [68].

For diagnosis, AI algorithms allow the identification of subtle patterns in retinal images, facilitating early detection of DME, before symptoms are evident. This anticipation facilitates a timely and effective approach that leads to the preservation of vision in diabetic patients.

In 2018, for the first time, the US Food and Drug Administration (FDA) approved an AI algorithm, called "IDx-DR," based on a non-mydriatic fundus photograph using a Topcon Fundus camera (Topcon Medical) for the identification and screening of diabetic retinopathy (DR) without interpretation by an ophthalmologist.

These algorithms were based on the initial studies by Abramoff et al., which showed that Deep Learning (DL), specifically the Convolutional Neural Network (CNN), achieved a high sensitivity rate of 96.8% in identifying DR from sets of images [69]. Since then, algorithms have been developed to identify DR from fundus photographs, with high sensitivity and specificity [70].

Optical coherence tomography (OCT) is the most widely used complementary study for the diagnosis and monitoring of this disease. It has been successfully coupled to AI, creating a large database and thanks to its machine learning capabilities, algorithms for the diagnosis and prognosis of the course of DME have been obtained.

De Fauw et al. conducted a study demonstrating the effectiveness of DL in identifying DME and other causes of macular edema using OCT as a diagnostic tool [71]. By analyzing 14,884 scans, they were able to develop an algorithm that showed an error rate lower than that performed by a group of trained retina specialists and optometrists. Tang et al. demonstrated similar findings using 73,746 OCT images to create a multitasking CNN to classify different types of DME. The results revealed an area under the receiver operating curve (ROC) greater than 0.93 [72], reinforcing the idea of the efficacy of the DL approach in this specific clinical application.

Optical coherence tomography angiography (OCT-A) is also a study widely used in recent years in the detection and monitoring of DME, because it can show changes in vascular density, decreased capillary permeability in superficial and deep capillary plexuses, and an increase in the foveal avascular area. Therefore, OCT-A DL algorithms are currently being designed for the diagnosis and monitoring of DME.

Le et al. demonstrated that a neural network trained with OCT-A diagnosed diabetic retinopathy with a sensitivity of 83.76% and a specificity of 90.82% [73]. Similarly, Ryu et al. designed a diagnostic algorithm that arrived at results with similar levels of predictability [74].

Concerning DME management, AI facilitates follow-up analysis to assess disease progression and adjust treatment plans in a continuous and personalized manner. This optimizes therapeutics, thus reducing the occurrence of large morphological variations, which are directly reflected in a poor final visual outcome [75].

In terms of treatment, AI has also influenced the development of more targeted and individual therapies. By better understanding the characteristics of each patient's DME, AI contributes to the optimization of drugs and procedures, maximizing benefits and minimizing side effects [76].

In summary, the integration of artificial intelligence in ophthalmology has revolutionized the way DME is approached, significantly improving early diagnosis, efficient management, and personalization of treatments, resulting in more effective care and more successful preservation of vision in diabetic patients.

8. Conclusion

Effective treatment of diabetic macular edema (DME) is a fundamental pillar in preserving visual acuity and improving the quality of life of affected patients. Advances in diagnostic methods now make it possible to provide patients with early diagnosis and targeted treatment.

Pharmacological advances have been extraordinary, as evidenced by the introduction of new agents such as Faricimab, which has significant potential in improving visual function and prolonging application intervals. Further advances in the pharmacological field are expected to offer even more effective treatments for patients. Ongoing research and development of drugs targeting different pathophysiological pathways in diabetic macular edema could expand the available therapeutic options, thereby improving anatomical and visual outcomes.

Retinal surgery has also undergone substantial progress, characterized by less invasive, more precise, and safer techniques. This progress is due to the development of specialized instrumentation and the constant improvement of surgical techniques, allowing surgeons to achieve better outcomes in patients with DME.

Finally, the incursion of artificial intelligence into the field of DME diagnosis, treatment, and monitoring promises to open new doors toward more efficient and accurate medical care.

In summary, the progress achieved in these various fields augurs new prospects for patients affected by this disease.

Author contributions

Author contributions according to CREdiT (Contributor Roles Taxonomy):

F.P.: Conceptualization, Supervision, Writing—Original Draft, Writing—Review and Editing;

L.M.R.: Conceptualization, Supervision, Writing—Original Draft, Writing—Review and Editing;

A.C.: Writing—Original Draft, Writing—Review and Editing, Formal analysis;

R.R.: Writing—Original Draft, Writing—Review and Editing, Formal analysis;

L.C.: Writing—Original Draft, Writing—Review and Editing, Formal analysis;

M.L.S.: Writing—Original Draft, Writing—Review and Editing, Formal analysis;

All authors have read and agreed to the published version of the manuscript.

Author details

Fabio Patelli*, Ana Lisa Carauni, Roberta Rissotto, Lily Chacra, Maria Laura Scopelliti and Luca M. Rossetti
ASST Santi Paolo e Carlo University Hospital, Milan, Italy

*Address all correspondence to: fabio@patelli.it

References

[1] International Diabetes Federation. Diabetes [Internet]. 2015. Available from: https://idf.org/about-diabetes/what-is-diabetes/

[2] Wilkinson CP, Ferris FL, Klein RE, Lee PP, Agardh CD, Davis M, et al. Proposed international clinical diabetic retinopathy and diabetic macular edema disease severity scales. Ophthalmology. 2003;**110**(9):1677-1682

[3] Romero-Aroca P, Baget-Bernaldiz M, Pareja-Rios A, Lopez-Galvez M, Navarro-Gil R, Verges R. Diabetic macular Edema pathophysiology: Vasogenic versus inflammatory. Journal of Diabetes Research. 2016;**2016**:1-17

[4] Funatsu H, Yamashita H, Sakata K, Noma H, Mimura T, Suzuki M, et al. Vitreous levels of vascular endothelial growth factor and intercellular adhesion molecule 1 are related to diabetic macular Edema. Ophthalmology. 2005;**112**(5):806-816

[5] Amoaku WM, Ghanchi F, Bailey C, Banerjee S, Banerjee S, Downey L, et al. Diabetic retinopathy and diabetic macular oedema pathways and management: UK consensus working group. Eye. 2020;**34**(S1):1-51

[6] Panozzo G, Cicinelli MV, Augustin AJ, Battaglia Parodi M, Cunha-Vaz J, Guarnaccia G, et al. An optical coherence tomography-based grading of diabetic maculopathy proposed by an international expert panel: The European School for Advanced Studies in ophthalmology classification. European Journal of Ophthalmology. 2020;**30**(1):8-18

[7] Sun JK, Lin MM, Lammer J, et al. Disorganization of the retinal inner layers as a predictor of visual acuity in eyes with center-involved diabetic macular edema. JAMA Ophthalmology. 2014;**132**:1309-1316

[8] Diabetic Retinopathy Clinical Research Network; Wells JA, Glassman AR, Ayala AR, Jampol LM, Aiello LP, et al. Aflibercept, bevacizumab, or ranibizumab for diabetic macular edema. The New England Journal of Medicine. 26 Mar 2015;**372**(13):1193-1203

[9] Halim MS, Afridi R, Hasanreisoglu M, Hassan M, Ibrahim-Ahmed M, Do DV, et al. Differences in the characteristics of subjects achieving complete, partial, or no resolution of macular edema in the READ-3 study. Graefe's Archive for Clinical and Experimental Ophthalmology. 2021;**259**(10):2941-2948

[10] Gerendas BS, Prager SG, Deak GG, Waldstein SM, Lammer J, Simader C, et al. Morphological parameters relevant for long-term outcomes during therapy of diabetic macular edema in the RESTORE extension trial. Investigative Ophthalmology & Visual Science. 2015;**56**:4686-4686

[11] Shin HJ, Lee SH, Chung H, Kim HC. Association between photoreceptor integrity and visual outcome in diabetic macular edema. Graefe's Archive for Clinical and Experimental Ophthalmology. 2012;**250**:61-70

[12] Bolz M, Lammer J, Deak G, Pollreisz A, Mitsch C, Scholda C, et al. SAVE: A grading protocol for clinically significant diabetic macular oedema based on optical coherence tomography and fluorescein angiography. The British Journal of Ophthalmology. 2014;**98**(12):1612-1617

[13] Schmidt-Erfurth U, Garcia-Arumi J, Bandello F, Berg K, Chakravarthy U,

Gerendas BS, et al. Guidelines for the Management of Diabetic Macular Edema by the European Society of Retina Specialists (EURETINA). Ophthalmologica. 2017;**237**(4):185-222

[14] De Barros Garcia JMB, Isaac DLC, Avila M. Diabetic retinopathy and OCT angiography: Clinical findings and future perspectives. International Journal of Retina and Vitreous. 2017;**3**(1):14

[15] Hwang TS, Jia Y, Gao SS, Bailey ST, Lauer AK, Flaxel CJ, et al. Optical coherence tomography angiography features of diabetic retinopathy. Retina. 2015;**35**(11):2371-2376

[16] Ishibazawa A, Nagaoka T, Takahashi A, Omae T, Tani T, Sogawa K, et al. Optical coherence tomography angiography in diabetic retinopathy: A prospective pilot study. American Journal of Ophthalmology. 2015;**160**(1):35-44

[17] Spaide RF, Klancnik JM Jr, Cooney MJ. Retinal vascular layers imaged by fluorescein angiography and optical coherence tomography angiography. JAMA Ophthalmology. 2015;**133**(1):45-50

[18] Couturier A, Mane V, Bonnin S, et al. Capillary plexus anomalies in diabetic retinopathy on optical coherence tomography angiography. Retina. 2015;**35**:2384-2391

[19] Wong TY, Sun J, Kawasaki R, Ruamviboonsuk P, Gupta N, Lansingh VC, et al. Guidelines on diabetic eye care. Ophthalmology. 2018;**125**(10):1608-1622

[20] Parodi Battaglia M, Iacono P, Cascavilla M, Zucchiatti I, Bandello F. A Pathogenetic classification of diabetic macular Edema. Ophthalmic Research. 2018;**60**(1):23-28

[21] Panozzo G, Parolini B, Gusson E, Mercanti A, Pinackatt S, Bertoldo G, et al. Diabetic macular edema: An OCT-based classification. Seminars in Ophthalmology. 2004;**19**(1-2):13-20

[22] Kim BY, Smith SD, Kaiser PK. Optical coherence tomographic patterns of diabetic macular edema. American Journal of Ophthalmology. 2006;**142**(3):405-412

[23] Diabetes Control and Complications Trial Research Group; Nathan DM, Genuth S, Lachin J, Cleary P, Crofford O, et al. The effect of intensive treatment of diabetes on the development and progression of long-term complications in insulin-dependent diabetes mellitus. The New England Journal of Medicine. 30 Sep 1993;**329**(14):977-986

[24] Everett LA, Paulus YM. Laser therapy in the treatment of diabetic retinopathy and diabetic macular Edema. Current Diabetes Reports. 2021;**21**(9):35

[25] Treatment techniques and clinical guidelines for photocoagulation of diabetic macular edema. Early Treatment Diabetic Retinopathy Study Report Number 2. Early Treatment Diabetic Retinopathy Study Research Group. Ophthalmology. Jul 1987;**94**(7):761-774

[26] Gross JG, Glassman AR, Jampol LM, Inusah S, Aiello LP, Antoszyk AN, et al. Panretinal photocoagulation vs intravitreous ranibizumab for proliferative diabetic retinopathy: A randomized clinical trial. Journal of the American Medical Association. 2015;**314**:2137-2146

[27] Miller JW, Adamis AP, Shima DT, PA DA, Moulton RS, MS OR, et al. Vascular endothelial growth factor/vascular permeability factor is temporally and spatially correlated with ocular angiogenesis In a primate model. Retina. 1995;**15**(2):174

[28] Aiello LP, Avery RL, Arrigg PG, Keyt BA, Jampel HD, Shah ST, et al. Vascular endothelial growth factor in ocular fluid of patients with diabetic retinopathy and other retinal disorders. The New England Journal of Medicine. 1994;**331**:1480-1487

[29] Antonetti DA, Barber AJ, Hollinger LA, Wolpert EB, Gardner TW. Vascular endothelial growth factor induces rapid phosphorylation of tight junction proteins Occludin and zonula Occluden 1. Journal of Biological Chemistry. 1999;**274**(33):23463-23467

[30] Wykoff CC, Abreu F, Adamis AP, Basu K, Eichenbaum DA, Haskova Z, et al. Efficacy, durability, and safety of intravitreal faricimab with extended dosing up to every 16 weeks in patients with diabetic macular oedema (YOSEMITE and RHINE): Two randomised, double-masked, phase 3 trials. Lancet. 2022;**399**(10326):741-755

[31] Cabrera F, Armadá F. Ensayos clínicos en el tratamiento del edema macular diabético. Archivos de la Sociedad Española de Oftalmología. 2012;**87**:27-37

[32] Brown DM, Emanuelli A, Bandello F, Barranco JJE, Figueira J, Souied E, et al. KESTREL and KITE: 52-week results from two phase III pivotal trials of Brolucizumab for diabetic macular Edema. American Journal of Ophthalmology. 2022;**238**:157-172

[33] Glassman AR, Wells JA 3rd, Josic K, et al. Five-year outcomes after initial Aflibercept, bevacizumab, or Ranibizumab treatment for diabetic macular edema (protocol T extension study). Ophthalmology. 2020;**127**:1201-1210

[34] Virgili G, Parravano M, Evans JR, et al. Anti-vascular endothelial growth factor for diabetic macular oedema: A network meta-analysis. Cochrane Database of Systematic Reviews. 2018;**10**:CD007419

[35] Veritti D, Sarao V, Soppelsa V, Lanzetta P. Managing diabetic macular Edema in clinical practice: Systematic review and meta-analysis of current strategies and treatment options. Clinical Ophthalmology. 2021;**15**:375-385

[36] Nauck M, Roth M, Tamm M, et al. Induction of vascular endothelial growth factor by platelet-activating factor and platelet-derived growth factor is downregulated by corticosteroids. American Journal of Respiratory Cell and Molecular Biology. 1997;**16**(4):398-406

[37] Elman MJ, Aiello LP, Beck RW, Bressler NM, Bressler SB, Edwards AR, et al. Randomized trial evaluating Ranibizumab plus prompt or deferred laser or triamcinolone plus prompt laser for diabetic macular Edema. Ophthalmology. 2010;**117**(6):1064-1077.e35

[38] Ip MS, Bressler SB, Antoszyk AN, Flaxel CJ, Kim JE, Friedman SM, et al. A randomized trial comparing intravitreal triamcinolone and focal/grid photocoagulation for diabetic macular edema: Baseline features. Retina. 2008;**28**:919-930

[39] Campochiaro PA, Hafiz G, Shah SM, Bloom S, Brown DM, Busquets M, et al. Sustained ocular delivery of fluocinolone acetonide by an intravitreal insert. Ophthalmology. 2010;**117**:1393-1399.e1393

[40] Fluocinolone acetonide envision TD implant. Fluocinolone acetonide ophthalmic- Bausch & Lomb. Drugs RD. 2005;**6**(2):116-119

[41] Montero JA, Ruiz-Moreno JM. Intravitreal inserts of steroids to treat diabetic macular edema. Current Diabetes Reviews. 2009;**5**(1):26-32

[42] Chang-Lin JE, Attar M, Acheampong AA, Robinson MR, Whitcup SM, Kuppermann BD, et al. Pharmacokineticsandpharmacodynamics of a sustained-release dexamethasone intravitreal implant. Investigative Ophthalmology & Visual Science. 2011;**52**:80-86

[43] Kuppermann BD, Blumenkranz MS, Haller JA, et al. Randomized controlled study of an intravitreous dexamethasone drug delivery system in patients with persistent macular edema. Archives of Ophthalmology. 2007;**125**(3):309-317

[44] Boyer DS, Faber D, Gupta S, et al. Dexamethasone intravitreal implant for treatment of diabetic macular edema in vitrectomized patients. Retina. 2011;**31**(5):915-923

[45] Avery RL, Gordon GM. Systemic safety of prolonged monthly anti-vascular endothelial growth factor therapy for diabetic macular edema: A systematic review and meta-analysis. JAMA Ophthalmology. 2016;**134**:21-29

[46] Nawaz IM, Rezzola S, Cancarini A, Russo A, Costagliola C, Semeraro F, et al. Human vitreous in proliferative diabetic retinopathy: Characterization and translational implications. Progress in Retinal and Eye Research. 2019;**72**:100756

[47] Diabetic Retinopathy Clinical Research Network Writing Committee; Haller JA, Qin H, Apte RS, Beck RR, Bressler NM, et al. Vitrectomy outcomes in eyes with diabetic macular edema and vitreomacular traction. Ophthalmology. Jun 2010;**117**(6):1087-1093.e3

[48] Stefansson E, Novack RL, Hatchell D. Vitrectomy prevents retinal hypoxia in branch retinal vein occlusion. Investigative Ophthalmology & Visual Science. 1990;**31**:284-289

[49] Figueroa MS, Contreras I, Noval S. Surgical and anatomical outcomes of pars plana vitrectomy of diffuse nontractional diabetic macular edema. Retina. 2008;**28**:420-426

[50] Kuhn F, Kiss G, Mester V, et al. Vitrectomy with internal limiting membrane removal for clinically significant macular oedema. Graefe's Archive for Clinical and Experimental Ophthalmology. 2004;**242**:402-408

[51] Otani T, Kishi S. A controlled study of vitrectomy for diabetic macular edema. American Journal of Ophthalmology. 2002;**134**:214-219

[52] Van Effenterre G, Guyot-Argenton C, Guiberteau B, Hany I, Lacotte JL. Macular edema caused by contraction of the posterior hyaloid in diabetic retinopathy. Surgical treatment of a series of 22 cases. Journal Français d'Ophtalmologie. 1993;**16**:602-610

[53] Massin P, Duguid G, Erginay A, Haouchine B, Gaudric A. Optical coherence tomography for evaluating diabetic macular edema before and after vitrectomy. American Journal of Ophthalmology. 2003;**135**:169-177

[54] Flaxel CJ, Edwards AR, Aiello LP, et al. Factors associated with visual acuity outcomes after vitrectomy for diabetic macular edema. DRCR.net. Retina. 2010;**30**:1488-1495

[55] Kumagai K, Furukawa M, Ogino N, Larson E, Iwaky M, Tachi N. Long term follow-up of vitrectomy for diffuse nontractional diabetic macular edema. Retina. 2009;**29**:464-472

[56] Tamura K, Yokoyama T, Ebihara N, Murakami A. Histopathologic analysis of the internal limiting membrane surgically peeled from eyes with diffuse diabetic macular edema. Japanese

Journal of Ophthalmology. May 2012;**56**(3):280-287

[57] Goebel W, Kretzchmar-Gross T. Retinal thickness in diabetic retinopathy: A study using optical coherence tomography (OCT). Retina. 2002;**22**:759-767

[58] Klein R, Klein BE, Moss SE, Linton KL. The beaver dam eye study. Retinopathy in adults with newly discovered and previously diagnosed diabetes mellitus. Ophthalmology. 1992;**99**:58-62

[59] Shah SP, Patel M, Thomas D, Aldington S, Laidlaw DA. Factors predicting outcome of vitrectomy for diabetic macular oedema: Results of a prospective study. The British Journal of Ophthalmology. 2006;**90**:33-36

[60] Otani T, Kishi S. Tomographic findings of foveal hard exudates in diabetic macular edema. American Journal of Ophthalmology. 2001;**131**:50-54

[61] Sorour OA, Levine ES, Baumal CR, Elnahry AG, Braun P, Girgis J, et al. Persistent diabetic macular edema: Definition, incidence, biomarkers, and treatment methods. Survey of Ophthalmology. 2023;**68**(2):147-174

[62] Sociedad Argentina de Oftalmología (SAO). Guía para el diagnóstico, tratamiento y complicaciones del edema macular diabético y la retinopatía diabética. Buenos Aires: SAO; 2022; 154p. : il col.; 28cm

[63] Rahimy E, Shahlaee A, Khan MA, et al. Conversion to aflibercept after prior anti-VEGF therapy for persistent diabetic macular edema. American Journal of Ophthalmology. 2016;**164**:118-127

[64] Bressler NM, Beaulieu WT, Glassman AR, Blinder KJ, Bressler SB, Jampol LM, et al. Persistent macular thickening following Intravitreous Aflibercept, bevacizumab, or Ranibizumab for central-involved diabetic macular Edema with vision impairment: A secondary analysis of a randomized clinical trial. JAMA Ophthalmology. 2018;**136**(3):257-269

[65] Rush RB, Rush SW. Faricimab for treatment-resistant diabetic macular Edema. OPTH. 2022;**16**:2797-2801

[66] Ohara H, Harada Y, Hiyama T, Sadahide A, Minamoto A, Kiuchi Y. Faricimab for diabetic macular Edema in patients refractory to Ranibizumab or Aflibercept. Medicina. 2023;**59**(6):1125

[67] Veiga Reis F, Dalgalarrondo P, Da Silva Tavares Neto JE, Wendeborn Rodrigues M, Scott IU, Jorge R. Combined intravitreal dexamethasone and bevacizumab injection for the treatment of persistent diabetic macular edema (DexaBe study): A phase I clinical study. International Journal of Retina and Vitreous. 2023;**9**(1):13

[68] Jin K, Ye J. Artificial intelligence and deep learning in ophthalmology: Current status and future perspectives. Advances in Ophthalmology Practice and Research. 2022;**2**(3):100078

[69] Abràmoff MD, Lou Y, Erginay A, Clarida W, Amelon R, Folk JC, et al. Improved automated detection of diabetic retinopathy on a publicly available dataset through integration of deep learning. Investigative Ophthalmology & Visual Science. 2016;**57**(13):52000-52006

[70] Li ZQ, Fu ZX, Li WJ, Fan H, Li SN, Wang XM, et al. Prediction of diabetic macular Edema using knowledge graph. Diagnostics (Basel). 2023;**26**(13):11

[71] De Fauw J, Ledsam JR, Romera-Paredes B, et al. Clinically

applicable deep learning for diagnosis and referral in retinal disease. Nature Medicine. 2018;**24**(9):1342-1350

[72] Tang F, Wang X, Ran AR, Chan CKM, Ho M, Yip W, et al. A multitask deep-learning system to classify diabetic macular edema for different optical coherence tomography devices: A multicenter analysis. Diabetes Care. Sep 2021;**44**(9):2078-2088

[73] Le D, Alam M, Yao CK, Lim JI, Hsieh Y-T, Chan RVP, et al. Transfer learning for automated OCTA detection of diabetic retinopathy. Translational Vision Science & Technology. 2020;**9**(2):35

[74] Ryu G, Lee K, Park D, Park SH, Sagong M. A deep learning model for identifying diabetic retinopathy using optical coherence tomography angiography. Scientific Reports. 2021;**11**(1):23024

[75] Arcadu F, Benmansour F, Maunz A, Willis J, Haskova Z, Prunotto M. Deep learning algorithm predicts diabetic retinopathy progression in individual patients. NPJ Digital Medicine. 2019;**2**:92

[76] Rasti R, Allingham MJ, Mettu PS, Kavusi S, Govind K, Cousins SW, et al. Deep learning-based single-shot prediction of differential effects of anti-VEGF treatment in patients with diabetic macular edema. Biomedical Optics Express. 2020;**11**(2):1139-1152

Chapter 3

Basement Membrane Alterations in Diabetic Retinopathy

Joobin Khadamy

Abstract

In diabetic retinopathy (DR), alterations in the basement membrane (BM) play a pivotal role in disease progression. This chapter reviews the intricate changes occurring in the BM, a critical structural and functional element in retinal integrity. Comprising collagen, laminin, nidogens, and proteoglycans, the BM orchestrates cell behavior, tissue compartmentalization, and vascular support. In diabetes, disruptions to BM composition lead to structural modifications and impact critical cellular functions, triggering a cascade of events in DR pathogenesis. Visualizing these alterations via histological stains, imaging, and in vitro models reveals BM thickening, glycation, and altered molecular composition. These changes compromise retinal architecture, vascular permeability, and neovascularization, contributing to DR's characteristic complications. Therapeutic approaches targeting BM alterations in DR primarily involve indirect interventions like anti-vascular endothelial growth factor (VEGF) therapy, while direct strategies such as gene therapy or siRNA-based methods show promise but require further exploration. Understanding these BM changes is crucial for devising precise therapeutic interventions to mitigate DR progression and associated ocular complications.

Keywords: basement membrane, diabetic retinopathy, pathophysiology, structural changes, chemical alterations, retinal basement membrane, vascular permeability, glycation, cross-linking, therapeutic interventions

1. Introduction

Diabetic retinopathy (DR) stands as one of the most severe complications of diabetes mellitus, posing a significant threat to vision and quality of life for millions worldwide. At the heart of its pathogenesis lies the intricate interplay of various molecular and cellular events, many of which converge on the basement membrane (BM), a fundamental structural component within the retinal microvasculature. The BM serves as a critical interface between endothelial cells, pericytes, and surrounding extracellular matrix (ECM), playing pivotal roles in vascular integrity, cellular signaling, and barrier function. However, in the setting of chronic hyperglycemia, the BM undergoes profound alterations, heralding the onset and progression of DR. These changes encompass a spectrum of biochemical, biophysical, and cellular modifications, ranging from abnormal thickening and cross-linking to dysregulated turnover and degradation. Importantly, these BM alterations not only disrupt the delicate balance of ECM homeostasis but also contribute to microvascular dysfunction, neurovascular coupling deficits, and ultimately, vision-threatening complications such as macular edema, ischemia, and neovascularization. Understanding the intricate sequences and consequences of these BM changes is paramount for unraveling the complexities of DR pathogenesis and devising targeted therapeutic strategies aimed at preserving BM integrity, restoring vascular function, and halting disease progression. In this chapter, we delve into the multifaceted roles of the BM in DR, exploring the mechanisms underlying its alteration, the implications for retinal vascular health, and the therapeutic avenues targeting BM pathology to combat this sight-threatening disease. Through a comprehensive examination of BM dynamics in the context of DR, we aim to provide insights into the pathophysiology of the disease and pave the way for innovative approaches to diagnosis, prevention, and treatment [1, 2].

2. Normal composition and physiologic role of basement membrane

The BM, a specialized extracellular matrix (ECM), has evolved from being perceived solely as a structural component to a pivotal regulator of cellular behavior and tissue microenvironment signaling. It typically consists of several key components:

- *Collagens:* Collagen IV is the most abundant collagen type found in BMs across species. It is distinguished as a unique protein matrix crucial for cellular function. Other collagen types, like Collagen XVIII and Collagen XV, are also present but to a lesser extent [3].

- *Laminins:* Laminins are glycoproteins that form cross-shaped structures and are crucial for BM assembly and stability. They interact with other BM components and cell surface receptors [4].

- *Nidogens (Entactins):* These glycoproteins help link laminin and collagen networks within the BM [5].

- *Heparan sulfate proteoglycans (HSPGs):* HSPGs, such as perlecan and agrin, contribute to the structural integrity of the BM and serve as binding sites for growth factors and other molecules [6].

- *Various glycoproteins and proteases* include fibronectin, thrombospondin, and various enzymes and proteases involved in the remodeling and maintenance of the BM [7].

The lens capsule, enveloping the eye's lens, ranks among the thickest BMs in the human body, offering robust structural support to lens fiber cells. Primarily comprised of collagen type IV, laminin, fibronectin, and other matrix proteins akin to other BMs, it plays a pivotal role in maintaining the lens' shape and stability. Although significant, the lens capsule is not the sole thick BM; Bruch's membrane in the eye, positioned between the retinal pigment epithelium and choroid, also holds substantial thickness and is crucial for supporting retinal function. Composed of collagen types IV and III, laminins, fibronectin, and additional components, Bruch's membrane serves as a vital structural element in maintaining retinal integrity [8–11].

Across different species, while the basic components of BMs are conserved, there can be variations in the specific composition and structure. For instance, some species may have unique isoforms or variations of certain proteins, which could influence the BM's properties and functions. The relative proportions or specific arrangements of components might also differ, contributing to species-specific characteristics in tissue structure and function. These variations often reflect adaptations to specific physiological or environmental needs within different species [12].

Across various tissues, including the retina, the BM orchestrates several fundamental functions:

- *Cell adhesion modulation:* Enabling cellular anchoring and interaction within the retinal microenvironment [13].

- *Cell signaling:* Influencing cellular behavior through interactions with receptors, thereby modulating growth, differentiation, and migration [14].

- *Structural scaffold:* Providing crucial support and organization to cellular components.

- *Tissue compartmentalization:* BMs partition different tissue compartments and communicate external microenvironment cues to epithelial or endothelial cells, guiding cellular responses. Separating different cellular regions contributes to retinal compartmentalization.

- *Vascular structural support:* Within blood vessels, the BM acts as an extracellular sensor for endothelial cells and pericytes, influencing their behavior and responses to external stimuli [15].

- *Regulating pericyte contractility:* BM provides structural support for pericyte attachment and function along capillary walls. It acts as a platform for signaling molecules that control pericyte contractility. It influences blood vessel stability and flow; changes in BM affect vessel contractility [16].

- *Selective barrier or blood-retinal barrier (BRB):* Regulating molecular and cellular transport between retinal compartments. Contributing significantly to maintaining retinal homeostasis by regulating substance exchange between blood vessels and the neural retina [17].

- *Tumor angiogenesis regulation/neovascularization:* Components of vascular BMs have emerged as potential targets for cancer therapies due to their involvement in regulating tumor angiogenesis [18–20].

- *Regulating apoptosis:* BM acts as a microenvironmental cue for cell survival and programmed cell death. It serves as a structural and signaling scaffold, guiding cells in apoptosis regulation. Changes in BM composition or integrity impact cellular signaling pathways involved in apoptosis [21].

In summary, the BM is pivotal in maintaining tissue integrity and regulating critical cellular functions like apoptosis, pericyte contractility, and vascular homeostasis. Any alterations in BM structure or composition can significantly impact these regulatory mechanisms, leading to pathological conditions or functional irregularities within tissues and organs.

3. Studying basement membrane changes in diabetic retinopathy

Studying BM's structures both *in vivo* (within living organisms) and *in vitro* (in controlled laboratory settings) involves various techniques tailored to the specific environment and objectives:

3.1 In vivo studies

- *Histology and immunohistochemistry:* Tissue samples obtained through biopsies or post-mortem examinations are stained and examined under a microscope to visualize BM components and changes.

- *Advanced imaging techniques:* Modalities like Optical Coherence Tomography (OCT) or Confocal Microscopy offer non-invasive, high-resolution visualization of BM in living tissues.

- *Molecular profiling:* Analyzing gene and protein expression in living tissues to understand alterations in BM components and associated genes.

- *Animal models:* Studying BM changes in live animal models, allowing for observation and manipulation under controlled conditions that partly mimic human physiology.

3.2 In vitro studies

- *Cell culture models:* Growing cells on specialized surfaces mimicking BM conditions to study cell-BM interactions, often using substrates like Matrigel or synthetic matrices.

- *Electron microscopy:* Ultrastructural analysis of BM components in cell cultures or isolated tissues to examine minute details.

- *Immunocytochemistry:* Labeling and visualization of specific BM proteins or components in cultured cells using fluorescent antibodies.

- *Functional assays:* Assessing cell behavior and responses to BM-like environments, including migration, adhesion, and signaling studies.

Each method offers distinct advantages and limitations in studying BM structures, providing complementary insights into their composition, organization, and functional roles in health and disease [22–27].

4. Stains for visualizing basement membrane

Utilizing these staining techniques in histology and cellular studies is crucial for understanding BM structure, integrity, and alterations in various pathologies. Accurate visualization of the BM aids in diagnosing and studying diseases like DR, glomerular diseases, and cancer metastasis, where BM changes are significant markers of disease progression. These stains and immunostaining methods offer valuable tools to uncover structural and molecular changes in BMs associated with different pathological conditions, enabling deeper insights into disease mechanisms and potential therapeutic interventions.

4.1 Histological stains

- *Periodic acid-Schiff (PAS) stain:* Commonly used to highlight carbohydrate-rich components in BMs, providing a pink to magenta coloration [28].

- *Jones' methenamine silver (JMS) stain:* Reveals the reticular fibers present in the BM, typically staining them black [29].

- *Hematoxylin and eosin (H&E) stain:* While not specific to the BM, this stain helps in visualizing tissue morphology and can indirectly indicate BM structure [30].

4.2 Immunohistochemical stains

- *Collagen IV antibodies:* Immunostaining with antibodies against collagen IV allows specific visualization of this major BM component [31].

- *Laminin antibodies:* Immunostaining against laminin proteins, particularly laminin 332 and 511, highlights their presence in the BM [31].

- *Fibronectin antibodies:* Staining with fibronectin antibodies aids in identifying fibronectin in the BM [32].

4.3 Cellular studies

- *Fluorescent probes:* Specific fluorescent markers can label BM components, allowing their visualization under fluorescence microscopy [33].

- *Immunocytochemistry:* Utilizing antibodies against various BM constituents for labeling and imaging in cell cultures [34].

- *Transmission electron microscopy (TEM)* provides ultrastructural details of the BM in cellular and tissue samples [35].

4.4 Visualizing basement membrane or basement membrane-like structures during ocular surgeries

Vital dyes like Trypan Blue and Indocyanine Green (ICG) play crucial roles in ocular surgeries, particularly in staining BM or BM-like structures such as the lens capsule and the internal limiting membrane (ILM) in various procedures.

- *Tripan blue in phacoemulsification:* Tripan Blue is often used in phacoemulsification surgery to stain the lens capsule in mature cataracts or complex surgeries. Its application helps surgeons visualize and precisely manipulate the capsule during cataract removal, ensuring accurate capsulorhexis and lens implantation [36].

- *Indocyanine green (ICG) or infracyanine green in vitrectomy:* During vitrectomy procedures, ICG is utilized to stain the ILM, a structure resembling the BM in the retina. It aids surgeons in delineating the ILM's boundary and facilitates its removal in surgeries addressing conditions like macular holes or diabetic macular edema. ICG's affinity for components like collagen type 4 and laminin in the ILM enables better visualization and manipulation [37].

These dyes' ability to interact with BM or BM-like structures provides valuable guidance for surgeons, ensuring meticulous handling and improved outcomes in ocular surgeries targeting these membranes.

5. Matrigel vs. retinal organoids in diabetic retinopathy studies

Matrigel, despite its widespread use as a basement membrane (BM) *in vitro* model in studies, has inherent limitations. Matrigel proves valuable in specific research contexts in exploring DR and potential cell therapies but needs more fidelity in replicating the complex composition of natural BM [38–40]. Matrigel, originating from a tumor, rich in laminin, collagen, and ECM proteins, offers a surrogate environment akin to BMs but does not entirely mirror the intricate alterations observed in DR's BM. This limitation profoundly impacts the interpretation and design of studies concerning DR and endothelial progenitor cell (EPC) defects. Researchers should acknowledge these limitations when using Matrigel for DR investigations, as it does not encompass the full spectrum of components, notably collagen IV, which is crucial for BM functionality [41]. Diversified study approaches, integrating Matrigel-based experiments with models capturing BM complexities seen in DR, such as animal models or ex vivo human tissue studies, become imperative. Additionally, validating findings in relevant clinical or physiologically representative models becomes crucial for the translational applicability of insights regarding human DR. Ultimately, while Matrigel serves as an initial tool in understanding cellular interactions and ECM responses, diversified study approaches are vital to unravel the complexities of DR-related BM alterations and optimize potential therapies [42, 43].

Indeed, retinal organoids have emerged as a promising alternative to Matrigel in ocular research. These three-dimensional structures, derived from stem cells, mimic the cellular organization and functionality of the retina. Unlike Matrigel, which serves as a general ECM surrogate, retinal organoids specifically replicate the complexity of retinal tissue, offering a more precise model for studying retinal diseases and treatments. Retinal organoids provide researchers with a closer representation of the retinal microenvironment, allowing for more accurate assessments of cellular interactions, disease mechanisms, and potential therapeutic interventions, marking a significant advancement in retinal research methodologies [44].

6. Structural and chemical changes in basement membrane in diabetic retinopathy

In DR, vascular BM thickening emerges as a pivotal histological alteration. Studies using high-resolution imaging establish BM thickening as a critical structural abnormality in retinal capillaries, likely resulting from excessive BM component accumulation induced by hyperglycemia. Preventing this thickening shows promise in mitigating DR-associated lesions, prompting the exploration of gene regulatory approaches to control BM component synthesis.

- *Thickening:* One of the hallmark alterations observed in DR involves BM thickening, impacting vascular permeability and cellular interactions [1, 2].

- *Glycation and cross-linking:* Increased glycation end products and cross-linking compromise BM flexibility and function [2].

- *Altered composition:* The elevated glucose levels causing increased expression of type IV collagen, fibronectin, and laminin genes, along with decreased matrix metalloproteinase (MMP) activities, significantly contribute to the alterations seen in the BM in DR [1]. Changes in matrix proteins and enzymes disrupt the normal BM architecture, affecting cell adhesion and migration.

7. Structural consequences of basement membrane changes

Understanding the temporal progression of basement membrane (BM) alterations in diabetic retinopathy (DR) is essential for elucidating the disease's pathophysiology and developing effective intervention strategies. While clinical manifestations of DR often manifest in advanced stages, accumulating evidence suggests that BM changes commence early in the disease course, long before overt signs of retinopathy emerge. Therefore, delineating the sequential stages of BM alteration is crucial for capturing the disease's evolution and identifying potential therapeutic targets. These stages typically encompass early biochemical modifications, including increased synthesis of BM components such as fibronectin, type IV collagen, and laminin, driven by chronic hyperglycemia and associated metabolic perturbations. After this, structural changes such as BM thickening, cross-linking, and dysregulation of turnover mechanisms ensue, leading to compromised BM integrity and functionality. Importantly, these early alterations pave the way for subsequent vascular abnormalities, including microaneurysm formation, capillary occlusion, and breakdown of the blood-retinal barrier. By elucidating the temporal sequence of BM alterations, researchers and clinicians can gain insights into the disease's natural history, identify biomarkers for early detection, and devise targeted interventions aimed at halting or reversing BM pathology before irreversible retinal damage occurs. Thus, a comprehensive discussion of the stages of BM alteration in DR is imperative for advancing our understanding of the disease's pathogenesis and improving clinical management strategies. This sequence outlines the progression from diabetes/hyperglycemia to the development of DR, illustrating the intricate cascade of events (**Figure 1**):

- *Diabetes/hyperglycemia:* Elevated glucose levels associated with diabetes trigger a series of changes.

- *Early changes:*

  - *Cx43 downregulation and reduced GJIC:* Connexin 43 (Cx43) downregulation reduces gap junctional intercellular communication (GJIC), impacting cellular signaling and coordination [45].

  - *Increased ECM synthesis:* This leads to BM thickening, a common occurrence in DR [1].

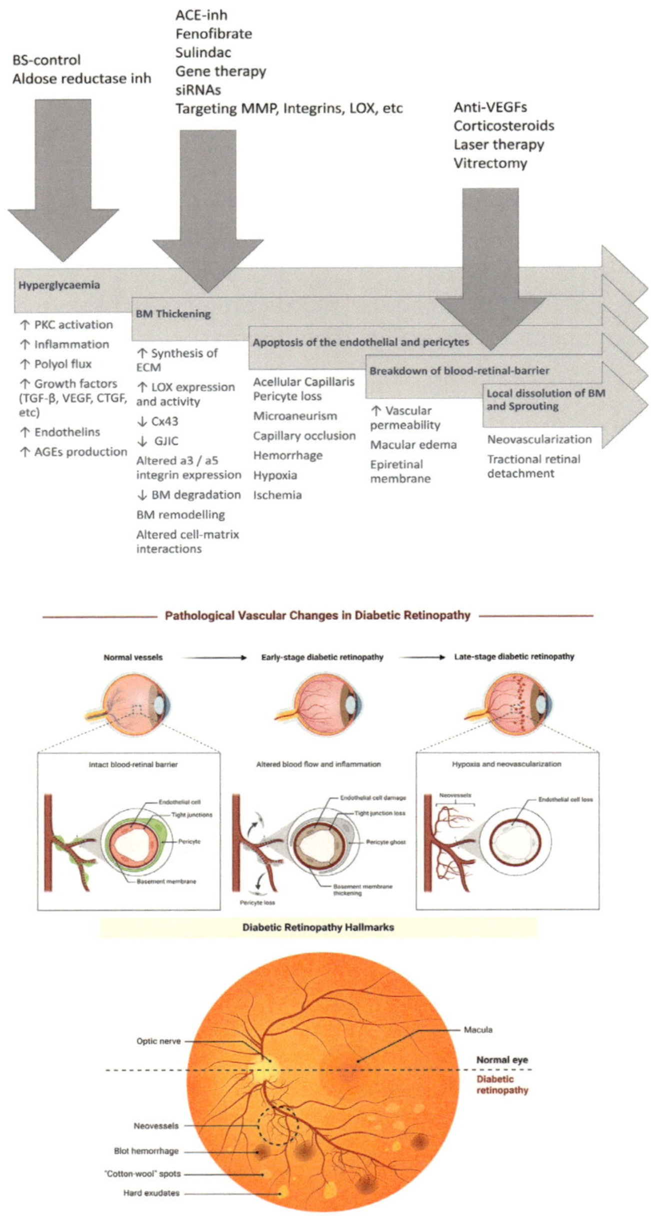

Figure 1.

The diagram depicts the intricate interplay of biochemical pathways driving diabetic retinopathy progression and potential therapeutic strategies. Hyperglycemia initiates a cascade of events, including PKC activation, inflammation, increased polyol flux, elevated growth factor levels, endothelin production, and AGE accumulation, ultimately leading to the thickening of the BM. This thickening, exacerbated by reduced BM degradation and altered cell-matrix interactions, contributes to endothelial and pericyte apoptosis, acellular capillaries, microaneurysms, and the breakdown of the blood-retina barrier, resulting in macular edema. Local dissolution of the BM promotes neovascularization. Potential therapeutic interventions targeting these pathways include blood sugar control, aldose reductase inhibitors, ACE inhibitors, fenofibrate, sulindac, gene therapy, siRNAs, MMP inhibitors, anti-VEGF agents, corticosteroids, laser therapy, and vitrectomy, offering diverse approaches to mitigate diabetic retinopathy progression. PKC: protein kinase C, TGF-β: transforming growth factor-beta, VEGF: vascular endothelial growth factor, CTGF: connective tissue growth factor, AGE: advanced glycation end products, ECM: extracellular matrix, LOX: lysyl oxidase, Cx43: Connexin 43, GJIC: gap junctional intercellular communication, BS-control: blood sugar control, Aldose reductase inh: aldose reductase inhibitors, ACE-inh: angiotensin-converting enzyme inhibitors.

- *Further progression:*

  - *Altered BM composition and integrin expression:* Changes in BM composition occur alongside altered expression of specific integrins (α3, α5), affecting cell-BM interactions and signaling [46].

  - *Acellular capillaries and pericyte loss:* As a consequence, there's the formation of acellular capillaries and loss of pericytes around blood vessels [47].

  - *Increased LOX expression and activity:* Elevated lysyl oxidase (LOX) expression and activity contribute to alterations in the BM's ultrastructural integrity [48].

  - *Loss of BM ultrastructural integrity:* These changes lead to compromised structural integrity of the BM, impacting its ability to maintain tissue architecture and cellular support [2].

  - *Apoptosis and breakdown of blood-retinal barrier:* Loss of BM integrity contributes to increased apoptosis and breakdown of the blood-retinal barrier (BRB) [49].

  - *Facilitate local dissolution of BM:* Weakened BM structure allows for local dissolution, further compromising BM integrity [2].

  - *Vascular permeability and sprouting:* This breakdown leads to increased vascular permeability and sprouting of new blood vessels [50].

- *Late stages:*

  This intricate sequence underscores how diabetes-induced changes in ECM synthesis and BM alterations set off a chain reaction of events leading to structural and functional abnormalities in the retina, culminating in the manifestation of DR and its associated complications.

  - *Vascular compromise and microaneurysms:* Disrupted integrity of the BM contributes to vascular abnormalities and microaneurysm formation characteristic of DR [51, 52].

  - *Diabetic macular edema (DME):* These changes may contribute to DME.

  - *Neovascularization:* Alterations in the BM architecture promote abnormal vessel growth, exacerbating retinal damage and progression of the condition [53, 54].

8. Impact on other basement membranes

- *Bruch's membrane:* In DR, Bruch's membrane, a crucial divider between the retinal pigment epithelium (RPE) and the choroid, experiences notable transformations. Thickening and structural modifications in Bruch's membrane can impair RPE function, disrupting the exchange of nutrients and waste materials between the retina and the underlying choroid. Moreover, the buildup of deposits within Bruch's membrane can hinder nutrient transport, potentially worsening retinal damage. These alterations compromise the integrity of the blood-retinal barrier (BRB), leading to heightened vascular permeability and potential leakage, thereby contributing to the advancement of DR. Investigating the dynamic relationship among Bruch's membrane, the RPE, and the BRB remains an active research area, aiming to comprehend the fundamental mechanisms driving DR and develop precise interventions to mitigate its progression [55, 56].

- *Corneal epithelial basement membrane (EBM):* In diabetic individuals, the corneal EBM undergoes significant changes, marked by heightened fragility, reduced hemidesmosomes, and altered adhesion. Hyperglycemia contributes to the resistance of stromal nerves entering the epithelium, forming nerve fiber loops alongside alterations in the corneal stromal ECM. Reduced corneal epithelial cell adhesion under high glucose conditions leads to fragile BM, which is susceptible to cell removal during manual debridement. Studies highlight increased MMP-10 and cathepsin F activity in diabetic corneas, potentially causing protein degradation and subsequent BM and integrin alterations. These structural and functional abnormalities in diabetic corneas elevate complications following surgeries like cataracts, refractive surgeries, vitrectomy, and panretinal photocoagulation (PRP), particularly impacting wound healing and corneal sensation post-epithelial debridement during vitrectomy and photorefractive keratectomy (PRK). Diabetic patients often experience increased corneal thickness, endothelial cell loss, and persistent edema post-cataract surgery, while refractive surgeries pose higher risks due to potential recurrent erosions, persistent defects, and slower healing, necessitating caution in recommending these procedures for diabetic individuals, especially those with DR [57, 58].

- *Lens capsule:* Similarly, in the lens capsule of diabetic patients, thickening alterations can contribute to opacity and capsular phimosis. These changes not only affect visual quality but may also pose challenges during subsequent retinal examinations following cataract surgery [59].

- *Internal limiting membrane (ILM):* The internal limiting membrane (ILM), while not a typical BM, shares several characteristics, acting as a boundary between the retina's neural tissue and the vitreous humor. Modifications in the ILM structure or composition might contribute to DR progression. Peeling the inner limiting membrane (ILM) and inducing a posterior vitreous detachment (PVD) have been explored as potential approaches to reduce neovascularization in DR. These techniques are commonly employed during vitrectomy surgery for DR. By meticulously removing the ILM, surgeons aim to eliminate residual fibrovascular tissue and cellular elements that could contribute to the progression of neovascularization or consequent epiretinal membrane (ERM) formation. Additionally, inducing a PVD, which is the separation of the vitreous from the retina, might reduce tractional forces and interrupt the signaling pathways that trigger abnormal vessel growth, potentially reducing the development of new blood vessels in the retina. While these strategies have shown promise in some cases, further research is needed to establish their efficacy and safety as interventions to specifically target and reduce neovascularization in DR [60–62].

9. Treatment approaches targeting basement membrane alterations

Treatment strategies addressing ECM or BM alterations lack direct medications tailored for these components. However, existing drugs used in various conditions can indirectly impact ECM/BM metabolism by influencing cell behavior and secretory activities (**Figure 1**). Anti-VEGF Therapy represents one such approach, where inhibiting vascular endothelial growth factor (VEGF) can address abnormal vascularization characteristic of DR, thereby impacting ECM/BM changes. Agents like ranibizumab, aflibercept, and bevacizumab are commonly employed to manage these vascular changes. Steroidal interventions play a crucial role in managing inflammation, which can indirectly affect BM integrity. By mitigating inflammation, steroids indirectly contribute to preserving BM integrity. Emerging Therapies are also being explored to target BM synthesis pathways directly, aiming to restore its normal architecture. These novel approaches hold promise for more targeted interventions in the future. Other approaches include strategies like tight glycemic control through insulin therapy, which has shown promise in preventing BM thickening in diabetic retinas. Matrix metalloproteinases (MMPs), known for their role in tissue remodeling and ECM degradation, have implications in BM changes and vascular damage in DR. While direct targeting of MMPs poses challenges due to their multifaceted functions, indirect strategies via upstream regulators or inflammation modulation are being investigated. Additionally, therapies like sulindac and aldose reductase inhibitors have shown potential in preventing retinal capillary BM thickening in experimental models. Gene therapy approaches, including CRISPR/Cas9 and antisense oligonucleotides targeting fibronectin, offer novel avenues for directly addressing ECM/BM alterations. Furthermore, siRNA approaches targeting fibronectin have shown promise in reducing BM thickening and preventing vascular cell loss. Fenofibrate, primarily used for hyperlipidemia, has also shown potential in blocking the progression of DR by reducing BM thickening and retinal vascular permeability. Prospective Directions include investigating the role of lysyl oxidase (LOX) alterations in classifying DR stages and its potential as a therapeutic target, as well as exploring the modulation of integrins, which mediate signals between ECM and cells, as a therapeutic approach. These prospective directions offer exciting avenues for further research and development in the field of diabetic retinopathy treatment.

- *Anti-VEGF therapy:* Mitigating BM alterations by inhibiting VEGF to address vascular changes. In conditions like DR, anti-VEGF agents (e.g., ranibizumab, aflibercept, and bevacizumab) are deployed to manage abnormal vascularization, inadvertently impacting ECM/BM changes [63].

- *Steroidal interventions:* Managing inflammation and its potential influence on BM integrity. Steroids are employed to mitigate inflammation, which can indirectly affect BM integrity [64].

9.1 Other approaches

- *Tight glycemic control:* insulin therapy prevented BM thickening in diabetic rat retinas.

- *Matrix metalloproteinases (MMPs):* These are key players in tissue remodeling and ECM degradation. In DR, MMPs like MMP-2 and MMP-9 are implicated in BM changes and vascular damage due to their ability to break down ECM components. Directly targeting MMPs in DR treatment remains challenging due to their multifaceted functions. Ongoing research explores MMP inhibitors to manage diabetic complications, but their broad impact on physiological processes and side effects limits their clinical use. Instead, indirect strategies are being investigated:

- *Inhibition via upstream regulators:* Therapies influencing factors regulating MMP activity, like anti-VEGF agents, indirectly impact MMP function by reducing inflammation and abnormal angiogenesis, potentially affecting MMP expression [65].

- *Inflammation modulation:* Anti-inflammatory therapies aim to control inflammation, indirectly impacting MMP function and, consequently, ECM degradation [66].

- *Gene therapy:* Gene therapy and RNA-based methods are exploring specific MMP expression modulation in diabetic complications, potentially offering more targeted interventions in the future [67]. While MMPs contribute to DR, targeting them directly encounters hurdles due to their diverse functions and potential side effects. Future strategies might focus on specific MMP isoforms or their regulatory mechanisms for more precise ECM remodeling [68, 69].

• *Sulindac:* An anti-inflammatory drug that prevents retinal capillary BM thickening in diabetic dogs [70].

• *Aldose reductase inhibitors (ARI):* Aldose reductase, an enzyme involved in the polyol pathway, has been implicated in the pathogenesis of DR due to its role in mediating glucose metabolism and oxidative stress. In diabetes, elevated levels of glucose lead to increased flux through the polyol pathway, resulting in the conversion of glucose to sorbitol by aldose reductase. Sorbitol accumulation within retinal cells can contribute to osmotic stress, oxidative damage, and altered cellular function, ultimately leading to retinal tissue damage characteristic of DR.

  Research suggests that ARIs may hold therapeutic potential for mitigating the development and progression of DR. By inhibiting aldose reductase activity, ARIs aim to reduce sorbitol accumulation, oxidative stress, and downstream pathological changes associated with DR. Preclinical studies have demonstrated the efficacy of ARIs in attenuating retinal vascular abnormalities, reducing inflammation, and preserving retinal function in diabetic animal models.

  However, clinical trials investigating the effectiveness of ARIs in diabetic patients have yielded mixed results. While some studies have reported beneficial effects of ARIs on slowing the progression of DR and preserving visual function, others have shown limited efficacy or adverse effects. Challenges in translating preclinical findings to clinical practice include variability in patient response, differences in study design and duration, and potential side effects of ARIs.

  Despite these challenges, ongoing research continues to explore novel ARIs with improved efficacy, safety, and tolerability profiles. Additionally, combination therapies targeting multiple pathways implicated in DR pathogenesis, including aldose reductase inhibition, may offer synergistic benefits for managing DR. Further clinical studies are needed to validate the therapeutic potential of ARIs and optimize their use as part of comprehensive management strategies for DR in diabetic patients [71].

- *Gene therapy:* Especially, CRISPR/Cas9, holds promise for directly addressing ECM/BM alterations by correcting genetic mutations affecting BM composition or function. Yet, these techniques are still nascent and require extensive exploration for clinical application [72].

- *Antisense oligonucleotides:* Targeting fibronectin overexpression using antisense oligonucleotides reduced BM thickness and vascular abnormalities. A combined antisense oligonucleotide approach against fibronectin, collagen IV, and laminin was more effective [73].

- *siRNA approach:* Short interfering RNAs (siRNAs) targeting fibronectin showed promise in reducing BM thickening and preventing vascular cell loss, offering longer efficacy than antisense oligonucleotides [74].

- *Angiotensin-converting enzyme (ACE) inhibitors:* The renin-angiotensin system (RAS) plays a crucial role in regulating blood pressure and fluid balance, but its components also have implications in the pathogenesis of DR, particularly in BM alterations. ACE inhibitors, commonly used to manage hypertension, have shown promise in mitigating BM changes associated with DR. The RAS, including angiotensin II, contributes to vascular abnormalities and BM thickening in DR through various mechanisms, including promoting inflammation, oxidative stress, and endothelial dysfunction. ACE inhibitors act by blocking the conversion of angiotensin I to angiotensin II, thereby attenuating its detrimental effects on the retinal vasculature and BM integrity. Studies have demonstrated that ACE inhibitors can reduce BM thickening and improve retinal microvascular function in diabetic animal models. Additionally, clinical trials have reported beneficial effects of ACE inhibitors in slowing the progression of DR and reducing the risk of vision loss in diabetic patients. These findings highlight the potential therapeutic role of ACE inhibitors in preserving BM integrity and mitigating the vascular complications associated with DR. However, further research is needed to elucidate the underlying mechanisms and optimize treatment strategies involving ACE inhibitors for the management of DR [53, 54].

- *Fenofibrate administration:* Fenofibrate, primarily used for hyperlipidemia, showed promise in blocking the progression of DR by reducing BM thickening and retinal vascular permeability. Further investigations are needed to understand fenofibrate's mechanism in preventing DR progression [75].

9.2 Prospective directions

- *LOX (lysyl oxidase):* LOX alterations could classify DR stages, potentially serving as a therapeutic target [76].

- *Integrin:* Integrins' role in mediating signals between ECM and cells suggests ECM modulation as a therapeutic approach [77].

9.3 Challenges and further research

Research continues to identify ECM/BM targets and develop treatments directly modulating their synthesis, assembly, or turnover. These evolving strategies might offer more precise interventions for conditions linked to ECM/BM abnormalities in the future. Complexities exist beyond BM thickening in DR, requiring an understanding of tissue-specific responses to hyperglycemia. Various tissues respond differently to hyperglycemia [78], indicating potential genetic protective factors against pathological changes. While BM thickening is pivotal in DR, additional pathological factors contribute to the characteristic lesions, necessitating further research. In essence, targeting BM thickening holds promise as a therapeutic avenue for DR treatment. However, complexities beyond BM thickening in DR necessitate comprehensive research to understand and develop effective therapeutic strategies.

Firstly, a key challenge lies in unraveling the precise mechanisms underlying BM alterations in DR. While BM thickening is a hallmark feature, understanding the sequence of events leading to this phenomenon and its implications for retinal pathology requires comprehensive investigation. Additionally, elucidating the cross-talk between BM changes and other pathological processes, such as inflammation, oxidative stress, and angiogenesis, is crucial for developing targeted interventions. Furthermore, there is a need to identify specific molecular targets within the BM matrix and explore innovative strategies for modulating their expression or activity. This may involve harnessing the potential of emerging technologies like gene editing or RNA-based therapeutics to precisely manipulate BM-related pathways. Another challenge is translating preclinical findings into clinically viable treatments. While promising results have been obtained in animal models, translating these findings to human patients poses significant hurdles, including safety concerns, efficacy in diverse patient populations, and long-term outcomes. Moreover, developing personalized treatment approaches that consider individual variations in BM composition and response to therapy represents a formidable challenge. Future research directions should also focus on evaluating combination therapies targeting multiple pathways implicated in BM alterations and DR progression. Collaborative efforts between basic scientists, clinicians, and pharmaceutical companies are essential to overcome these challenges and drive forward the development of effective treatments for DR targeting the BM. Additionally, clinical trials assessing the efficacy and safety of novel therapeutics targeting BM alterations are needed to validate their potential clinical utility and guide evidence-based treatment strategies. Overall, addressing these challenges and advancing further research in this field holds the promise of revolutionizing DR management and improving outcomes for affected individuals.

10. Conclusions

The intricate changes in the BM within the context of DR underscore the pivotal role of this structure in maintaining tissue integrity and regulating essential cellular functions.

The BM, initially recognized as a structural element, has evolved into a critical regulator of cellular behavior and tissue microenvironments. Composed of various components like collagens, laminins, nidogens, and proteoglycans, the BM acts as a scaffold, influencing cellular behavior, compartmentalizing tissues, and regulating critical functions like apoptosis and vascular permeability.

In diabetic conditions, alterations in BM composition and structure disrupt its integrity, leading to a cascade of events culminating in retinal complications characteristic of DR. This progression from early changes like reduced gap junctional communication and increased ECM synthesis to advanced stages involving neovascularization and diabetic macular edema highlights the intricate sequence of events triggered by diabetes-induced alterations in the BM.

Understanding these changes is crucial for devising effective therapeutic strategies. Techniques ranging from histological stains to advanced imaging modalities aid in visualizing BM alterations both in vivo and in vitro. However, challenges persist in replicating the complexity of BM alterations observed in DR, particularly in in vitro models like Matrigel.

Structural and chemical changes in the BM, notably thickening, glycation, and altered composition, significantly impact retinal integrity, vascular permeability, and neovascularization. These alterations also extend their impact to other BMs in the eye, such as Bruch's membrane, the corneal epithelial BM, the lens capsule, and the internal limiting membrane, affecting various ocular functions and surgical outcomes in diabetic individuals.

Therapeutic approaches targeting BM alterations in DR remain indirect, utilizing agents like anti-VEGF therapy, steroidal interventions, and emerging strategies to mitigate vascular changes and inflammation. Direct interventions targeting specific BM components, gene therapies, or siRNA-based approaches show promise but require extensive exploration for clinical application.

While targeting BM thickening holds therapeutic promise, the complexities beyond this aspect in DR necessitate comprehensive research for effective interventions. Understanding tissue-specific responses to hyperglycemia, identifying ECM/BM targets, and developing precise treatments are essential for mitigating the progression of DR and its associated complications. Future research should aim to unravel these complexities and bridge the gap between bench findings and clinical applicability for improved management of DR.

Acknowledgements

The authors acknowledge the use of ChatGPT for language polishing of the manuscript.

Conflict of interest

The authors declare no conflict of interest.

Author details

Joobin Khadamy
Department of Ophthalmology, University Hospital of Umea, Umea, Sweden

*Address all correspondence to: joobin.khadamy@regionvasterbotten.se

References

[1] Sankaramoorthy A, Roy S. Vascular basement membrane thickening: Basis of disease pathology in diabetic retinopathy. In: Prakash G, Iwata T, editors. Advances in Vision Research, Volume III: Genetic Eye Research around the Globe. Singapore: Springer Singapore. pp. 275-287

[2] Roy S, Kim D. Retinal capillary basement membrane thickening: Role in the pathogenesis of diabetic retinopathy. Progress in Retinal and Eye Research. 2021;**82**:100903

[3] Timpl R, Martin GR. Components of basement membranes. In: Immunochemistry of the Extracellular Matrix. Boca Raton, FL, USA: CRC Press eBooks. DOI: 10.1201/9781351073424-5

[4] Martin GR, Timpl R. Laminin and other basement membrane components. Annual Review of Cell Biology. 1987;**3**:57-85

[5] Breitkreutz D, Koxholt I, Thiemann K, et al. Skin basement membrane: The foundation of epidermal integrity—BM functions and diverse roles of bridging molecules nidogen and perlecan. BioMed Research International. 2013;**2013**:179784. Epub ahead of print 21 March 2013. DOI: 10.1155/2013/179784

[6] McCarthy KJ. The basement membrane proteoglycans perlecan and agrin: Something old, something new. Current Topics in Membranes. 2015;**76**:255-303

[7] Sonbol HS. Extracellular matrix remodeling in human disease. Journal of Microscopy and Ultrastructure. 2018;**6**:123-128

[8] Lee CJ, Vroom JA, Fishman HA, et al. Determination of human lens capsule permeability and its feasibility as a replacement for Bruch's membrane. Biomaterials. 2006;**27**:1670-1678

[9] Rankenberg J, Rakete S, Wagner BD, et al. Advanced glycation end products in human diabetic lens capsules. Experimental Eye Research. 2021;**210**:108704

[10] Halfter W, Moes S, Halfter K, et al. The human Descemet's membrane and lens capsule: Protein composition and biomechanical properties. Experimental Eye Research. 2020;**201**:108326

[11] Fields MA, Del Priore LV, Adelman RA, et al. Interactions of the choroid, Bruch's membrane, retinal pigment epithelium, and neurosensory retina collaborate to form the outer blood-retinal-barrier. Progress in Retinal and Eye Research. 2020;**76**:100803

[12] Karsdal MA, Nielsen MJ, Sand JM, et al. Extracellular matrix remodeling: The common denominator in connective tissue diseases. Possibilities for evaluation and current understanding of the matrix as more than a passive architecture, but a key player in tissue failure. Assay and Drug Development Technologies. 2013;**11**:70-92

[13] O'Leary F, Campbell M. The blood-retina barrier in health and disease. The FEBS Journal. 2023;**290**:878-891

[14] Streuli C. Extracellular matrix remodelling and cellular differentiation. Current Opinion in Cell Biology. 1999;**11**:634-640

[15] Wang D, Brady T, Santhanam L, et al. The extracellular matrix mechanics in the vasculature. Nature Cardiovascular Research. 2023;**2**:718-732

[16] Beltramo E, Porta M. Pericyte loss in diabetic retinopathy: Mechanisms and consequences. Current Medicinal Chemistry. 2013;**20**:3218-3225

[17] Klaassen I, Van Noorden CJF, Schlingemann RO. Molecular basis of the inner blood-retinal barrier and its breakdown in diabetic macular edema and other pathological conditions. Progress in Retinal and Eye Research. 2013;**34**:19-48

[18] Kalluri R. Basement membranes: Structure, assembly and role in tumour angiogenesis. Nature Reviews. Cancer. 2003;**3**:422-433

[19] Katz S. Role of Basement Membrane and Extracellular Matrix Proteins in the Adhesion and Spreading of Immortalized Human Corneal Epithelial Cells. 2007. Available from: https://play.google.com/store/books/details?id=IOy9OgAACAAJ

[20] Yurchenco PD, Amenta PS, Patton BL. Basement membrane assembly, stability and activities observed through a developmental lens. Matrix Biology. 2004;**22**:521-538

[21] Bissell MJ. The central role of basement membrane in functional differentiation, apoptosis, and cancer. In: Tilly JL, Strauss JF, Tenniswood M, editors. Cell Death in Reproductive Physiology. New York, NY: Springer New York. pp. 125-140

[22] Kelley LC, Lohmer LL, Hagedorn EJ, et al. Traversing the basement membrane in vivo: A diversity of strategies. The Journal of Cell Biology. 2014;**204**:291-302

[23] Smits D, Khalil AA. Multimodal techniques to study tumor growth, basement membrane breaching, and invasion in 3D matrices. Methods in Molecular Biology. 2023;**2608**:281-303

[24] Baluk P, Morikawa S, Haskell A, et al. Abnormalities of basement membrane on blood vessels and endothelial sprouts in tumors. The American Journal of Pathology. 2003;**163**:1801-1815

[25] Snorradottir AO, Isaksson HJ, Ingthorsson S, et al. Pathological changes in basement membranes and dermal connective tissue of skin from patients with hereditary cystatin C amyloid angiopathy. Laboratory Investigation. 2017;**97**:383-394

[26] Wu P, Cortes D, Li J, et al. Epithelial basement membrane dystrophy: A study with in vivo confocal microscopy and high-resolution anterior segment optical coherence tomography. Investigative Ophthalmology & Visual Science. 2013;**54**:564-564

[27] Pozzi A, Yurchenco PD, Iozzo RV. The nature and biology of basement membranes. Matrix Biology. 2017;**57-58**:1-11

[28] Rambourg A, Leblond CP. Staining of basement membranes and assocated structures by the periodic acid-Schiff and periodicacid-silver methenamine techniques. Journal of Ultrastructure Research. 1967;**20**:306-309

[29] Kalof AN, Evans MF, Cooper K. Special diagnostic techniques in surgical pathology. In: Gattuso P, Reddy VB, David O, Spitz DJ, editors. Differential Diagnosis in Surgical Pathology. 2nd ed. Philadelphia, PA, USA: Saunders; 2010. pp. 156-157. DOI: 10.1016/B978-1-4160-4580-9.00001-0

[30] Pujar A, Pereira T, Tamgadge A, et al. Comparing the efficacy of hematoxylin and eosin, periodic acid Schiff and fluorescent periodic acid Schiff-Acriflavine techniques for demonstration of basement membrane in oral lichen planus: A histochemical study. Indian Journal of Dermatology. 2015;**60**:450-456

[31] Vega JA, Esteban I, Naves FJ, et al. Immunohistochemical localization of laminin and type IV collagen in human cutaneous sensory nerve formations. Anatomy and Embryology. 1995;**191**:33-39

[32] Hahn E, Wick G, Pencev D, et al. Distribution of basement membrane proteins in normal and fibrotic human liver: Collagen type IV, laminin, and fibronectin. Gut. 1980;**21**:63-71

[33] Futaki S, Horimoto A, Shimono C, et al. Visualization of basement membranes by a nidogen-based fluorescent reporter in mice. Matrix Biology Plus. 2023;**18**:100133

[34] Debnath J, Muthuswamy SK, Brugge JS. Morphogenesis and oncogenesis of MCF-10A mammary epithelial acini grown in three-dimensional basement membrane cultures. Methods. 2003;**30**:256-268

[35] Barry Carter C, Williams DB. Transmission Electron Microscopy: Diffraction, Imaging, and Spectrometry. Germany: Springer International Publishing; 2016. DOI: 10.1007/978-3-319-26651-0

[36] Abdelmotaal H, Abdelazeem K, Hussein MS, et al. Safety of trypan blue capsule staining to corneal endothelium in patients with diabetic retinopathy. Journal of Ophthalmology. 2019;**2019**:4018739

[37] Rodrigues EB, Meyer CH, Farah ME, et al. Intravitreal staining of the internal limiting membrane using indocyanine green in the treatment of macular holes. Ophthalmologica. 2005;**219**:251-262

[38] Li X, Zhang L, Tang F, et al. Corrigendum: Retinal organoids: Cultivation, differentiation, and transplantation. Frontiers in Cellular Neuroscience. 2021;**15**:810268

[39] Kozlowski MT, Crook CJ, Ku HT. Towards organoid culture without Matrigel. Communications Biology. 2021;**4**:1387

[40] Shaw LC, Neu MB, Grant MB. Cell-based therapies for diabetic retinopathy. Current Diabetes Reports. 2011;**11**:265-274

[41] Brown KC, Light RS, Modi KJ, et al. An improved protocol for the Matrigel duplex assay: A method to measure retinal angiogenesis. Bio-Protocol. 2023;**13**:e4899

[42] Valdoz JC, Johnson BC, Jacobs DJ, et al. The ECM: To scaffold, or not to scaffold, that is the question. International Journal of Molecular Sciences. 2021;**22**:12690

[43] Sadikan MZ, Abdul Nasir NA, Lambuk L, et al. Diabetic retinopathy: A comprehensive update on in vivo, in vitro and ex vivo experimental models. BMC Ophthalmology. 2023;**23**:421

[44] Sharma K, Krohne TU, Busskamp V. The rise of retinal organoids for vision research. International Journal of Molecular Sciences;**21**:8484. Epub ahead of print 11 November 2020. DOI: 10.3390/ijms21228484

[45] Andrysík Z, Procházková J, Kabátková M, et al. Aryl hydrocarbon receptor-mediated disruption of contact inhibition is associated with connexin43 downregulation and inhibition of gap junctional intercellular communication. Archives of Toxicology. 2013;**87**:491-503

[46] Ljubimov AV, Huang Z-S, Huang GH, et al. Human corneal epithelial basement membrane and integrin alterations in diabetes and diabetic retinopathy. The Journal of Histochemistry and Cytochemistry. 1998;**46**:1033-1041

[47] Ejaz S, Chekarova I, Ejaz A, et al. Importance of pericytes and mechanisms of pericyte loss during diabetes retinopathy. Diabetes, Obesity & Metabolism. 2008;**10**:53-63

[48] Chronopoulos A, Tang A, Beglova E, et al. High glucose increases lysyl oxidase expression and activity in retinal endothelial cells: Mechanism for compromised extracellular matrix barrier function. Diabetes. 2010;**59**:3159-3166

[49] Bai X, Luo J, Zhang X, et al. MicroRNA-126 reduces blood-retina barrier breakdown via the regulation of VCAM-1 and BCL2L11 in ischemic retinopathy. Ophthalmic Research. 2017;**57**:173-185

[50] Goddard LM, Iruela-Arispe ML. Cellular and molecular regulation of vascular permeability. Thrombosis and Haemostasis. 2013;**109**:407-415

[51] An D, Tan B, Yu D-Y, et al. Differentiating microaneurysm pathophysiology in diabetic retinopathy through objective analysis of capillary nonperfusion, inflammation, and pericytes. Diabetes. 2022;**71**:733-746

[52] Ramos D, Carretero A, Navarro M, et al. Mimicking microvascular alterations of human diabetic retinopathy: A challenge for the mouse models. Current Medicinal Chemistry. 2013;**20**:3200-3217

[53] Mukwaya A, Jensen L, Lagali N. Relapse of pathological angiogenesis: Functional role of the basement membrane and potential treatment strategies. Experimental & Molecular Medicine. 2021;**53**:189-201

[54] Roy S, Ha J, Trudeau K, et al. Vascular basement membrane thickening in diabetic retinopathy. Current Eye Research. 2010;**35**:1045-1056

[55] Wang X-N, Li S-T, Li W, et al. The thickness and volume of the choroid, outer retinal layers and retinal pigment epithelium layer changes in patients with diabetic retinopathy. International Journal of Ophthalmology. 2018;**11**:1957-1962

[56] Booij JC, Baas DC, Beisekeeva J, et al. The dynamic nature of Bruch's membrane. Progress in Retinal and Eye Research. 2010;**29**:1-18

[57] Ljubimov AV. Diabetic complications in the cornea. Vision Research. 2017;**139**:138-152

[58] Zhao H, He Y, Ren Y-R, et al. Corneal alteration and pathogenesis in diabetes mellitus. International Journal of Ophthalmology. 2019;**12**:1939-1950

[59] Kelkar A, Kelkar J, Mehta H, et al. Cataract surgery in diabetes mellitus: A systematic review. Indian Journal of Ophthalmology. 2018;**66**:1401-1410

[60] Rush RB, Gomez PL, Rush SW, et al. Internal limiting membrane peeling in patients undergoing vitrectomy for tractional retinal detachment secondary to diabetic retionpathy. Retina. 2023;**43**:1282-1290

[61] Tagawa H, McMeel JW, Furukawa H, et al. Role of the vitreous in diabetic retinopathy. I. Vitreous changes in diabetic retinopathy and in physiologic aging. Ophthalmology. 1986;**93**:596-601

[62] Akiba J, Arzabe CW, Trempe CL. Posterior vitreous detachment and neovascularization in diabetic retinopathy. Ophthalmology. 1990;**97**:889-891

[63] Zhao H. Pericyte-Endothelial Cell Interactions during Blood Vessel Formation and in Diabetic Scenarios.

2019. Available from: https://vtechworks.lib.vt.edu/handle/10919/100112

[64] Pouw AE, Greiner MA, Coussa RG, et al. Cell–Matrix Interactions in the Eye: From Cornea to Choroid. Cells. 2021;**10**:687

[65] Biswas A, Choudhury AD, Agrawal S, et al. Recent insights into the etiopathogenesis of diabetic retinopathy and its management. Journal of Ocular Pharmacology and Therapeutics. 2024;**40**(1):13-33. Epub ahead of print 21 September 2023. DOI: 10.1089/jop.2023.0068

[66] Cox JH, Overall CM. Cytokine substrates: MMP regulation of inflammatory signaling molecules. In: Edwards D, Høyer-Hansen G, Blasi F, et al., editors. The Cancer Degradome: Proteases and Cancer Biology. New York, NY: Springer New York. pp. 519-539

[67] Tanwar VS, Reddy MA, Natarajan R. Emerging role of long non-coding RNAs in diabetic vascular complications. Frontiers in Endocrinology. 2021;**12**:665811

[68] Wang X, Khalil RA. Matrix metalloproteinases, vascular remodeling, and vascular disease. Advances in Pharmacology. 2018;**81**:241-330

[69] Kowluru RA, Zhong Q, Santos JM. Matrix metalloproteinases in diabetic retinopathy: Potential role of MMP-9. Expert Opinion on Investigational Drugs. 2012;**21**:797-805

[70] Gardiner TA, Anderson HR, Degenhardt T, et al. Prevention of retinal capillary basement membrane thickening in diabetic dogs by a non-steroidal anti-inflammatory drug. Diabetologia. 2003;**46**:1269-1275

[71] Kirchain WR, Rendell MS. Aldose reductase inhibitors. Pharmacotherapy. 1990;**10**:326-336

[72] Zhai Y, Yang L, Zheng W, et al. A precise design strategy for a cell-derived extracellular matrix based on CRISPR/Cas9 for regulating neural stem cell function. Biomaterials Science. 2023;**11**:6537-6544

[73] Roy S, Nasser S, Yee M, et al. A long-term siRNA strategy regulates fibronectin overexpression and improves vascular lesions in retinas of diabetic rats. Molecular Vision. 2011;**17**:3166-3174

[74] Kokil GR, Veedu RN, Ramm GA, et al. Type 2 diabetes mellitus: Limitations of conventional therapies and intervention with nucleic acid-based therapeutics. Chemical Reviews. 2015;**115**:4719-4743

[75] Simo R, Roy S, Behar-Cohen F, et al. Fenofibrate: A new treatment for diabetic retinopathy. Molecular mechanisms and future perspectives. Current Medicinal Chemistry. 2013;**20**:3258-3266

[76] Wang W, Wang X, Yao F, et al. Lysyl oxidase family proteins: Prospective therapeutic targets in cancer. International Journal of Molecular Sciences. 2022;**23**:12270. Epub ahead of print 14 October 2022. DOI: 10.3390/ijms232012270

[77] Cooper J, Giancotti FG. Integrin signaling in cancer: Mechanotransduction, stemness, epithelial plasticity, and therapeutic resistance. Cancer Cell. 2019;**35**:347-367

[78] González P, Lozano P, Ros G, et al. Hyperglycemia and oxidative stress: An integral, updated and critical overview of their metabolic interconnections. International Journal of Molecular Sciences. 2023;**24**:9352. Epub ahead of print 27 May 2023. DOI: 10.3390/ijms24119352

Chapter 4

Prevalence and Associated Factors of Diabetic Retinopathy among Cameroonians Patients Followed in Two Hospitals in the City of Garoua – North Cameroon

Josiane Mare Njoya, Balkissou Adamou Dodo, Inna Hadja, Patrice Esame and Godefroy Koki

Abstract

This study aims to fill this gap by conducting a cross-sectional and analytical investigation within the ophthalmology departments of Garoua General Hospital and Garoua Regional Hospital. By focusing on type 2 diabetic patients, we endeavor to elucidate the factors contributing to the presence of DR in our local context over a period of 1 year from January 3rd, 2023 to January 15th, 2024. Demographic data (age, sex, and profession) and clinical information were collected. Ocular examinations included measurement of visual acuity, slit lamp examination, and fundus examination. Additional tests, such as macular optical coherence tomography and ocular ultrasound, were conducted when necessary. Diagnosed ocular pathologies were documented. The mean age of our patients is 53.9 years with a standard deviation of 13.2 years. Notably, there is a predominant representation of females. Regarding ocular health, 8.8% of patient exhibit blindness. The prevalence of diabetic retinopathy (DR) in our cohort is 24.5% with a 95% confidence interval ranging from 16.16 to 32.86%. It is noteworthy that all patients diagnosed with DR have a glycated hemoglobin level exceeding 7%. We have observed a prevalent occurrence of diabetic retinopathy within our community. Notably, all individuals diagnosed with diabetic retinopathy exhibit abnormal levels of glycated hemoglobin.

Keywords: diabetic retinopathy, associated factors, Northern Cameroon, prevalence – Cameroonians patients, type 2 diabetic patients

1. Introduction

Diabetes constitutes a significant and escalating public health concern worldwide, affecting an estimated 463 million individuals globally, with over 19 million cases recorded in Africa alone [1]. Remarkably, this number is projected to surge to

55 million by 2045, marking a 34% increase from 2021 figures [2]. Of grave concern is that a substantial portion of affected individuals remain undiagnosed, with an estimated 70% unaware of their diabetic status [2]. Type 2 diabetes, predominant in developing nations, has undergone a notable rise across Africa since 1980, with prevalence rates escalating in various regions. For instance, Tanzania witnessed an increase from 2.3% in 1980 to 4.6% in 1996, while in Central Africa, prevalence rates soared to 7.1% in Guinea, 10.2% in Zimbabwe, and 14.5% in the Democratic Republic of Congo. The Maghreb region has also experienced a surge, with prevalence rates recorded at 10% in Tunisia, 9.3% in Egypt, and 8.1% in Morocco [2].

The ocular complication of diabetes, known as diabetic retinopathy (DR), stems from elevated blood sugar levels, instigating a cascade of biochemical and histological changes in the retina [3]. These changes, including thickening of capillary basal membranes and subsequent breakdown of the blood-retinal barrier, culminate in severe visual impairments, including macular edema and neovascularization, leading to blindness [4].

In Africa, the burden of DR is palpable, with prevalence rates varying across countries. Abouki Coa and al in Cotonou reported a prevalence of 30.5% in 2019 [3], whereas recent studies in Cameroon documented frequencies ranging from 12.3 to 45.5% [4, 5]. Identifying risk factors associated with DR is crucial for effective management and prevention strategies. A meta-analysis conducted by Jie Xuan et al. in 2022 outlined several risk factors, including the duration of diabetes, systolic blood pressure, body mass index, HbA1c levels, and lipid profile abnormalities [6]. In the world and specially in Morocco there are underscored associations between DR and chronic hyperglycemia, arterial hypertension, dyslipidemia, and diabetic neuropathy [7, 8].

Despite the pressing need for comprehensive studies on DR risk factors in Africa, limited research exists, particularly in countries, such as Cameroon. Thus, this study aims to fill this gap by conducting a cross-sectional and analytical investigation within the ophthalmology departments of Garoua General Hospital and Garoua Regional Hospital. By focusing on type 2 diabetic patients within these centers, we endeavor to elucidate the factors, contributing to the presence of DR in our local context.

2. Patients and methods

A cross-sectional and analytical study over a period of 1 year from January 3rd, 2023 to January 15th, 2024 was conducted in the main two hospitals unit in Garoua-North Cameroon:

- The Garoua General Hospital, a collaborative effort between Cameroon and South Korea, which has swiftly become a vital healthcare hub, caters to a diverse patient base hailing from Garoua and beyond, including various localities in northern Cameroon, as well as neighboring regions in TChad and Nigeria [9]. The hospital hosts a noteworthy department. The department is equipped with advanced diagnostic and surgical capabilities and attends to approximately 60 patients each month; it offers a range of services, including consultations, eye surgeries, and diagnostic procedures such as perimetry, ocular ultrasound, and retinal angiography.

- The Garoua Regional Hospital

With an average monthly patient load of around 3000 individuals, the Garoua Regional Hospital received 4990 ophthalmology consultations in 2023 alone. Among the most prevalent conditions treated were ametropia, allergic conjunctivitis, cataracts, infectious conjunctivitis, glaucoma, pterygium, and corneal ulcerations, indicative of the diverse range of eye health issues addressed by the hospital. Within a hospital, there exists a diabetes clinic housed at the voluntary prevention and screening Center (VPSC).

2.1 Procedure

Following administrative and ethical approvals, the study included all type 2 diabetic patients who consented to participate and received care at the ophthalmology departments of Garoua General Hospital (GGH) and Garoua Regional Hospital (GRH) during the study period. Patients with complete data available were included, while those who did not consent or had incomplete information were excluded.

Using an anonymous technical form, demographic data (age, sex, and profession) and clinical information were collected. This included general cardiovascular history (such as dyslipidemia, nephropathy, heart disease, hyperuricemia, obesity/overweight, and hypertension), duration of diabetes, prescribed antidiabetic treatment, treatment compliance, reasons for noncompliance if applicable, and diabetes-related complications (including infections, ketoacidosis, polyneuropathy, kidney damage, diabetic foot, retinopathy, cardiopathy, and stroke).

Therapeutic compliance was assessed using the French-translated Morisky Green questionnaire, with a score below six indicating poor compliance. Obesity was defined as a body mass index (BMI) of 30 or above and overweight as a BMI greater than 25.

Ocular examinations included measurement of corrected distance visual acuity, slit lamp examination, and fundus examination using a 90-diopter Volk lens. Additional tests, such as macular optical coherence tomography and ocular ultrasound, were conducted when necessary. Diagnosed ocular pathologies were documented, including cataracts, glaucoma, ametropia, and diabetic retinopathy (DR). They were classified according to the simplified Alfediam classification, which distinguishes between no diabetic retinopathy, non-proliferative DR (with varying severity), and proliferative DR (with varying severity and complications). Diabetic maculopathy was classified as either edematous or ischemic.

This study aimed to comprehensively assess the ocular health of diabetic patients and their adherence to treatment protocols, providing valuable insights for their management and care.

2.2 Sample size

We determined the minimum sample size using OpenEpi software version 3 (revised April 2013). Considering the combined active queues of type 1 and type 2 diabetic patients at GGH (200 patients) and VPSC of GRH (603 patients), our study population was estimated at 803 patients in 2023. Based on a 90% confidence interval and a diabetic retinopathy prevalence of 12.3% in Cameroon according to Bediang et al. [10], the minimum sample size was calculated to be 101 patients.

2.3 Statistical analyses

Data were analyzed using IBM SPSS Statistics for Windows, Version 23 (IBM Corp., Armonk, New York, United States, 2015). Quantitative variables were presented as means and standard deviations, while qualitative variables were expressed as counts and percentages. Univariate analysis was utilized to assess the association between qualitative variables (such as age, sex, duration of diabetes, type of treatment, therapeutic compliance, and cardiovascular pathologies) and the presence of diabetic retinopathy (DR) observed during fundus examinations. The chi-square test was employed for comparing qualitative variables, while quantitative variables were compared using either the Student's t-test or the Mann-Whitney U test for non-parametric data. Variables found to be associated with DR in univariate analysis were included in a logistic regression model to identify independent factors associated with DR. A significance threshold of 5% was applied.

3. Results

In total, we examined 102 type 2 diabetic patients or 204 eyes.

3.1 Sociodemographic data

The mean age was 53.9 ± 13.2 years with a minimum age of 30 years and a maximum of 90 years. We had 59(57.8%) women and 43(42.2%) men for a sex ratio of 1.4 in favor of women (**Figure 1**).

3.2 Clinical data

- Blindness was found in 09(8.8%) (**Figures 2** and **3**) (**Tables 1** and **2**).
  The prevalence of diabetic retinopathy in our setting was 24.5 95% CI [16.16;32.86].
  The average duration of diabetes in our patients was 6.8± 6.1 years with (33) 32.4% of patients having a history of diabetes for more than 10 years (**Figures 4** and **5**).

- The compliance to treatment was found in 62 (60.8%) patients (**Figures 6** and **7**).

- Overweight or obesity was found in 45(44.1%) patients.

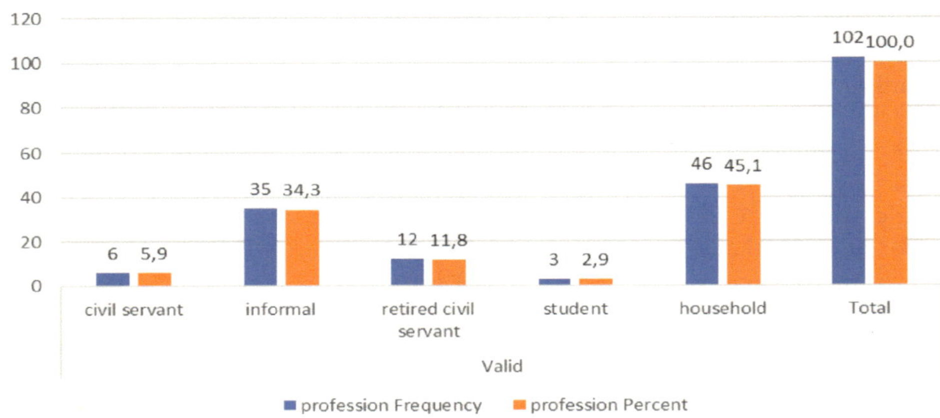

Figure 1.
Distribution of patients according to their profession.

- Glycated hemoglobin greater than 7% was found in 83 (81.4%) patients (**Table 3**).

The factor, which seems to influence the occurrence of diabetic retinopathy in our patients, seems to be the glycated hemoglobin level greater than 7%. ($p < 0.05$).

Visualacuityof right eye	Effective n	Percentage %
No light perception	1	1
Light perception	2	2
<1/10	6	5.9
<5/10	41	40.2
5/10–8/10	40	39.2
>8/10	12	11.7
Total	102	100

Table 1.
Distribution of patients according to the visual acuity of the right eye.

Visual acuity of left eye	Effective n	Percentage %
No light perception	2	2
Light perception	3	2.9
<1/10	3	2.9
<5/10	41	40.2
5/10–8/10	40	39.2
>8/10	13	12.8

Table 2.
Distribution of patients according to the visual acuity of the left eye.

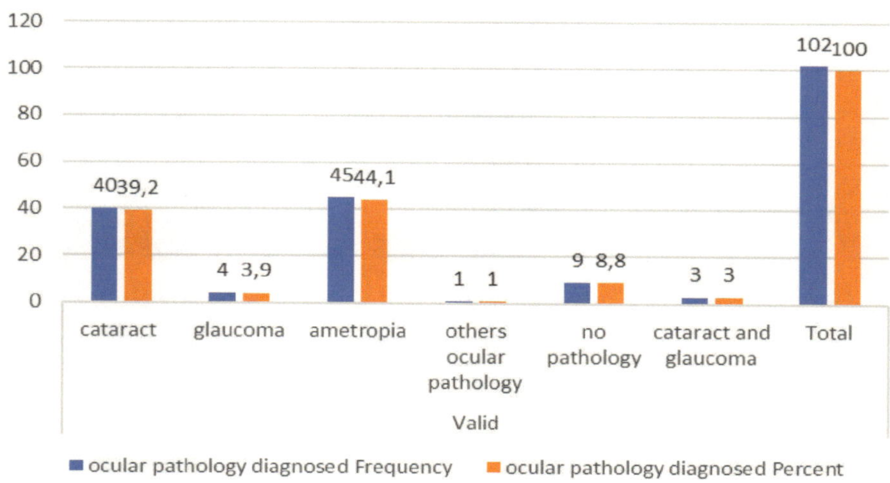

Figure 2.
Distribution of ocular pathologies diagnosed in type 2 diabetic patients.

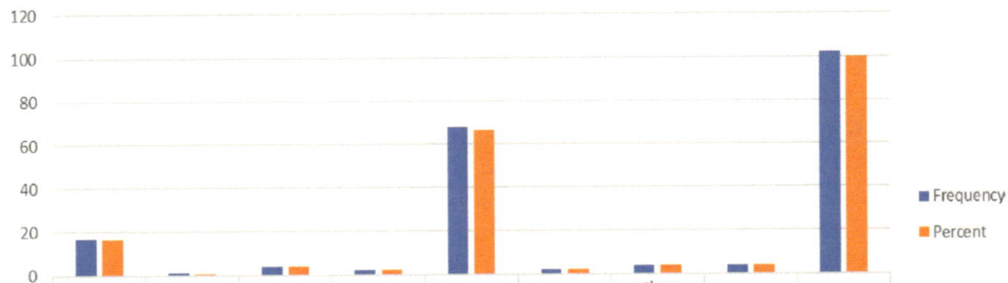

	Mild NPDR	Moderate NPDR	macula oedema	DRcomplicated by IVH	normal fundus examination	ischemic maculopathy	others anomalies of fundus examination	fundus examination inacessible	Total
Frequency	17	1	4	2	68	2	4	4	102
Percent	16,7	1,0	3,9	2,0	66,7	2,0	3,9	3,9	100,0

Figure 3.
Distribution of results of fundus examination of the right eye. NPDR = non-proliferative diabetic retinopathy, IVH=IntraVitreal hemorrhage, DR = diabetic retinopathy.

	Mild NPDR	Moderate NPDR	macula oedema	DR complicated by vitreoretinal tractions	PVD	normal examination of fundus	others anomalies of fundus examination	fundus examination inacessible	Total
Frequency	7	9	3	1	1	74	4	3	102
Percent	6,9	8,8	2,9	1,0	1,0	72,5	3,9	2,9	100,0

Frequency Percent

Figure 4.
Distribution of results of fundus examination of the left eye. NPDR = non-proliferative diabetic retinopathy, PVD=posterior vitreous detachment, DR = diabetic retinopathy.

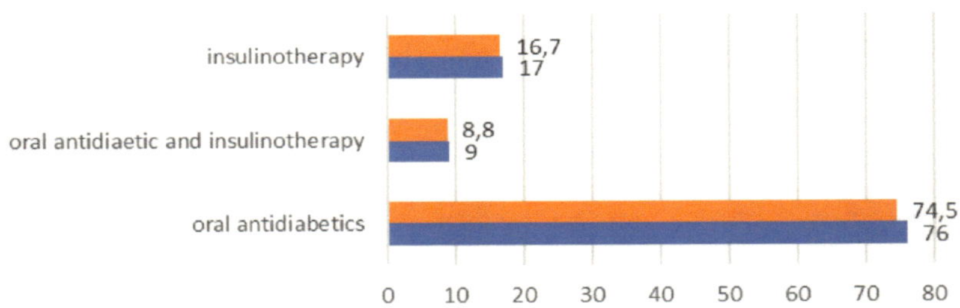

	oral antidiabetics	oral antidiaetic and insulinotherapy	insulinotherapy
Percent	74,5	8,8	16,7
Frequency	76	9	17

Percent Frequency

Figure 5.
Distribution of the type of treatment taken by patients.

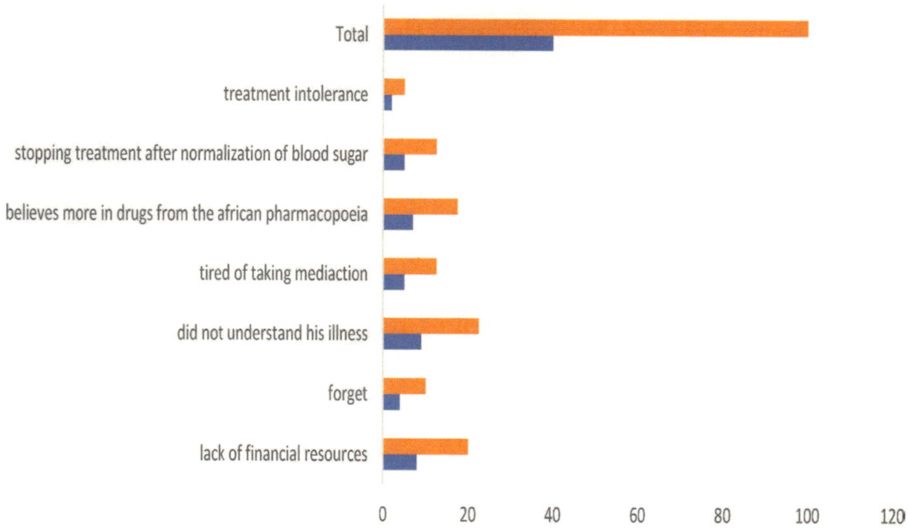

	lack of financial resources	forget	did not understand his illness	tired of taking mediaction	believes more in drugs from the african pharmacopoeia	stopping treatment after normalization of blood sugar	treatment intolerance	Total
Percent	20.0	10.0	22.5	12.5	17.5	12.5	5.0	100.0
Frequency	8	4	9	5	7	5	2	40

Figure 6.
Reasons for noncompliance to treatment.

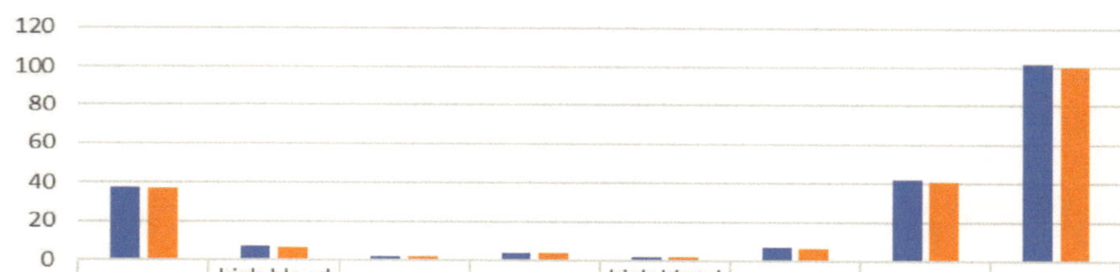

	high blood pressure	high blood pressure and hyperuricemia	hyperuricemia	kidney damage	high blood pressure and dyslipidemia	dyslipidemaia	None	Total
Frequency	38	7	2	4	2	7	42	102
Percent	37,3	6,9	2,0	3,9	2,0	6,9	41,2	100,0

Figure 7.
Distribution of metabolic disorders among our patients.

4. Discussion

Several key findings are presented in this study. Firstly, the mean age of our patients is 53.9 years with a standard deviation of 13.2 years. Notably, there is a predominant

Associated factors		Diabetic retinopathy		Total	p value
		Present	Absent	28	0.3
Duration of Diabetes equal or more than 10 years	YES	5	23		
	NO	20	54	74	
Therapeutic Compliance	YES	14	48	62	0.6
	NO	11	29	40	
Metabolic disorders	YES	18	41	59	0.09
	NO	7	36	43	
Neuropathy	YES	9	23	32	0.6
	NO	16	54	70	
Nephropathy	YES	3	6	9	1.0
	NO	23	71	94	
Glycate hemoglobin superior to 7%	YES	25	58	83	0.001
	NO	0	19	19	

Table 3.
Cross table showing associated factors with diabetic retinopathy.

representation of females, accounting for 57.8% of the study population compared to 42.2% of males. On average, our patients have been living with diabetes for 6.8 years, with 27.5% of them having a disease duration exceeding 10 years. Regarding ocular health, 12.7% of patients exhibit blindness, while pathologies, such as cataracts and glaucoma, which can potentially lead to blindness, are present in 43.1% of cases. The prevalence of diabetic retinopathy (DR) in our cohort is 24.5% with a 95% confidence interval ranging from 16.16% to 32.86%. It is noteworthy that all patients diagnosed with DR have a glycated hemoglobin level exceeding 7%. Moreover, adherence to treatment measures is observed in 56% of patients. Metabolic syndrome is prevalent in 72% of those diagnosed with DR, indicating a significant comorbidity. Additionally, neuropathy is identified in 36% of patients presenting with DR, while nephropathy is present in 8% of cases. These findings underscore the multifaceted nature of diabetes and its associated complications within our patient population.

4.1 Characteristics of the study population

The demographic profile of the study population mirrors findings from Bediang et al. [10] conducted in Yaoundé, Central Cameroon, where the mean age was 53.5 ± 14.7 years, with females constituting 56.9% of participants [11]. Similarly, in our study conducted in North Cameroon, the mean age was 53.9 ± 13.2 years, with 57.8% being female. This trend of female predominance is also observed in Cotonou, as evidenced by Abouki C et al., who reported a sex ratio of 0.57 in favor of women [3]. Conversely, an Ethiopian study on 331 diabetic patients reported a slightly lower mean age of 45.48 (SD ± 16.88) years, with men comprising around 54.7% of the participants [12].

4.2 Clinical data

The prevalence of diabetic retinopathy in our study stands at 24.5%, slightly higher than the 12.3% reported by Bediang et al. in Yaoundé but lower than the 34.1%

found in Ethiopia [13]. The variation in prevalence rates may be attributed to differences in sample sizes and methodologies employed. Notably, a French study highlights diabetic retinopathy as the leading cause of low vision in individuals under 50 years old, with affluent populations experiencing a decreasing trend in prevalence due to advancements in screening, diagnostics, and therapeutic interventions, including intravitreal pharmacological treatments [14].

In our community, all patients diagnosed with diabetic retinopathy have a glycated hemoglobin level exceeding 7%, with 81.4% exhibiting poorly controlled diabetes. Nonadherence to treatment is observed in 39.2% of patients, often attributed to financial constraints, forgetfulness, treatment fatigue, and the use of traditional African remedies. Studies conducted in Cameroon emphasize the necessity of implementing effective management strategies for diabetes and its complications, highlighting low awareness levels and inappropriate attitudes toward disease prevention among diabetic patients [15, 16]. In China, the prevalence of diabetic retinopathy is about 9.9% [10]. Patients who have diabetic retinopathy in our community all have a glycated hemoglobin level greater than 7%. In addition, 81.4% of patients in our study have poorly controlled diabetes. Nonadherence is observed in 39.2% of patients. This noncompliance can be explained by the lack of financial means, forgetfulness, fatigue in taking the treatment, and the use of the plants of the African pharmacopeia. Cameroonian study to evaluate systems and services for the management of diabetes and diabetic retinopathy shows that a suitable implementation strategy is necessary in our context [4]. Abah Abah shows in 2023 concerning diabetic patients followed at the diabetic clinic in the center region of Cameroon that diabetic patients have a poor level of awareness and a non-appropriated attitude toward preventing the outcome of disease complications [5].

Regarding associated factors, our study identifies a high glycated hemoglobin level (>7%) as the sole independent determinant of diabetic retinopathy. However, studies conducted elsewhere reveal additional determinants such as poor medication adherence, older age, illiteracy, high systolic blood pressure, family history of diabetes, other microvascular complications, poor glycemic and cholesterol control, anemia, arterial hypertension, dyslipidemia, diabetes imbalance, and prolonged disease duration [17–20]. On a slightly larger sample, Ouazzani and al in Morocco add as another associated factor the imbalance of diabetes. In South Africa, Mjwara shows that proliferative diabetic retinopathy is associated with higher HbA1c in type 2 diabetes mellitus in all races and age groups and was independent of duration of disease [6, 12]. In 2019, a study conducted in Benin revealed that the presence of long-standing nephropathy, glycated hemoglobin, age of discovery of diabetes, and its duration were the factors associated with diabetic retinopathy [3]. Ahmadou et al. in 2014 in a large sample of 408 patients with 88% of type 2 patients noticed a strong correlation between the duration of diabetes and retinopathy status ($p < 0.001$, $r = 0.9541$) [6].

Burgees PI et al. about DR in sub-Saharan African patients said poor glycemic and blood pressure control lead to rapid progression of DR [14].

The limitations of our study are the small number of our patients.

5. Conclusion

In summary, we have observed a prevalent occurrence of diabetic retinopathy within our community. Notably, all individuals diagnosed with diabetic retinopathy exhibit abnormal levels of glycated hemoglobin. The issue of therapeutic adherence emerges as a critical concern in the management of diabetes, often stemming from financial constraints, limited awareness, misconceptions about the disease, and the burden of chronic medication intake.

Therefore, we recommend the following actions:

To healthcare facilities: It is imperative to institute counseling initiatives and incorporate counseling and psychological support into healthcare professionals' training programs. This approach aims to enhance patient adherence to treatment regimens.

To the Ministry of Public Health: Efforts should be directed toward enhancing patient access to endocrinologists and antidiabetic medications. This can be achieved through the establishment of subsidized pathways to ensure the affordability and availability of essential drugs.

To the Ministry of Scientific Research: Encourage and financially support research endeavors focusing on diabetes, particularly exploring the potential of African pharmacopoeia derived from plants. This avenue is of interest as some patients within our community express a preference for traditional remedies over conventional medications. Such research could lead to the development of effective treatments aligned with local preferences and practices.

Acknowledgements

The author wishes to thank their dear family for the support and all co-authors of this study for their contributions. The author would also like to thank Dr. Aminou Mohamadou for proofreading the manuscript. The author is grateful to all the patients, who consented to participate, and all the staff of the ophthalmology department of the health facilities.

Conflict of interest

All authors of this work do not declare any conflicts of interest.

Author details

Josiane Mare Njoya[1*], Balkissou Adamou Dodo[1], Inna Hadja[1], Patrice Esame[2] and Godefroy Koki[3]

1 Faculty of Medicine and Biomedicals Sciences, Garoua University, Cameroon

2 Garoua Regional Hospital Center, Cameroon

3 Faculty of Medicine and Biomedicals Sciences, Yaoundé 1 University, Cameroon

*Address all correspondence to: marenjoya@gmail.com

References

[1] WHO. Le fardeau de plus en plus lourd du diabète en Afrique. Afrique Renouveau; WHO. Decembre 2021. Available from: https://www.un.org/africarenewal/fr/magazine/décembre-2021/le-fardeau-de-plus-en-plus-lourd-du-diabète-en-afrique

[2] Idemyor V. Diabetes in sub-Saharan Africa: Health care perspectives, challenges, and the economic burden of disease. Journal of the National Medical Association. 2010;**102**(7):650-653. ISSN 0027-9684

[3] Ling C, Groop L. Epigenetics: A molecular link between environmental factors and type 2 diabetes. Diabetes. 2009;**58**(12):2718-2725

[4] Jingi AM, Noubiap JJN, Ellong A, Bigna JJR, Mvogo CE. Epidemiology and treatment outcomes of diabetic retinopathy in a diabetic population from Cameroon. BMC Ophthalmology. 2014;**14**(1). DOI: 10.1186/1471-2415-14-19

[5] Xuan J, Wang L, Fan L, Ji S. Systematic review and meta-analysis of the related factors for diabetic retinopathy. Annals of Palliative Medicine. 2022;**11**(7):2368-2381

[6] Ouazzani FZC, Lazar N, Salhi H, El Ouahabi H. Facteurs associés à la rétinopathie diabétique chez 746 patients diabétiques marocains. Annales d'Endocrinologir. 2020;**81**(4):419. ISSN 003-4266

[7] Khalaf R, Khamassi S, Boukhayatia F, Mehrez A, Marrakchi M, Ben Brahim A, et al. Observance thérapeutique chez le patient diabétique: evaluation et facteurs associés. Annales d'endocrinologie. 2023;**84**(1):186-187. DOI: 10.1016/j.ando.2022.12.279

[8] Hammoudi J, Nour El Houda B, El Habri C, Yassamine B, Hamid N, Abdelkhaleq L, et al. Diabetic retinopathy in the Eastern Morocco: Different stage frequencies and associated risk factors. Saudi J Biol SCI. 2021;**28**(1):775-784

[9] 9 – Portail web du ministère de la santé publique du Cameroun publié le 17 Octobre 2022

[10] Bediang G, Abbou Panpom V, Koki G, Epee E. Utilisation d'un Logiciel d'Aide à la Décision pour le Dépistage de la rétinopathie diabétique au Cameroun. Health Sciences and Diseases. 2020;**21**(3). DOI: 10.5281/hsd.v21i3.1855

[11] Abah Aristide Stephane A, Etienne Philemon A, Bernadette Flaure K, Farida Oumarou H, Nwaha Marcel Wilfried N, Ohana Joseph Alain A, et al. Diabetes awareness and complications in patients from clinics in the Centre region, Cameroon. World Journal of Public Health. 2023;**8**(1):23-28

[12] Mjwara M, Khan M, Kruse CH, Sibanda W, Connolly C. Significance of HbA1c levels in diabetic retinopathy extremes in South Africa. South African Medical Journal. 2021;**111**(9):886-890

[13] Garoma D, Merga H, Hiko D. Determinants of diabetic retinopathy in Southwest Ethiopia: A facility-based case-control study. BMC Public Health. 2020;**20**(1):503. DOI: 10.1186/s12889-020-08652-2

[14] Burgess PI, Msukwa G, Beare NAV. Diabetic retinopathy in sub-Saharan Africa: Meeting the challenges of an emerging epidemic. BMC Medicine. 2013;**11**:157. Available from: https://

bmcmedicine.biomedcentral.com/articles/10.1186/1741-7015-11-157

[15] Amoaku WM, Ghanchi F, Bailey C, Banerjee S, Banerjee S, Downey L, et al. Diabetic retinopathy and diabetic macular oedema pathways and management: UK consensus working group. Eye. 2020;**34**:1-51

[16] Bella AL, Koki G, Djouma NF, Aboubakar H, Nomo A, Noa G, et al. Assessment of systems and Services for Management of diabetes and diabetic retinopathy in Cameroon. Ophthalmic Epidemiology;**28**(2):114-121

[17] Bertelsen G, Peto T, Lindekleiv H, Schirmer H, Solbu MD, Toft I, et al. Tromsø eye study: Prevalence and risk factors of diabetic retinopathy. Acta Ophthalmologica. 2013;**91**(8):716-721

[18] Mersha GA, Alimaw YA, Woredekal AT. Prevalence of diabetic retinopathy among diabetic patients in Northwest Ethiopia-a cross sectional hospital based study. PLoS One. 2022;**17**(1 January):e0262664. DOI: 10.1371/journal.pone.0262664

[19] Delyfer MN, Delcourt C. Épidémiologie De La Rétinopathie Diabétique Dans Les Données Internationales Et Françaises. Médecine des Maladies Métaboliques. 2018;**12**(7):553-558

[20] Ma Y, Wang H, Jiang J, Han C, Lu C, Zeng S, et al. Prevalence of and risk factors for diabetic retinopathy in residents with different types of abnormal glucose metabolism with or without hypertension: A suburban community-based cross-sectional study. Frontiers in Endocrinology. 2022;**13**:966619. DOI: 10.3389/fendo.2022.966619

Section 2

Clinical and Cellular Alteration Associated with Diabetic Retinopathy

Chapter 5

Postoperative Evaluation of Retinal and Choroidal Perfusion in Diabetic Tractional Retinal Detachment

Miguel A. Quiroz-Reyes, Erick A. Quiroz-Gonzalez and Miguel A. Quiroz-Gonzalez

Abstract

Optical coherence tomography angiography (OCT-A) is useful for quantitative analyses of different choroidal and retinal vascular plexuses. Highlighting postoperative choroidal and retinal perfusion outcomes in patients who have undergone successful tractional retinal detachment (TRD) repair is crucial for understanding the impact of this condition on postoperative visual acuity. This chapter describes postoperative perfusion outcomes, such as vessel density (VD) quantified in the superficial and deep capillary plexuses of the retina and choroidal perfusion markers, such as the choroidal vascularity index (CVI) and choriocapillaris flow area (CFA). In this analysis, superficial and deep capillary plexuses were quantified, and the CVI and CFA were significantly lower in the surgical group ($P = 0.0011$), with median CVIs of 57.95% and 2.28 mm^2 in the control group and 44.41% and 1.38 mm^2 in the surgical group, respectively. Definitive correlations were shown between alterations in the structure of the retina and choroid after surgery and visual dysfunction in diabetic individuals. The CVI and CFA can be used as quantitative measures to evaluate choroidal damage in postoperative patients with traction retinal detachment. The CVI serves as a dependable quantitative biomarker for evaluating the progression of diabetic retinopathy (DR) or for tracking postoperative eyes.

Keywords: choroidal vascularity index, deep capillary plexus, disorganization of the retinal inner layers, tractional retinal detachment, optical coherence tomography angiography, macular perfusion indices, ischemic macula, superficial vascular plexus, vessel density

1. Introduction

The prevalence of diabetes mellitus (DM) is increasing worldwide, affecting an estimated 285 million adults (6.4%) in 2010 [1]. It is considered to be the main cause of preventable visual morbidity and blindness worldwide. Until 2008, the prevalence of vision-threatening proliferative diabetic retinopathy (PDR) was 4.4%, with a general prevalence of diabetic retinopathy (DR) of 28.5% among adults with diabetes in the United States. DR is caused by chronic microangiopathy, which induces progressive uncontrollable ischemic changes in the inner and outer retina, damaging the permeability of the blood-retinal barrier (BRB) [2].

The main causes of vision loss in the diabetic population include various clinical types of diabetic macular edema (DME) and severe complications of high-risk PDR, including active recurrent vitreous hemorrhage (VH) and tractional retinal detachment (TRD) of different configurations and extensions as the final fibroproliferative stage of PDR; which require surgical repair because of the high risk of severe vision loss [3–5]. Chronic nonresponsive macular edema associated or not associated with vitreomacular traction and the occurrence of epiretinal membrane (ERM) proliferation are also common causes of vision loss and visual disability and constitute the most prevalent challenges in ophthalmology and diabetic eye care [3–5].

An approach used to manage DR-related bleeding complications involves repetitive injectable intervention protocols consistent with intravitreal injection of different specific target agents against signaling proteins involved in the angiogenesis cascade called vascular endothelial growth factors (anti-VEGFs) to improve BRB stability [6]. They are widely available for use worldwide, especially for the treatment of aggressive proliferative DR [6]. Similarly, some patients are boosted with steroids, periocular injections, or intravitreal extended-release devices to improve long-term visual outcomes. Panretinal photocoagulation (PRP) is the gold standard of care, but currently approved practices in developed countries prefer this approach as second-line treatment [7].

Sivaprasad et al. [8] defined a protocol for diabetic retinopathy titled Clinical efficacy and mechanistic evaluation of aflibercept for proliferative diabetic retinopathy (CLARITY) and the Research Network Protocol, which has guided medical approaches for treating DME and PDR bleeding complications. TRD involving the macula is considered a late and severe sight-threatening complication, and surgical approaches such as advanced updated control-perfusion pars plana vitrectomy (PPV) have been routinely performed [7]. Extensive research has failed to predict the factors associated with better visual outcomes after PPV [9–12].

Optical coherence tomography angiography (OCT-A), a novel noninvasive digital advanced imaging technology, has emerged to facilitate the visualization of blood flow in the most critical eye tissues. OCT-A technology exploits moving red blood cells based on the diffractive particle movement principle to critically resolve vessel location and characterize the different vascularized tissues of the eye. OCT-A imaging produces three-dimensional composites of the layers of the vascular choroid and the different retinal capillary plexuses without the use of contrast agents, which can be visualized with high-definition depth-encoded and en-face slabs; the different vascularized tissue slabs merged along with the structural OCT B scans to be analyzed, and detailed blood flow imaging of the superficial and deep retinal vascular plexuses and choriocapillaris flow can be obtained with quantified options, which were not well visualized with previous imaging modalities [13]. Because this imaging technique overcomes several significant limitations of previous dye-based techniques for evaluating the choroid, OCT-A has become a key tool for evaluating the choroid, offering new and important insights into the pathogenesis of many retinal and choroidal disorders. This technology has increased the sensitivity of detailed imaging of different manually or digitally selected choriocapillaris submacular regions and specific areas of interest at the level of the deep and superficial retinal capillary networks [13]. OCT-A perfusion analysis uses motion as a contrast mechanism to visualize the location of moving intravascular cells [13]. OCT-A is a novel, noninvasive, free-dying technology capable of avoiding indocyanine green dye (ICG) dark artifacts of retinal and choroidal vascular features that are present owing to the leakage of dye molecules [14–16]. This high-resolution technique provides capillary-level details such as histological information [17–20].

OCT-A has been useful for assessing DR and clear media PDR, as it delineates foveal avascular zone (FAZ) abnormalities, microvascular occlusions, end-vascular-occluded fine vascular segments, the presence of saccular or fusiform microaneurysms and clearly demonstrates the characteristics of the deep capillary plexus (DCP) and superficial capillary plexus (SCP). In addition to OCT-A, the Optovue AngioVue system enables quantitative analysis of the different capillary plexuses of the retina and choroid, serving as a marker for the diagnosis and surveillance of medical or surgical approaches [21]. Fundus fluorescein angiography (FFA) cannot visualize the details of peripapillary radial vascular or deep capillary networks [16, 17, 22]. OCT-A has been demonstrated to be a superior digital technique for the quantitative analysis of different vessel density (VD) metrics and objectively evaluates choroidal and retinal perfusion patterns to detect all vascular-relevant findings in the eyes of patients with DR [22, 23]. OCT-A techniques also reliably detect abnormal vascularization at any level in choroidal or retinal tissue (**Figure 1**) [24–26].

OCT-A is a potentially valuable imaging tool for improving DR treatment outcomes and monitoring injectable intervention protocols. In addition, deleterious changes in retinal and choroidal perfusion markers and patterns that occur after vitrectomy for TRD or due to the progression of diabetic microangiopathy may be detected and consequently treated with injectable interventions such as sustained anti-VEGF therapy [19].

This chapter examines the importance of retinal and choroidal perfusion evaluations in diabetic patients with DR and TRD who have undergone PPV and their role in guiding treatment to improve functional outcomes. We explored the influence of surgical approaches on postoperative superficial and deep retinal perfusion plexuses and the correlation of the choroidal vascularity index (CVI) and choriocapillaris flow area (CFA) with final best-corrected visual acuity (BCVA). After a thorough analysis of PubMed and scholarly literature, complemented by the authors' experience, we aimed to increase the comprehension of TRD management and ultimately improve patient visual outcomes for this serious sight-threatening condition by detecting postoperative retinal and choroidal ischemic alterations using sophisticated OCT-A imaging technology.

1.1 Preoperative and postoperative functional and structural evaluation protocol

Surgical patients must be evaluated by recording BCVA values, biomicroscopy, fundus examination with different fundoscopic lenses, indirect ophthalmoscopy (different TRD clinical cases with clear media are presented in **Figures 2** and **3**), and high-resolution vitreoretinal mode B-scan ultrasonography. Horizontal and vertical cross-sectional images of the macular region should be obtained using SD-OCT in eyes with clear media. In this study, OCT images were captured using a Ret-Vue-3.4 OCT (Optovue, Inc., Fremont, CA, USA). The measurement of axial length using coherence laser interferometry (IOL Master 700; Carl Zeiss Meditec AG, Oberkochen, Germany) is highly recommended. In eyes with opaque media, TRD should be confirmed and characterized by high-resolution B-scan ultrasonography. Postoperative microstructural evaluations should be performed using an SD-OCT device (images shown in this chapter were obtained using a Spectralis OCT; Heidelberg Engineering,

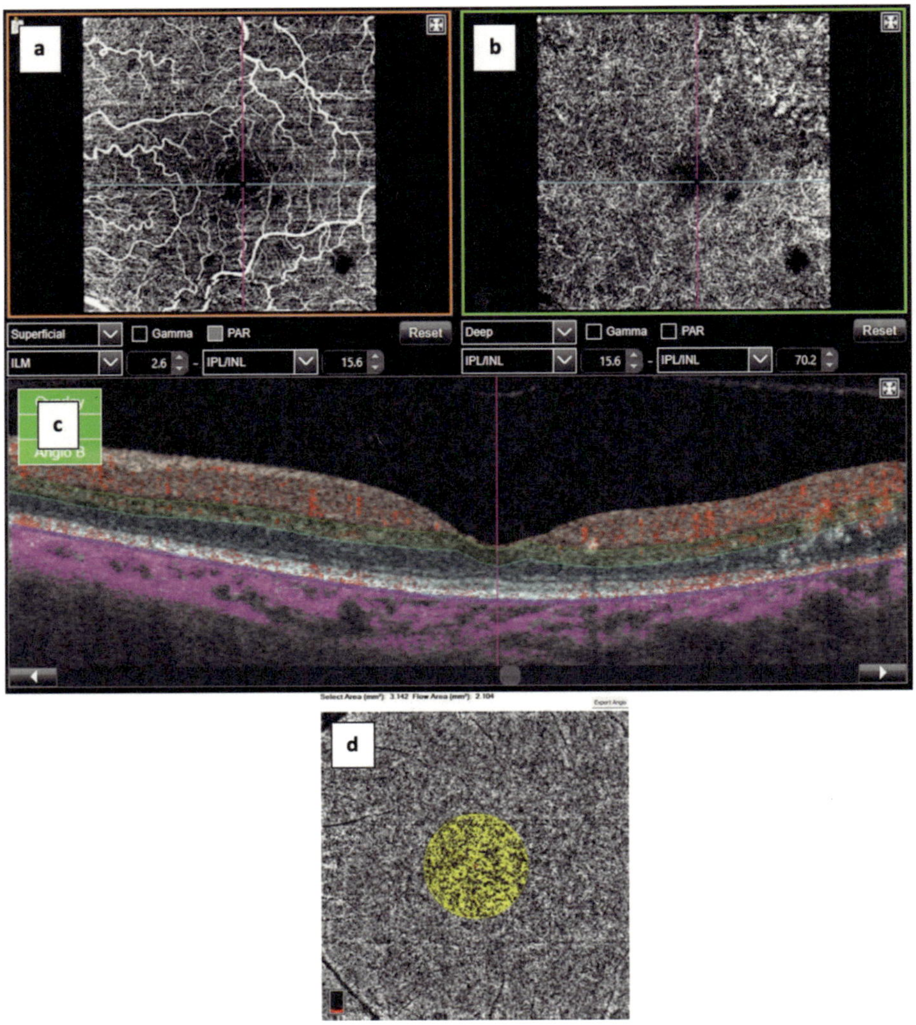

Figure 1.
OCT-A image of the superficial capillary plexus (SCP) (a) and deep capillary plexus (DCP) (b) showing fine vessel abnormalities and vessel tortuosity (VT) in a diabetic eye. Multiple small vascular areas of nonperfused areas are observed throughout the macula in both plexuses. (c) In the bottom image, a corresponding structural high-definition (HD) image shows some degree of disorganization of the retina inner layers (DRIL) with well-demarcated outer retina structures pinpointed by automatic segmentation of the green lines. The purple and red dots represent vascular structures in the choroid and retina, respectively. (d) Corresponding binarizing processing of the choriocapillaris flow area (CFA) of 2.104 mm² in the selected protocol for a total area of 3.142 mm². This modified multipanel figure was obtained from a previous publication [27] by Quiroz-Reyes et al. and is used under the Creative Commons Attribution 4.0 International License (https://creativecommons.org/licenses/by/4.0/).

Heidelberg, Germany) and a swept-source DRI OCT Triton device (Topcon Medical Systems, Inc.). We regularly performed postoperative perfusion evaluations, quantitative VD measurements, and quantitative perfusion evaluations of the choriocapillaris flow using an OCT-A device (images in this chapter were captured using RTVue XR OCT Avanti with AngioVue Software; OptoVue Inc., Fremont, CA, USA). This equipment uses a specialized split-spectrum amplitude-decorrelation angiography software algorithm to acquire 70,000 A-scans/s to construct OCT-A volumes consisting of 304 Å–304 A-scans, achieving a high axial resolution at depths of up to 5 μm

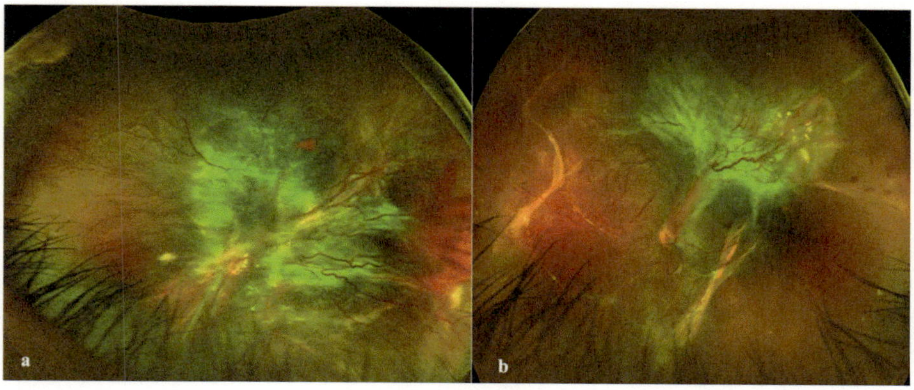

Figure 2.
Different types of diabetic tractional retinal detachment (TRD). (a) Magnified wide-field Optos color image of exuberant fibrovascular tissue proliferation over the posterior pole and along the vascular arcades that contract and detach the macula. (b) Another image of diabetic TRD with macular involvement. The TRD extends to the nasal equator of the retina with vertical subretinal demarcation lines. This modified multipanel figure was obtained from a previous publication [27] and was generated under the Creative Commons Attribution 4.0 International License (https://creativecommons.org/licenses/by/4.0/).

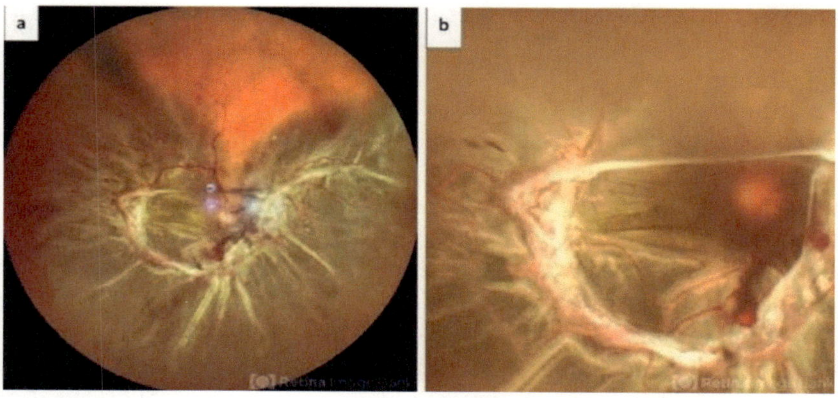

Figure 3.
Different types of diabetic tractional retinal detachment TRD. (a) Macula-off combined with tractional and rhegmatogenous retinal detachment (RRD). 57082. (b) Combined tractional and RRD in a patient with proliferative diabetic retinopathy (PDR). 57083. The images in this modified figure were originally published on the Retina Image Bank® website. Manish Nagpal, MD. Photographer Gayathri Mohan. Retina Foundation. Retina Image Bank. Jun 10, 2020. © The American Society of Retina Specialists.

and minimizing motion artifacts. Each OCT-A cube scan comprised 304 Å–304 A-scans within a 3 mm × 3 mm square centered around the fovea, which yielded 304 B-scans. Each B-scan output displays an average of at least two scans. Segmentation of the SCP, DCP, outer retinal layer, and CFA slabs is obtained using AngioVue software. The central subfield thickness (CSFT) is automatically calculated using standardized algorithms contained in the device software. Perfusional choroidal measurements were obtained following a previously published protocol using the aforementioned OCT-A device [27]. CFA should be performed by segmenting the choriocapillaris subfoveal plexus (CSP) slabs using an OCT-A instrument that can manually locate an area of interest and digitally calculate the VD in a preselected area. Only high-quality images with a standard signal strength index (SSI) > 46 provided by the software for scan quality are used for perfusion analysis.

1.1.1 Image binarization for CVI quantification and the CFA measurement protocol

CVI values are calculated by quantifying the luminal area (LA) and total choroidal area (TCA) from SD-OCT images of the macula using ImageJ analysis software (version 1.53; USA, public domain). High-definition (HD) 9-mm OCT-B images are converted into an 8-bit format (**Figure 4a**) and adjusted using the autothreshold technique (Niblack autothreshold). Using the polygon tool, the area of the subfoveal choroid is then digitally selected on the map of the total choroidal area (TCA) 750 μm nasally and 750 μm temporally from the foveal center in the direction of the horizontal plane and vertically from the RPE-Bruch's membrane region to the inner scleral border in the direction of the vertical plane (demarcated by the dotted red line in **Figure 4b**). The stromal vascular tissue area is determined by the number of white pixels, and the luminal area (LA) at the choroid is determined by applying the threshold tool and quantifying the number of dark pixels once the binarized image is obtained (**Figure 4c**). The dark-to-light pixel ratio is then expressed as a percentage and defined as the CVI, as previously described by Agrawal et al. [29, 30]. The protocol study method for binarization was validated in a previous study [28]. The CFA is obtained by automated binarization and segmentation of the CSP slabs using the RTVue XR OCT Avanti with AngioVue Software (OptoVue Inc., Fremont, CA, USA) and automatically calculated from a 3.142 mm^2 evaluation area (**Figure 4d**).

1.2 Surgical approaches

A technique using a standard 25-gauge, self-sealed, three-port, control-perfused PPV is recommended by the authors in this section. Local sedation is recommended when using this approach. In addition to central vitrectomy, triamcinolone acetonide (Kenalog 40 mg/mL; Bristol-Myers, New York, NY, USA)-assisted removal of the cortical vitreous from the surface of the retina should be performed, with a focus on the detection of preretinal fibrovascular tissue bands. Detaching or peeling condensed hyaloids in cases of complex vitreoretinal interfaces requires a combination of delamination with segmentation maneuvers and with visco-delamination techniques for epiretinal fibrovascular tissue to avoid iatrogenic retinal breaks. Any foci of bleeding from the fibrovascular tissue should be endodiathermized throughout the procedure. Following previously described steps, the fibrovascular membranes are dissected using membrane stripping techniques, and the residual epiretinal tissue is peeled to release macular traction. The focus of the surgery should be on tangential traction, and surgical macular evaluation and revision should be performed using 0.15% trypan blue ophthalmic solution (Membrane Blue; Dutch Ophthalmic, USA) to stain the cortical vitreous remnants or epiretinal membrane (ERM) proliferation. A 0.25 mg/mL (0.025%) diluted isomolar solution (pH 7.4) of Brilliant Blue G (BBG) dye is recommended for ILM staining when ILM traction is suspected. If there are any rhegmatogenous lesions, the lesion should be diathermally marked, macular reattachment should be achieved, and argon laser-assisted scatter panretinal photocoagulation (PRP) should be performed. In retinal zones with shallow RD due to the presence of subretinal fluid without rhegmatogenous lesions, PRP should be avoided or cautiously applied because the laser may induce small retinal breaks (**Figures 5** and **6**). A selected gas tamponade, such as a long-acting nonexpandable perfluoropropane (C_3F_8) gas mixture at 15%, sulfur hexafluoride (SF_6), or silicone oil (SO) lighter than water 1000 or 5000 Cks (centistokes), should be administered at the end of the surgical procedure based on the surgeon's preference.

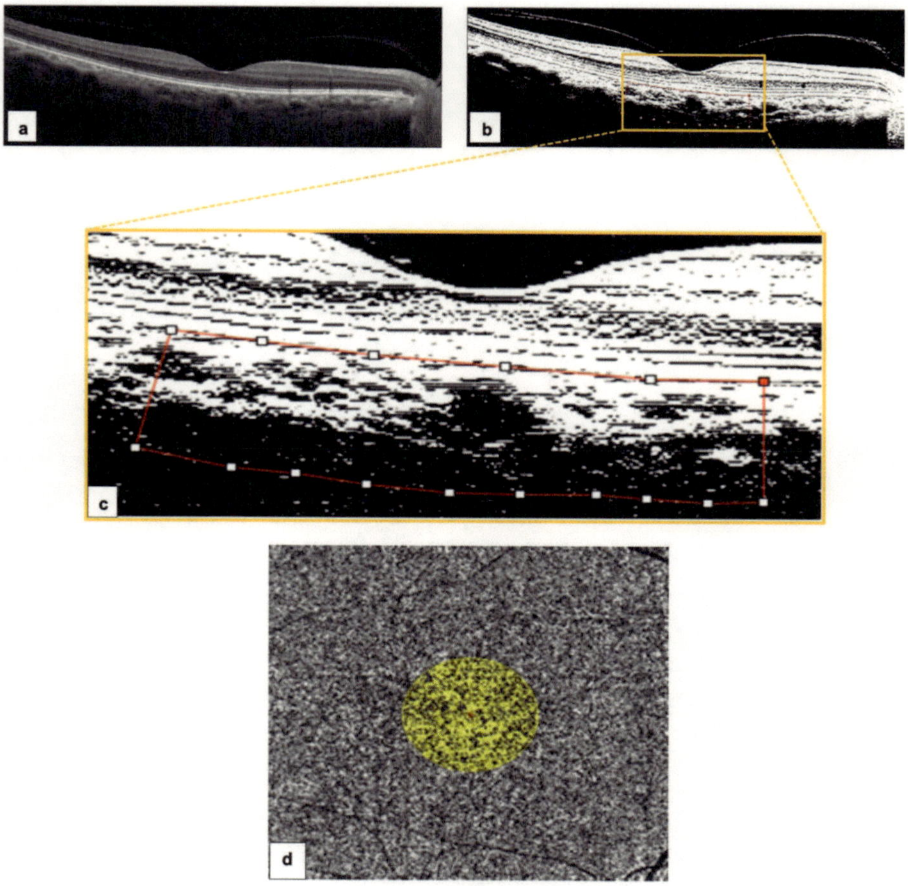

Figure 4.
A figure depicting the method used for quantifying the CVI in healthy eyes. (a) Binarized image designed to depict the intraretinal structure and choroidal layers in greater detail in a healthy emmetropic eye. (b) Binarizing processing in a 9-mm HD image. (c) Magnified image within the yellow square showing binarized processing of the subfoveal choroidal stroma and luminal vascular visualization of the subfoveal choroidal vessels to obtain a choroidal vascularity index (CVI) of 62.8%. The selected subfoveal area of choroidal flow is clearly delineated by the red-white dotted line. (d) Binarizing processing of the normal choriocapillaris flow area (CFA). This modified multipanel figure was obtained from a previous publication [28] and was generated under the Creative Commons Attribution 4.0 International License (https://creativecommons.org/licenses/by/4.0/).

1.3 Postoperative structural and perfusion outcomes in patients with TRD

Postoperative SD-OCT findings (**Figures 5–7**) revealed foveal contour profile abnormalities, retinal nerve fiber thickness (RNFT) alterations, disorganization of the retinal inner layers (DRIL), diffuse retinal layer thinning with central subfield thickness (CSFT) abnormalities, ellipsoid zone (EZ) disruption, and external limiting membrane (ELM) line abnormalities in a subset of surgical eyes. Based on the OCT-A perfusion data, both the SCP and DCP exhibited extensive perfusion abnormalities, and subfoveal CVI and CFA analyses revealed subnormal values in all the examined patients, with an enlarged and irregular perifoveal capillary network (PCN) with lower-than-normal VD values in the analyzed capillary plexuses (**Figures 5–7**). A summary of the postoperative structural and perfusion outcomes is shown in **Table 1**.

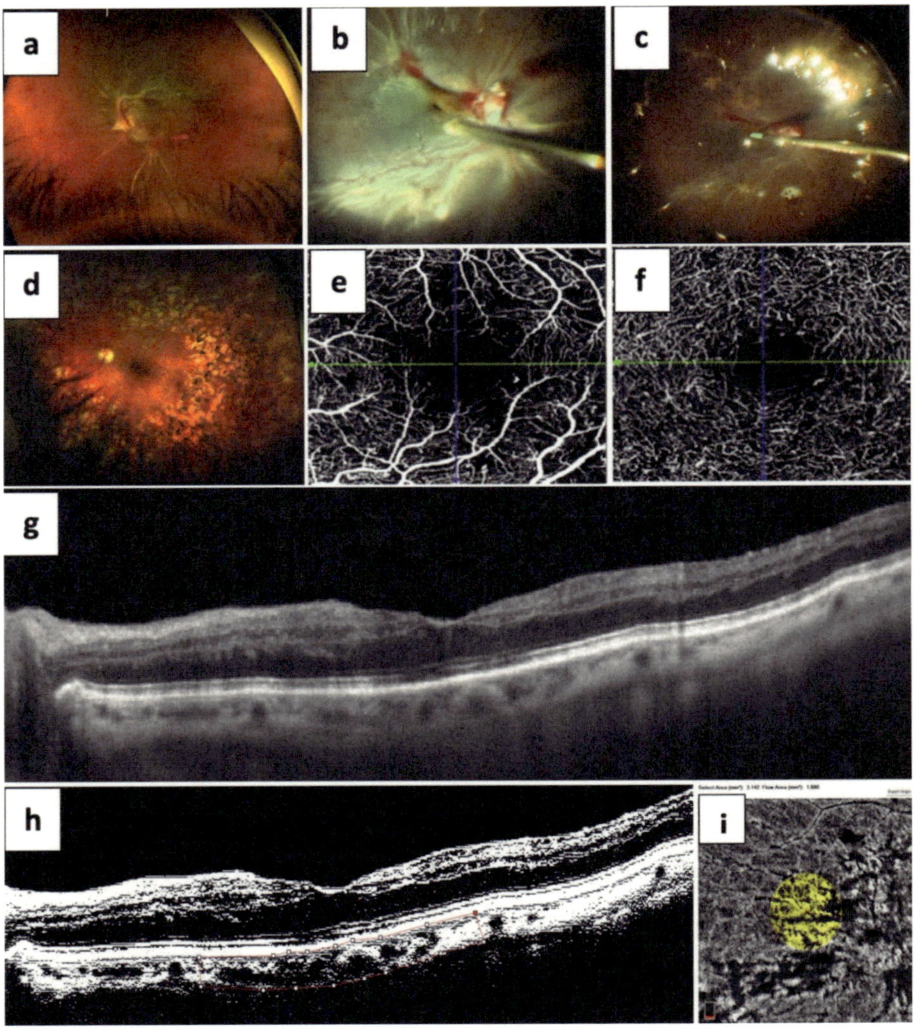

Figure 5.
Surgical approach and postoperative structural and perfusion findings. (a) Wide-field Optos color fundus image of an eye with long-term type 2 diabetes mellitus and abundant proliferative fibrovascular preretinal tissue that detached the retina involving the macula. (b) Surgical image showing a severe TRD; the macula is off, and fibrovascular tissue emerges from the optic nerve, detaching the retina and temporal vascular arcades. The detached macula is released when trypan blue dye is used to stain vitreous or fibrovascular remnants and facilitate membrane stripping. This surgical image also depicts a distorted and stained macular surface with evidence of dragged macular tissue due to proliferative fibrous tissue remnants over the optic nerve and along the inferior temporal arcade. (c) Surgical magnified image showing clear reattachment of the macula after air-fluid exchange. (d) Corresponding final long-term fundus photo showing an attached retina and extensive panretinal photocoagulation (PRP) scars. (e) Long-term postoperative superficial capillary plexus (SCP) showing end-vessel abnormalities and an enlarged foveal avascular zone (FAZ) with multiple capillary dropouts. (f) Corresponding deep capillary plexus (DCP) with ischemic changes and vascular deficiencies. (g) Long-term postoperative 9-mm HD horizontal B-scan depicting an abnormal foveal profile, disorganization of the retinal inner layers (DRIL), and abnormal outer retina layer markers. (h) The image within the red-white dotted line clearly delineates a low CVI of 54.4%. (i) Abnormal CFA of 1.880 mm^2. This modified multipanel figure was obtained from a previous publication [27] and was generated under the Creative Commons Attribution 4.0 International License (https://creativecommons.org/licenses/by/4.0/).

CFA, choriocapillaris flow area; CSFT, central subfield thickness; CVI, choroidal vascularity index; Deep capillary plexus; DRIL, disorganization of the retinal inner layers; EZ, ellipsoid zone; ELM, external limiting membrane; OCT-A, optical coherence

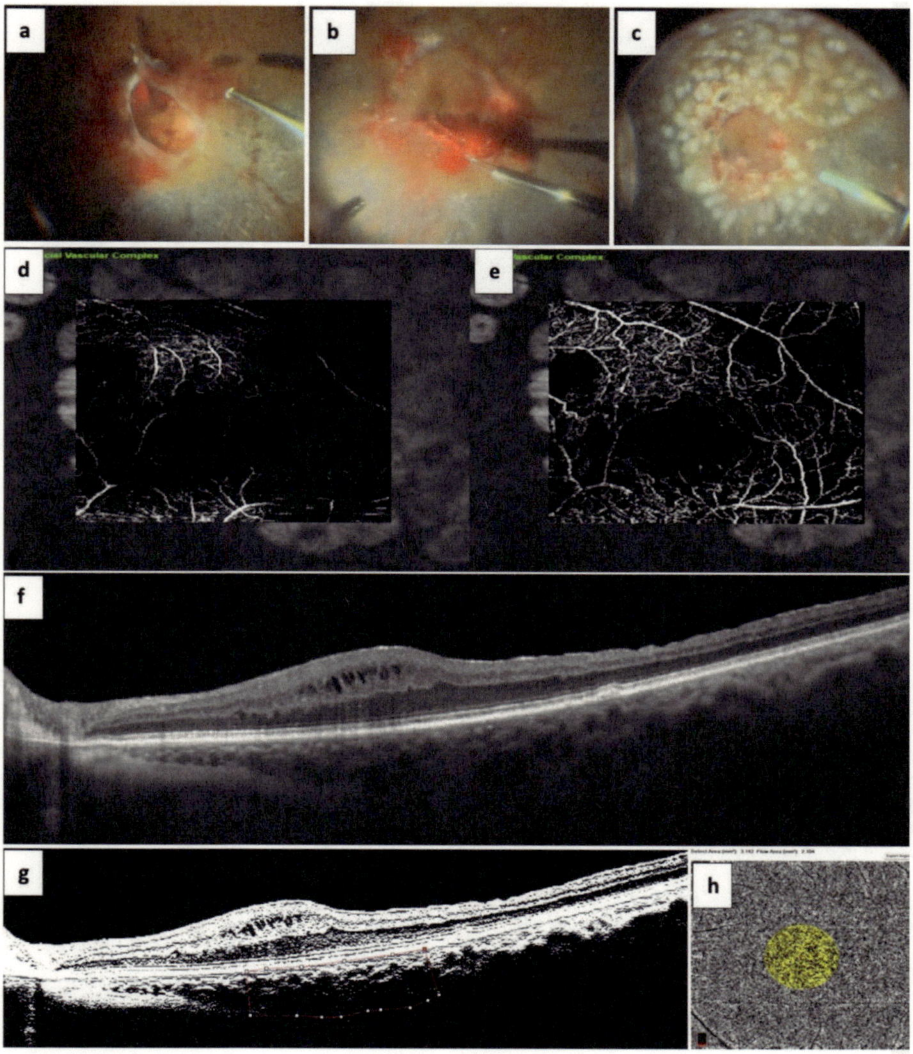

Figure 6.
Surgical approach and postoperative structural and perfusion findings. (a) Surgical view of a very complex diabetic TRD involving the macula in a hammock configuration. (b) The macula was traction-released, and passive blood aspiration and retinal exploration were mandatory. (c) Image of the final surgical step depicting air-fluid exchange with a completely reattached retina and extensive PRP. (d) and (e) Postoperative en-face OCT-A images depicting irregular filling at the level of the SCP and DCP insufficiently filled due to low vessel density (VD) and capillary dropout with an irregular and enlarged perifoveal capillary network (PCN). (f) Long-term postoperative image showing diffuse retinal thinning on the temporal macular side; the macular contour is indistinguishable, indicating severe nasal macular cystic edema, DRIL, and external limiting membrane (ELM) subfoveal discontinuities. (g) Postoperative binarizing processing of this image showed an abnormal CVI of 57.6% within the red-white dotted line. (h) Close to normal CFA of 2.104 mm^2. This modified multipanel figure was obtained from a previous publication [27] and was generated under the Creative Commons Attribution 4.0 International License (https://creativecommons.org/licenses/by/4.0/).

tomography angiography; PCN, perifoveal capillary network; SD, standard deviation; SD-OCT, spectral-domain optical coherence tomography; SCP, superficial capillary plexus; TRD, tractional retinal detachment; VD, vessel density These modified data were published previously [27] by Quiroz-Reyes et al. and is used under the Creative Commons Attribution 4.0 International License (https://creativecommons.org/licenses/by/4.0/).

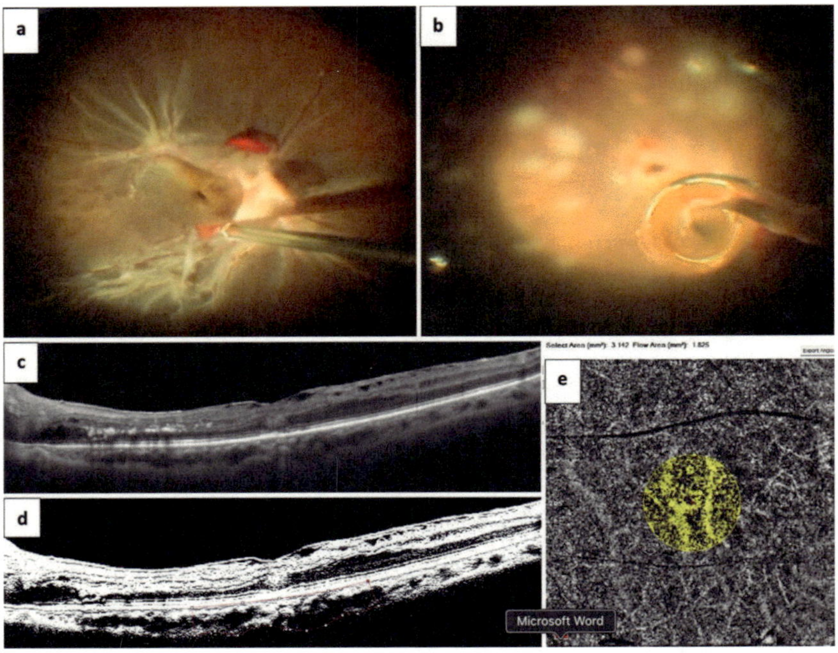

Figure 7.
Surgical approach and postoperative structural and perfusion findings. (a) Surgical magnified image depicting a combined tractional and RRD. (b) Transoperative image after intraocular silicone oil (SO) injection at the end of the surgical procedure. (c) Postoperative cross-sectional horizontal SD-OCT B-scan image showing an irregular macular profile with some mild superficial wrinkling of the temporal region along with extrafoveal cystic chronic residual edema with deep hyperreflexive dots, mainly over the nasal side of the macula. ELM line discontinuities were observed, and the subfoveal ellipsoid zone (EZ) was disrupted. (d) Corresponding long-term postoperative binarized image where the red-white dotted line clearly delineates an abnormal CVI of 56.2%. (e) Binarizing of the choriocapillaris to obtain an abnormal CFA of 1.825 mm^2. This modified multipanel figure was obtained from a previous publication [27] by Quiroz-Reyes et al. and is used under the Creative Commons Attribution 4.0 International License (https://creativecommons.org/licenses/by/4.0/).

1.4 Postoperative functional performance in patients with TRD

The final TRD resolution and final visual acuity (VA) correlated with the OCT-A outcomes are shown in **Figures 8** and **9**, respectively. In **Figure 10**, comparisons between the preoperative, 3-month, and final postoperative BCVA values are shown. In **Figure 11**, the BCVA repeated measures that estimated marginal mean values are explained, and the figure shows the mean points for each stage (pre, 3 months, and final) with a 95% confidence interval. In **Figure 12**, comparisons of preoperative, 3-month, and final postoperative BCVA between eyes that underwent more than one surgery and eyes that underwent only one surgery are shown. In **Figure 13**, a total of 44 eyes were plotted, including 14 postoperative TRD patients and 30 age-matched healthy control eyes. The Mann-Whitney nonparametric test did not reveal significant differences in age between the control and diabetes cohorts ($P = 0.125$). The final BCVA, as represented by the logMAR scale, was significantly greater in the diabetes group ($P < 0.0001$), with a median logMAR of 0.000 in the control group and 0.480 in this subset of the diabetic group. As shown in **Figure 14**, the CVI values calculated from OCT measurements were significantly lower in the diabetic group ($P = 0.0011$), with a median CVI of 57.95% in the control group and 44.41% in the diabetic group. A

SD-OCT (n = 30) and OCT-A (n = 14) findings	Mean	SD
Preoperative evolution of TRD	11.6 weeks	±2.3 weeks
Mean postoperative TRD resolution	3.6 weeks	±1.7 weeks
Mean postoperative follow-up	11.4 weeks	±5.7 weeks
SD-OCT marker	n	Percentage
Postoperative CSFT abnormalities	9	30%
Presence of DRIL	13	43.3%
EZ abnormalities	23	76.6%
ELM line abnormalities	21	70.1%
Plexus		
SCP and DCP abnormalities	14	87.5%
PCN abnormalities	12	75%
Decreased VD	10	62.5%
Decreased CVI	14	100%
Decreased CFA	14	100%

Table 1.
Preoperative and postoperative TRD evolution. Postoperative structural and perfusion outcomes.

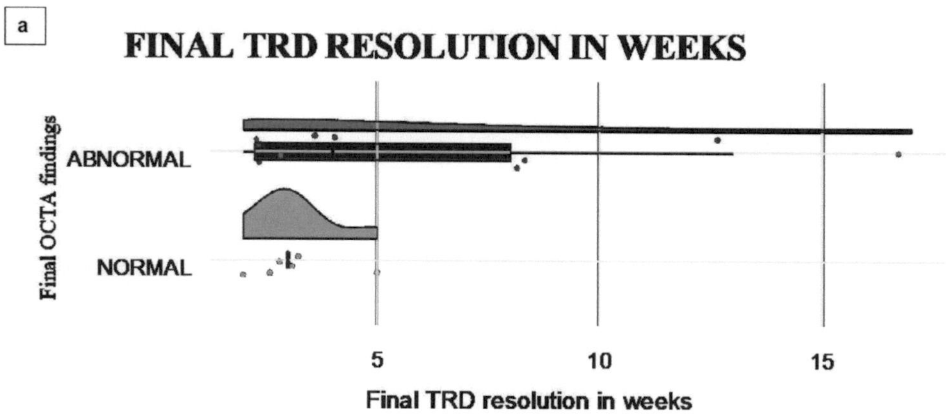

Figure 8.
Final TRD resolution correlated with OCT-A findings. This modified figure was published previously [27] by Quiroz-Reyes et al. and is used under the Creative Commons Attribution 4.0 International License (https://creativecommons.org/licenses/by/4.0/).

moderately positive correlation was found between the CVI and BCVA in the control cohort (r = 0.535) (P = 0.015). The correlation between the CVI and BCVA in the diabetes cohort was close to zero (r = −0.005) and was not significant (P = 0.986). The BCVA and CVI exhibited broader distributions in the diabetes cohort than in the control cohort, indicating greater variations in visual function and retinal morphology in diseased eyes. **Figures 8–14** summarize the structural, functional, and perfusional outcomes previously published by the authors [27].

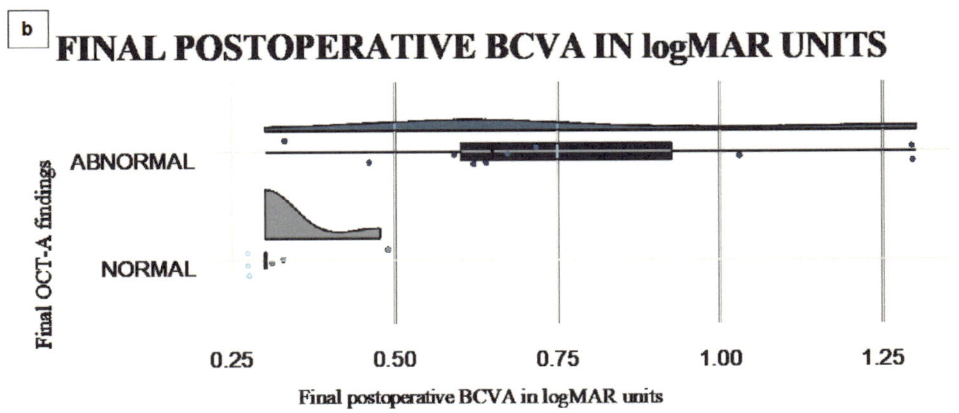

Figure 9.
Final postoperative BCVA correlated with OCT-A findings. This modified figure was published previously [27] by Quiroz-Reyes et al. and is used under the Creative Commons Attribution 4.0 International License (https://creativecommons.org/licenses/by/4.0/).

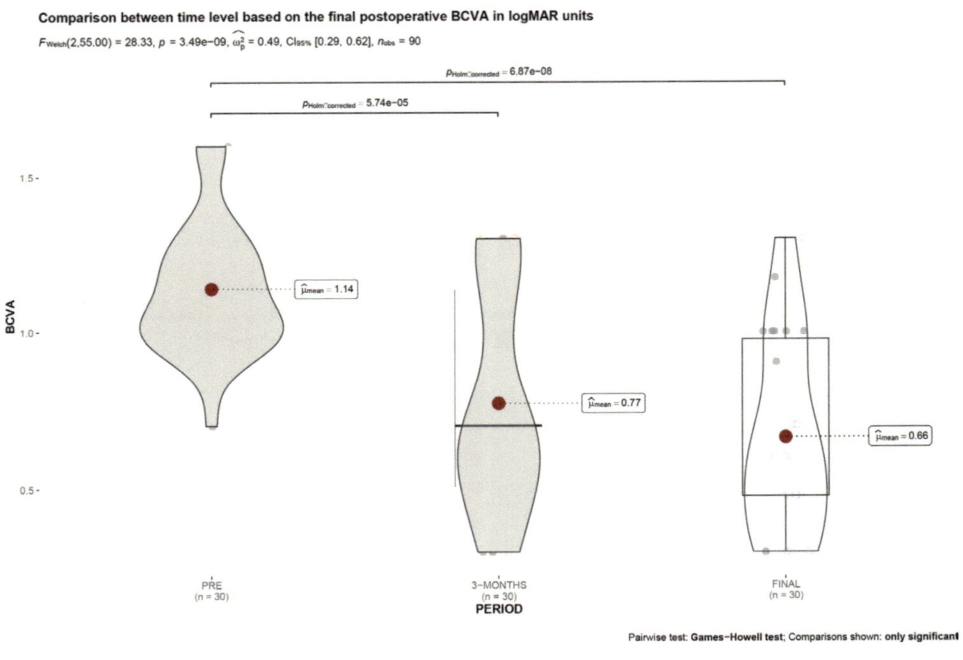

Figure 10.
Comparison of the preoperative, 3-month, and final postoperative BCVA values. This figure was published previously [27] by Quiroz-Reyes et al. and is used under the Creative Commons Attribution 4.0 International License (https://creativecommons.org/licenses/by/4.0/).

1.4.1 CVI and CFA measurements

Compared to those of the control eyes, the surgically treated TRD eyes had significantly smaller LA, TCA, CVI, and CFA values (all $P < 0.0001$) (**Table 2**). No significant differences were found in LA or TCA values in the PPV group (both $p > 0.05$). However, the PPV group had significantly lower CVI ($P = 0.0125$) and CFA ($P = 0.0003$) values than those in the control group.

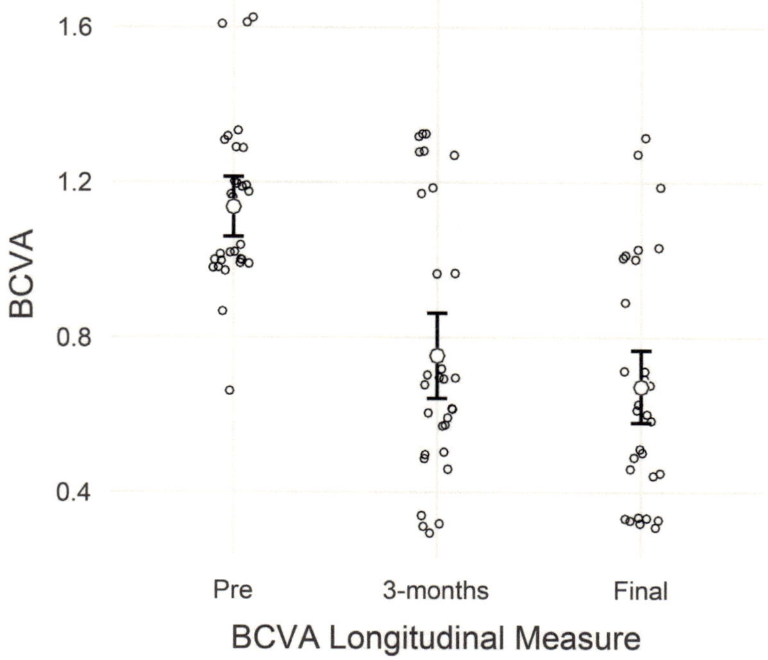

Figure 11.
BCVA repeated measures estimated marginal means. The figure shows the mean points for each stage (preoperative, 3-month, and final) with the 95% confidence interval. This figure was published previously [27] by Quiroz-Reyes et al. and is used under the Creative Commons Attribution 4.0 International License (https://creativecommons.org/licenses/by/4.0/).

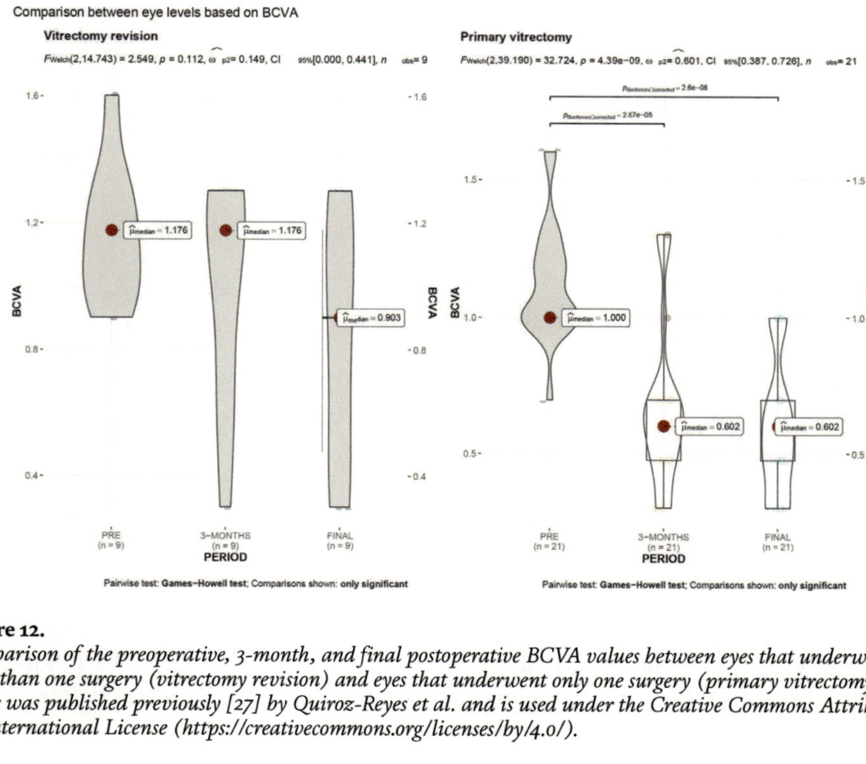

Figure 12.
Comparison of the preoperative, 3-month, and final postoperative BCVA values between eyes that underwent more than one surgery (vitrectomy revision) and eyes that underwent only one surgery (primary vitrectomy). This figure was published previously [27] by Quiroz-Reyes et al. and is used under the Creative Commons Attribution 4.0 International License (https://creativecommons.org/licenses/by/4.0/).

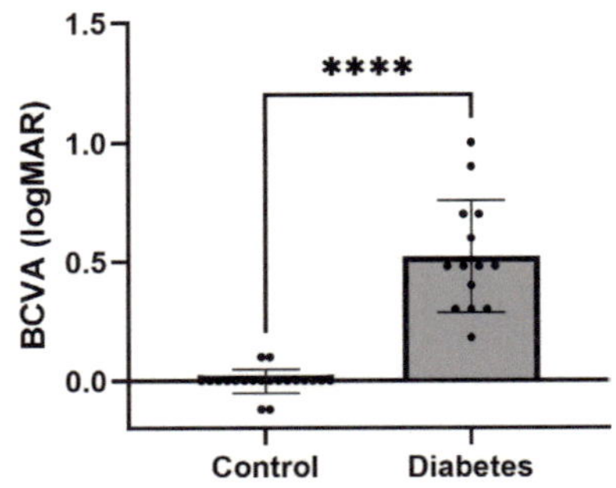

Figure 13.
*Final BCVA across study cohorts. The BCVA values collected on the Snellen scale were converted to logMAR units and evaluated across study cohorts. The control eyes had significantly lower BCVA values in logMAR units than did the diabetic eyes. The P value is indicated by * (**** = $P \leq 0.0001$). The bars represent the means and standard deviations; the data for each patient are plotted as dots. BCVA, best-corrected visual acuity.*

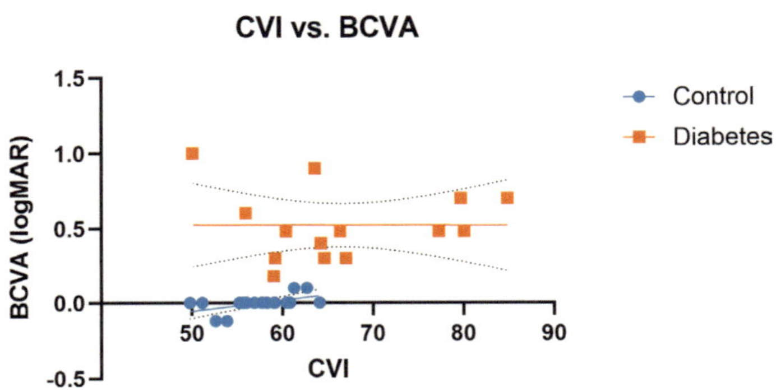

Figure 14.
Distribution of the CVI and BCVA. Individual patient data were plotted with points colored according to the study cohort. Linear regression lines are shown as solid-colored lines, with 95% intervals shown as dotted lines.

Parameters	Vitrectomy group (mean values)	Control group (mean values)
LA (mm^2)	0.189	0.198
TCA (mm^2)	0.312	0.342
CVI (%)	44.41	57.95
CFA (mm^2)	1.38	2.28

CFA, choriocapillaris flow area; CVI, choroidal vascularity index; LA, luminal area; TCA, total choroidal area.

Table 2.
Mean choroidal measurements across treated eyes (n = 14).

As the state of the choroid and retinal postoperative perfusion may influence visual function, a correlation analysis between the choroidal parameters (CVI and CFA) and BCVA was performed. Positive correlations were observed among BCVA, the CVI, and the CFA (**Table 3**). Because BCVA was measured in logMAR units, these findings suggested a positive correlation between the two choroidal perfusion parameters and visual function; that is, a lower CVI and CFA correlated with a worse BCVA ($P = 0.0003$ and $P = 0.0037$, respectively).

Choroidal parameters	Control eyes (n:30)	TRD eyes (n:14)
CVI	−0.124	−0.117
CFA	−0.211	−0.355

CFA, choriocapillaris flow area; CVI, choroidal vascularity index; TRD, traction retinal detachment.

Table 3.
Correlation coefficients between BCVA and choroidal parameters.

1.5 Representative surgical cases

Based on the surgical experience of the authors, representative and complex surgical cases of diabetic macula-off TRD in which vitreous surgery was performed at different stages of TRD, with the estimation of the corresponding long-term postoperative and enhanced binarized OCT imaging CVI and CFA calculations, are shown in multipanel **Figures 15–17**.

2. Role of the postoperative CVI in assessing choroidal vascular changes in TRD patients

The CVI has proven to be informative in determining the condition of choroidal perfusion across various treatment scenarios [31, 32]. Quantitative metrics, such as the CVI and CFA, have been used to diagnose, categorize, and guide treatments for retinal diseases [33]. Hayreh demonstrated that the submacular choroidal supply is affected by chronic ischemic conditions such as age-related macular degeneration (AMD) and PDR because of the multiple zones of altered perfusion at the level of the short posterior ciliary arteries. A decrease in the CVI at baseline is indicative of choroidal ischemia in patients with DR. Moreover, the CVI is a useful postoperative indicator for monitoring disease incidence, surgical influence, and treatment response [34]. Employing noninvasive techniques, such as CVI estimation [35] and OCT-A perfusion indices [36], to monitor disease and treatment outcomes could significantly enhance the management of different conditions, such as postoperative TRD.

3. Postoperative CVI and CFA alterations in TRD patients

Studies have determined the relationship between CVI and CFA in the development and progression of various diseases, including genetic, retinal, and vascular conditions [34, 37, 38]. The CVI can be used as an indicator of retinal and choroidal vascular disease. Since retinal diseases involve multiple factors, such as inflammation, edema, and leakage, the CVI and CFA have been suggested as potential markers because they reflect vascular perfusion changes of paramount and critical importance that affect the postoperative integrity and recovery of the vascular network within the highly blood-supplied structure known as the choroid [39–41].

Our study showed that postoperative OCT-A perfusion values were lower in surgical patients with a longer preoperative duration of TRD and in those who underwent more than one surgical procedure (see **Figure 12**). Surgical intervention with TRD reapplication significantly improved visual acuity in all patients (see **Figure 13**). Nevertheless, postoperative perfusion outcomes revealed that the CVI was

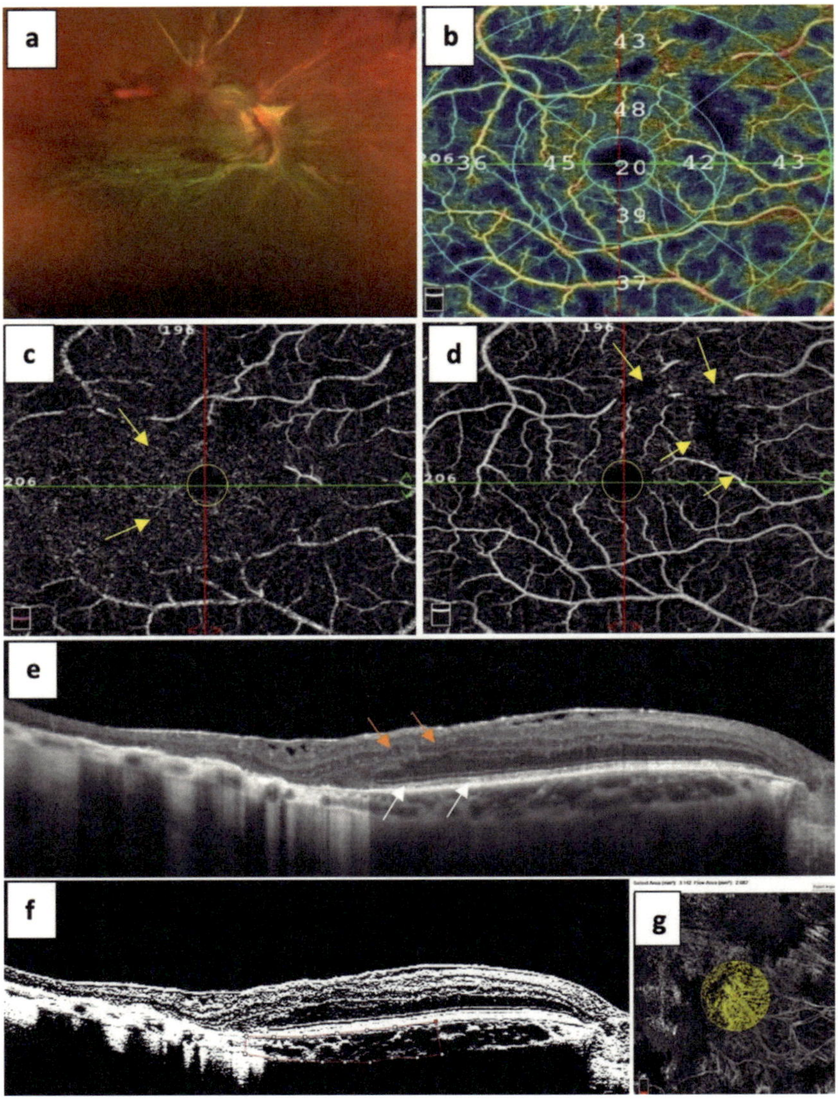

Figure 15.
Surgical Patient 1. A 42-year-old male patient with 18 years of type 2 diabetes had irregular metabolic control. His last glycosylated hemoglobin level was 7.7. The patient had PDR and panretinal photocoagulation (PRP) in both eyes. The patient presented with progressive visual acuity (VA) loss in his right eye after 12 weeks of evolution. Ophthalmological examination revealed a pseudophakic RE with cloudy media. The TOA was 16 mmHg, with no manifestations of anterior segment neovascularization, signs of moderate vitreous bleeding, or evidence of a fibrovascular tissue stalk that detached the posterior pole, mainly at the level of the macula and inferotemporal vascular arcade (a). B-mode ultrasonography confirmed a diagnosis of TRD with macular involvement. The patient underwent an uneventful vitrectomy and endophotocoagulation-like PRP, during which macular reapplication was achieved. Long-term postoperative quantitative VD evaluation of the SCP was considered to be lower than normal, as shown by white numbers on the different subfoveal regions on the ETDRS-like grid (b). Postoperative final evaluation at 14 months showed an abnormal FAZ area on the DCP and SCP slabs (c) and (d) (yellow arrows). DRIL (orange arrows) and postoperative cystic macular edema were detected via B-scan OCT, and white arrows pinpoint outer retina layer markers (e). The binarized image showed a low CVI of 56.2% (f). (g) The CFA was abnormal with a value of 1.887 mm^2. The final BCVA was 20/80 (0.60 logMAR units). This modified multipanel figure was obtained from the International Journal of Ophthalmology & Visual Science. 2021;6(4):187–198. DOI: 10.11648/j.ijovs.20210604.12 and is used under the Creative Commons Attribution 4.0 International License (https://creativecommons.org/licenses/by/4.0/).

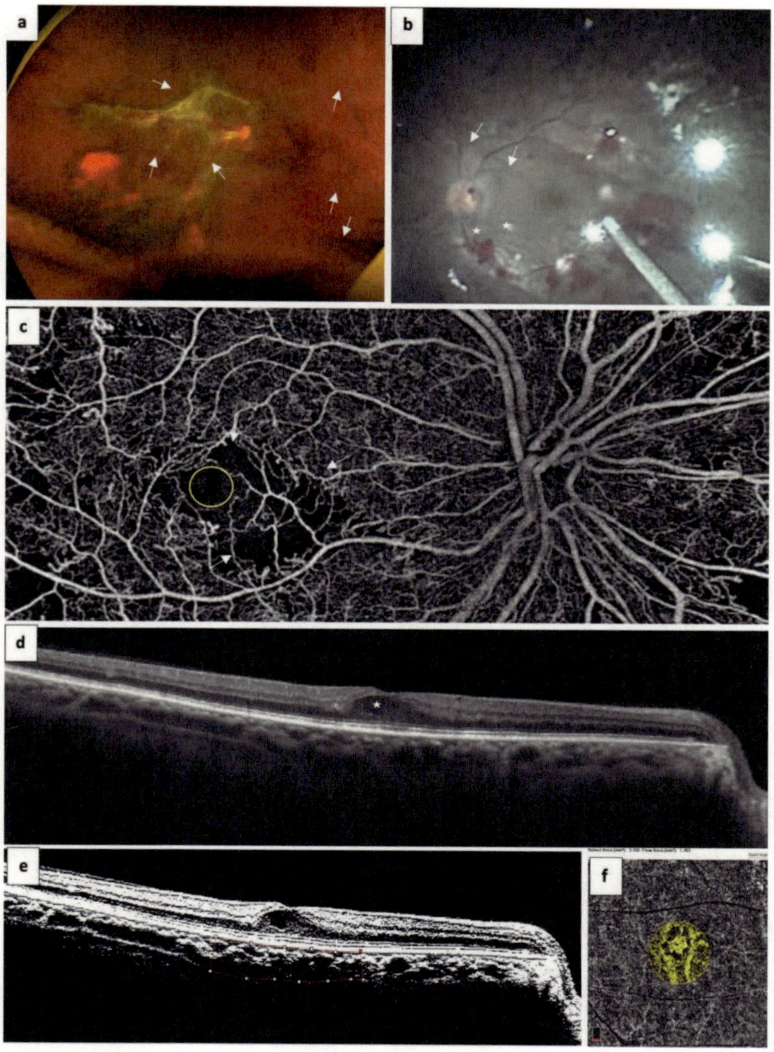

Figure 16.
Surgical Patient 2. A 59-year-old female patient with chronic complications of PDR presented evidence of vitreous hemorrhage on several occasions (a). She was unable to satisfactorily undergo laser PRP, and because of the presence of fibroglial tissue, the patient was not managed preoperatively with intravitreal bevacizumab. She had experienced a significant decrease in her VA for 3 weeks, and ultrasound examination revealed complex TRD of the posterior pole, complex vitreoretinal interface, and macular involvement. She underwent an uneventful vitrectomy, as depicted in the surgical image (b). Fifteen months after vitrectomy, the patient was evaluated using OCT-A. An angiogram of the papilla and macula showed restored perfusion close to normal but still with extensive yuxtafoveal capillary dropouts, an irregular and enlarged FAZ (yellow circle), and interruptions of the capillary margin at the SCP level (c) (white arrows). Postoperative OCT-A evaluation revealed a quantitative VD pattern that was considered lower than normal, which indicated important capillary dropout in the vicinity of the FAZ area. The pericapillary net (PCN) was abnormal, with a lower-than-normal VD. Long-term postoperative horizontal B-scan SD-OCT showed irregular foveal contours and diffuse irregular macular thickening due to the presence of macular edema with a large intraretinal subfoveal cyst (white asterisk), evidence of DRIL, and abnormal outer retinal biomarkers on the SD-OCT scan (d). The binarizing process showed a very low CVI of 53.7%, which was clearly defined in the red-white dotted selected area (e). (f) An abnormal CFA of 1.783 mm^2 is shown. The final BCVA was 20/120 (0.78 logMAR units). This modified multipanel figure was obtained from the International Journal of Ophthalmology & Visual Science. 2021;6(4):187–198. DOI: 10.11648/j.ijovs.20210604.12 and is used under the Creative Commons Attribution 4.0 International License (https://creativecommons.org/licenses/by/4.0/).

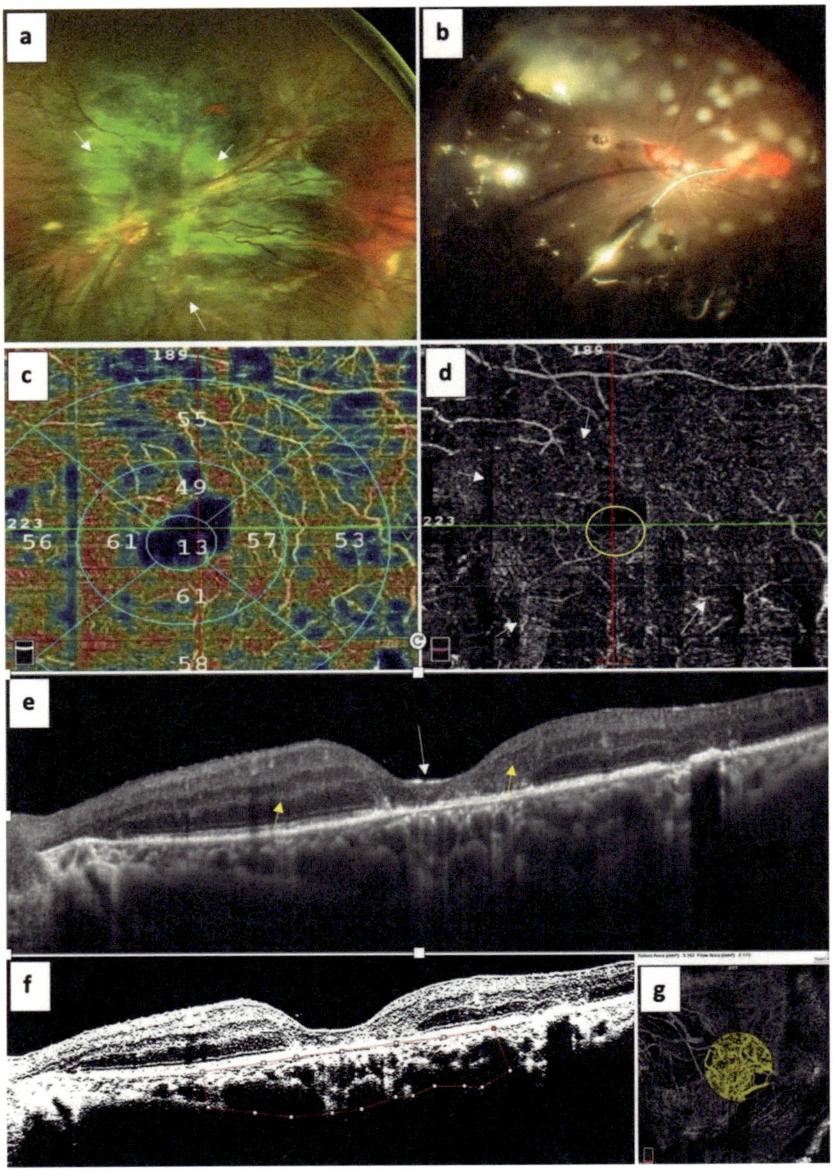

Figure 17.
Surgical Patient 3. A 57-year-old male patient with diabetes mellitus for 22 years presented with progressively decreasing vision in the left eye with 14 weeks of disease evolution and no history of laser PRP or antiangiogenic therapy. Ophthalmoscopic examination and B-mode ultrasonography revealed severe and extensive macula-off TRD, as shown in panel (a). The patient underwent uneventful PPV and phacoemulsification with surgical reattachment of the macula without complications, as shown in the corresponding surgical image (b). At 19 months postsurgery, perfusion evaluation was performed using OCT-A, which revealed an SCP with multiple vascular deficiencies in the VD evaluation, an abnormally enlarged FAZ area, and loss of shape of the corresponding PCN, as shown in the binarizing image with the ETDRS grid quantified with white numbers in its subregions (c). OCT-A evaluation of the DCP showed extensive and diffuse capillary dropouts (white arrows) (d). Long-term postoperative OCT examination revealed severe diffuse irregular thickening of the macula, intraretinal microcysts in the middle layers of the retina, and the presence of extrafoveal DRIL; biomarkers of the outer retinal layers were not recognizable, and atrophic subfoveal tissue was detected (e). (f) Binarized image processing showed a very low CVI of 46.8%. (g) An abnormal CFA of 1.775 mm^2 was quantified. The final BCVA of this eye was 20/200 (1.00 logMAR units). This modified multipanel figure was obtained from a previous publication [27] by Quiroz-Reyes et al. and is used under the Creative Commons Attribution 4.0 International License (https://creativecommons.org/licenses/by/4.0/).

significantly lower in the surgical group than in the control group (see **Figure 14**). The CVI and CFA may indicate disease progression in DR patients, and a lower CVI in postoperative eyes could be linked to the absence of recovered choroidal ischemic vascular defects caused by DR or tractional flow deprivation, the impact of surgical procedures or the influence and effects of antiangiogenic therapies. In conclusion, choroidal and retinal perfusion evaluations highlight the potential of the CVI and CFA as biomarkers for RD and their significance in differentiating healthy eyes from eyes with surgically resolved TRD and poor final BCVA. However, further research is needed to explore and better quantify CVI and CFA values in diabetic patients without DR, those with high-risk PDR, and those with resolved TRD to better understand their implications as prognostic markers for DR.

4. Literature review and discussion

Small-gauge instrumentation, control-perfusion techniques, bimanual PPV, wide-field viewing, improved fluidics, longitudinal pre- and postcutting endodiathermy, and precise tissue control techniques have all improved the anatomical outcomes of TRD surgical approaches. However, functional outcomes continue to be disappointing. Other injectable interventions using medical intravitreal antiangiogenic agents have been shown to alleviate postoperative residual DME, postoperative bleeding, and ischemic tissue complications due to severe BRB damage in TRD-associated PDR patients. The analysis of the results in this chapter was based on the surgical experience published by the authors [27] and its correlation with the literature review up to the publication date of this chapter.

It has been demonstrated that visual improvement is better in patients with DR who are receiving anti-VEGF therapy than in those who have received laser treatment [24]. The different options for clearing dense VH in patients who cannot undergo laser treatment include waiting and monitoring for the hemorrhage to reabsorb, performing additional laser treatment, administering injectable intervention with anti-VEGF in the absence of TRD, or performing vitrectomy. Recurrent bleeding with membrane formation and TRD occurrence were risk factors associated with the former method. The Writing Committee for Diabetic Retinopathy for the Clinical Research Network compared the clinical efficacy of intravitreal ranibizumab with that of PRP in clearing VH [9]. They concluded that patients with PDR and high-risk characteristics of severe vision loss treated with injectable intervention using sustainable intravitreal ranibizumab had better visual outcomes at 1 year than those treated with standard PRP care. Protocol S, based on injectable intervention using an anti-VEGF algorithm for PDR, assessed neovascularization status for 2 years in patients with high-risk PDR without prior PRP [42]. These authors concluded that the Diabetic Retinopathy Clinical Research Network (DRCR.net) protocol provided excellent outcomes for 2 years in patients who received intravitreal antiangiogenic treatment for PDR following the protocol guidelines [42].

Decreased perifoveal capillary blood flow caused by microangiopathy results in chronic ischemia of retinal tissue. According to a comprehensive assessment of the long-term postoperative macular perfusion indices, in functional eyes with a BCVA better than 20/200 (1.0 logMAR unit equivalent), retinal capillary nonperfusion was observed to be associated with photoreceptor damage according to the SD-OCT biomarkers, with evident alterations in EZ continuity and the presence of subfoveal DRIL. Macular ischemia is reflected in profound capillary deficiencies in the DCP, low CVI, and CFA VD deficiencies that cause choriocapillaris and outer retinal changes, and deleterious perfusion defects in central photoreceptors. When the central retina remains detached from the RPE, the risk of outer retinal layer ischemia increases because of capillary dropout at the DCP and choriocapillaris reflected in the low VD in the CFA slabs. Postoperative TRD eyes showed outer retinal layer abnormalities that colocalized with areas of enlargement in the FAZ area with a very irregular and ischemic PCN, and diffuse or localized macular capillary nonperfusion areas were detected with VDs lower than the mean VD in the SCP and DCP [27]. Therefore, photoreceptor damage with EZ abnormalities, DRIL, and macular ischemia are the most common factors contributing to limited improvement in vision after successful diabetic TRD surgical reattachment [27].

The current literature does not provide much information on the potential of quantitative retinal and choroidal OCT-A markers to predict visual outcomes in patients undergoing vitrectomy for TRD. There are many technical difficulties in quantitatively assessing pre- and early postoperative retinal and choroidal perfusion in patients with TRD. Cloudy media due to hemorrhage, the presence of preretinal fibrovascular complexes, and media opacities with complexities in the vitreoretinal interface are not technically allowed for preoperative evaluation via OCT-A perfusion imaging. We routinely evaluated the postoperative correlation of six OCT-A perfusion indices, the FAZ area, the FAZ shape, the VD in the SCP and DCP, the CVI, and the CFA, with the final BCVA and structural biomarkers such as the CSFT, EZ, and ELM line characteristics. The presence of subfoveal DRIL also determines how these SD-OCT and OCT-A perfusion biomarkers change longitudinally over time and how they are correlated with BCVA.

Unlike FFA, OCT-A evaluations facilitate in-depth analyses of vascular alterations in individuals with DR [17–20], acting as a key technological tool for evaluating perfusion in the different vascular layers in the choroid [43]. Patients with macular ischemia exhibit structural changes in both retinal capillary plexuses. In these patients, postoperative assessment of perfusional indices using OCT-A may be a useful predictor of the final VA [44–46].

Recent reports [25, 44–47] have shown that a poorer VD in both the superficial and deep capillary networks is correlated with DRIL appearance, EZ abnormalities, and CSFT with a poorer final BCVA. Freiberg et al. [45] quantified FAZ area dimensions and symmetry in patients with DR compared to normal controls using OCT-A. These authors found that OCT-A imaging could pinpoint the abnormal integrity of the capillary network surrounding the FAZ area, which corresponds to the PCN [44, 45]. Other researchers have reported that outer parafoveal VD in the superficial layer may predict improvement in VA after injectable intervention with ranibizumab injection. VD perfusion indices may be useful for evaluating the perfusion status of the macular area after surgery and predicting final vision. Several authors have previously reported that an increased FAZ area or contour irregularities in the PCN contour, an increased nonperfusion area, and decreased VD perfusion indices at the central macula in OCT-A may predict worsening DR [46–48]. Here, we report the potential of evaluating both retinal capillary plexus-quantified values and choroidal perfusion indices as indicators of complementary treatment for improving postoperative macular ischemia.

Photoreceptor disruption due to macular ischemia contributes to poor visual outcomes. The impaired blood flow associated with subfoveal DRIL generated by decreased blood perfusion combined with cell apoptosis due to retinal ischemia, which is mainly associated with lower-than-normal VD values in the SCP, CVI, and CFA, contributes to poor postoperative visual results. A large FAZ area associated with poor visual acuity (VA) recovery is a common outcome [27, 28, 49].

The analyzed data indicate that DRIL resolves over time and that DRIL resolution is a good predictor of visual improvement [14]. Spontaneous or pharmacologic (antiangiogenic) postoperative improvement in the appearance of subfoveal DRIL represents an anatomical marker of more normal morphology and potentially better visual recovery [27]. Researchers have not determined whether reversibility potentially decreases with increasing DRIL duration or whether this change can be induced. However, these findings have important implications for the timing of TRD [49].

We presumed that DRIL may be a biomarker of tissue damage. Therefore, further histological assessments are needed to determine the mechanisms by which the ischemic GCL-IPL complex, RNFL thickness, and neurodegenerative damage affect VA. However, the functional outcomes in a case series [27] and literature review [20, 21, 26, 45–50] suggested that increased subfoveal DRIL length, indicating less viable remaining tissue, is associated with worse visual outcomes.

Reports on PDR have shown that disruption of the outer retina, mainly of the EZ and ELM line markers, is a significant predictor of visual prognosis [46, 48, 51]. We found that subfoveal DRIL, ELM line integrity, and EZ characteristics correlated well with postoperative evolution and predicted final visual outcomes [27].

Moreover, certain perfusion indices, such as VD at different subregions of the macula according to the ETDRS grid, and structural biomarkers, such as DRIL, are important for postoperative monitoring once the retina has been successfully reattached and the eye is tamponade-free, which precludes detailed structural and perfusion evaluation. An important issue is that when the retina becomes detached along the macula, it must be managed in a timely manner to ensure that perfusion, mainly to the outer layers, resumes. Postoperative multimodal evaluation is mandatory for better evaluation and improvement of functional outcomes [6, 27] using injectable interventions or sustained anti-VEGF agents [21, 52].

The choroid is the vascularized layer of tissue that provides the most important blood supply to the RPE and outer retinal layers. A restricted blood supply to the choroid adversely affects the outer retinal layers, potentially disrupting tissue homeostasis and causing diabetic choroidopathy and, consequently, different degrees of ischemic chorioretinal tissue damage [43].

The CVI is a recently introduced quantification parameter that represents the vascular status of the choroid based on OCT images [29]. The CVI is a more precise and robust measurement of choroidal vascular characteristics than previous measurements, such as choroidal vessel diameter and choroidal thickness (CT), both of which have important limitations [53]. CVI abnormalities can be used as indicators of choroidal vasculature disease; however, the CVI cannot capture choriocapillaris flow, which is also an important characteristic of the inner choroidal vasculature and can be quantified using OCT-A binarized imaging [54].

The CVI reveals the status of the choroidal vasculature in a variety of diseases and allows treatment monitoring [31, 52, 55–58]. *In vivo*, noninvasive imaging of the choroid is relevant for both disease diagnosis and treatment monitoring but can be challenging because this structure is located beneath multiple layers of tissue. Recent advancements in enhanced depth OCT and rapidly evolving OCT-A technology have proven to be useful tools for evaluating retinal and choroidal circulation without the need for dye injection [43, 59].

Improved visualization of the vascular choroid has resulted in quantitative evaluation of the choroidal vasculature. The CVI was first described by Agrawal et al. [29] in 2016 as a relatively new and reliable biomarker of the choroidal vasculature. This imaging technology was developed for a more accurate assessment of choroidal vascular layers [53]. Since its introduction, the CVI has gained popularity; additionally, the CVI has been applied in diabetic choroidopathy, uveitis, central serous chorioretinopathy, retinal vein occlusion, myopic traction maculopathy (MTM), and many other conditions [29, 34, 56, 60–63]. Recent reports have shown that CVI is a promising biomarker for the diagnosis and follow-up evaluation of retinal diseases, among which diabetic retinopathy and postoperative perfusion evaluation are important for patients with severe resolved TRD [64]. At the molecular level, recent reports have suggested that retinal cell apoptosis due to DR is related to neurofilament deposition in the RNFL accompanied by a high level of extracellular glutamate, which results in Müller cell damage and is likely generated by alterations in retrograde flux, an increase in neurotoxic debris [65], and uncontrolled hyperglycemia causing GCC-IPL disturbances and RNFL thinning [66].

In recent research, some authors have concluded that DME in patients with a higher CVI, higher EZ reflectivity, the presence of SRF, and the absence of DRIL at baseline are more likely to gain visual acuity after anti-VEGF treatment. The CVI may serve as a novel biomarker for visual response to anti-VEGF treatment in DME patients [67].

Quiroz-Reyes et al. have shown how critical CVI and CFA are used to evaluate perfusion in different pathologies, such as GRT-related RRD postoperative evaluation, and surgically resolved MTM eyes, which generally exhibit larger superficial postoperative FAZs, smaller CFAs, lower VDs, more structural macular defects, and thinner CSFTs [35, 68]. Better functional, structural, and perfusion index outcomes were observed in highly myopic eyes that underwent early surgery. However, the postoperative perfusion changes in patients with TRD are somewhat disappointing and do not correlate well with the functional outcomes, as shown in this chapter.

Currently, there are few and conflicting data on the predictive indicators for diabetic retinopathy available. The choroidal thickness (CT) is a characteristic that is unstable and dependent on numerous circumstances. Furthermore, the results of earlier research on choroidal thickness were inconsistent. Regardless of whether they have DR or not, diabetic patients often have a lower CVI than healthy controls. Additionally, DR patients had a lower CVI than non-DR individuals. The CVI is a sensitive and early biomarker for the onset of DR [69].

Jing et al. [70] have described a noteworthy correlation between declining BCVA and CVI in individuals with DR. A reduction in CVI was the factor most strongly associated with visual impairment, according to multivariate regression analysis. This study revealed a correlation between the CVI and BCVA. Thus, we propose that tracking CVI changes could offer a new target for interventions meant to stop the worsening of visual impairment in DR patients as well as a reliable measure for predicting future loss of visual acuity.

This chapter was subject to some constraints that are typical of retrospective analyses with a small sample size. We observed that this was a result of implementing rigorous exclusion criteria, which were specifically designed to restrict our trial to patients who had effectively undergone surgical treatment for diabetic TRD. Nevertheless, it effectively utilized a meticulously controlled group design and employed SD-OCT and OCT-A for pre- and postoperative evaluations. Additionally, we examined the visual outcomes and their correlation with perfusion markers. We anticipate that the scientific retina community will find our paper valuable and timely, considering the scarcity of published literature on perfuse macular assessment in this situation.

The merits of this study lie in its comprehensive data collection on the occurrence of diseases in a substantial number of colleague eyes, as well as its ability to detect postoperative perfusional alterations to be improved with some kind of anti-VEGF injectable interventions. The study revealed that the contralateral eyes exhibited notable changes in perfusion that were strongly correlated with BCVA values. Crucially, all eyes underwent vitrectomy surgery promptly after the development of TRD, resulting in documented detrimental functional and perfusional outcomes.

5. Future prospects

The study of DR and its connection to choroidal perfusion through the CVI and CFA has provided vital knowledge about the fundamental mechanisms and clinical features of this disorder. However, there are other areas that need to be investigated more in order to improve our understanding and improve patient care.

1. Longitudinal investigations involve conducting research over an extended period to examine how DR progresses and its connection with changes in the CVI and CFA values. These studies can offer vital insights into the natural development of the disease and help uncover the possible factors that contribute to its advancement.

2. Exploring the effects of genetic and environmental factors on the development and progression of DR and surgical forms of PDR and their connection to the CVI and CFA values can offer valuable information about an individual's vulnerability and potential preventive actions.

3. Utilizing developments in imaging technology, such as OCT-A, could provide new opportunities for researching choroidal perfusion and its impact on enhancing the postoperative functional outcomes in PDR. By integrating several imaging techniques, it is possible to obtain extensive information regarding alterations in the choroidal blood vessels.

4. Examining the impact of various treatment modalities, such as medications, injections into the eye, and surgical procedures, on the advancement of CVI and DR could result in the creation of more successful therapeutic approaches.

5. Collaborative large-scale investigations involve numerous sites and patient cohorts. These efforts can result in larger studies, increase the statistical significance of the findings, and enhance the generalizability of the conclusions.

6. Developing animal models that replicate the pathophysiology of DR and allow for the evaluation of choroidal perfusion can offer further understanding of the causes of the disease and potential targets for treatment.

7. When comparing the changes in choroidal perfusion in DR with other retinal disorders such as AMD or MTM, it might be useful in identifying distinct patterns of choroidal perfusion that are specific to DR.

8. Examining the functional correlations between the modifications in CVI and CFA values and visual acuity as well as other functional outcomes after surgery should assist doctors in predicting results and determining treatment decisions.

6. Conclusions

The choroidal vasculature provides the outer retina with its circulatory supply. Even before clinical symptoms appear, the choroidal vascularity index (CVI) assessment may be a useful early indicator of DR. There is a correlation between the degree of retinopathy and CVI in diabetic patients. As the severity of the retinopathy grows, the CT and CVI decrease. The CVI is a more accurate measure of disease development. In the eyes of patients with DR, DME, and those who are successfully reattached, the CVI and CFA biomarkers dramatically changed. In addition to alterations in the retinal vasculature, changes in the choroid also contribute to changes in DR.

Significant associations were observed between postoperative changes in the structure of the choroid and visual impairment in diabetic patients. The CVI can serve as a quantitative metric for assessing choroidal damage in patients with DR. The CVI can be used as a reliable quantitative biomarker to track the progression of DR or for monitoring postoperative eyes. Healthcare professionals should carefully observe alterations in the blood vessels of the choroid in patients with DR and acknowledge that preserving the CVI may be a crucial treatment objective in order to impede the advancement of DR. Patients with DR experience choroidal vascular changes, including a decrease in the CVI. The CVI decreased as the length of DM increased and showed a correlation with visual impairment. This finding suggests that the CVI could serve as a reliable imaging biomarker for monitoring the progression of DR.

Our results suggest severe and remarkable postoperative detrimental structural and perfusion changes in resolved TRD, which correlate with disappointing long-term visual results and may be aggravated by persistent chronic ischemic damage to the macula. The correlations among DRIL resolution, SD-OCT structural findings, other OCT-A perfusion markers, and functional outcomes yielded significant conclusions. Some eyes showed recovery of structural biomarkers with improved VD indices and capillary remodeling at the level of the deep and superficial vascular plexuses in the macula and lower-than-normal CVI and CFA values. The FAZ remained irregular and enlarged without recovery data, indicating that the FAZ may be a prognostic indicator of the worst final visual acuity. Postoperative diabetic macular ischemia of the photoreceptor and the outer and inner retinal layers is responsible for poor visual outcomes, possibly because of the low vascular perfusion in the visual photoreceptor cells in retina and mainly because of low choroidal indices with consequent cellular ischemic damage. The structural and perfusion data described here expand our knowledge of DRIL and other biomarkers obtained using SD-OCT and OCT-A, suggesting that perfusion indices such as the CVI and CFA could be used as clinical and prognostic biomarkers for TRD. Further research to determine the optimal timing for surgical intervention in patients with TRD involving the macula secondary to PDR is needed to minimize irreversible damage to retinal tissue and to vision. Careful longitudinal ophthalmological structural and perfusion evaluations, especially in patients with early-stage active PDR, are highly recommended to prevent tractional complications. Postoperative functional results are often disappointing, even in cases of successful anatomical reapplication of the macula, as described by the authors and the extensive literature reviewed in this chapter.

Acknowledgements

We express our deep appreciation to the technical staff of the Retina Department at Oftalmologia Integral ABC (Nonprofit Medical and Surgical Organization), Mexico City, Mexico, which is affiliated with The Postgraduate Study Division at the National Autonomous University of Mexico.

Funding

No funding or grant support was received for this study.

Conflict of interest

The authors declare no conflicts of interest.

Patient consent

Written informed consent was obtained from all patients in accordance with the institutional guidelines.

Disclaimer

All the scientific comments issued in this chapter are solely the responsibility of the authors and not of the institutions with which they are affiliated.

List of abbreviations

AVC	average vessel caliber
BCVA	best-corrected visual acuity
BRB	blood-retina barrier
CFA	choriocapillaris flow area
CME	cystoid macular edema
CSFT	central subfield thickness
CT	choroidal thickness
CVI	choroidal vascularity index
C_3F_8	perfluoropropane
Cks	centistokes
DM	diabetes mellitus
DME	diabetic macular edema
DRIL	disorganization of the retinal inner layers
DR	diabetic retinopathy
DCP	deep capillary plexus
ELM	external limiting membrane
ERM	epiretinal membrane
EZ	ellipsoid zone
FFA	fundus fluorescein angiography
FAZ	foveal avascular zone
GCL-IPL	ganglion cell layer-inner plexiform layer
HD	high-definition
ICG	indocyanine green dye
INL	inner nuclear layer
logMAR	logarithm of the minimum angle of resolution
MTM	myopic traction maculopathy

OCT-A	optical coherence tomography angiography
OPL	outer plexiform layer
PDR	proliferative diabetic retinopathy
PCN	perifoveal capillary network
PPV	pars plana vitrectomy
PFO	perfluoro-n-octane
PRP	panretinal photocoagulation
RNFL	retinal nerve fiber layer
RRD	rhegmatogenous retinal detachment
RPE	retinal pigment epithelium
SO	silicone oil
SSI	signal strength index
SCP	superficial capillary plexus
SF_6	sulfur hexafluoride
SRF	subretinal fluid
TRD	traction retinal detachment
VA	visual acuity
VD	vessel density
VEGF	vascular endothelial growth factor
VH	vitreous hemorrhage
VT	vessel tortuosity

Author details

Miguel A. Quiroz-Reyes*, Erick A. Quiroz-Gonzalez and Miguel A. Quiroz-Gonzalez
Retina Department, Oftalmologia Integral ABC, Medical and Surgical Institution, Affiliated with the Postgraduate Studies Division at the National Autonomous University of Mexico, Mexico City, Mexico

*Address all correspondence to: drquiroz@prodigy.net.mx

References

[1] Echouffo-Tcheugui JB, Dagogo-Jack S. Preventing diabetes mellitus in developing countries. Nature Reviews Endocrinology. 2012;**8**:557-562. DOI: 10.1038/nrendo.2012.46

[2] Kempen JH, O'Colmain BJ, Leske MC, Haffner SM, Klein R, Moss SE. The prevalence of diabetic retinopathy among adults in the United States. Archives of Ophthalmology. 2004;**122**:552-563. DOI: 10.1001/archopht.122.4.552

[3] Cruz-Iñigo YJ, Acabá LA, Berrocal MH. Surgical management of retinal diseases: Proliferative diabetic retinopathy and traction retinal detachment. Developments in Ophthalmology. 2014;**54**:196-203. DOI: 10.1159/000360467

[4] Sharma S, Mahmoud TH, Hariprasad SM. Surgical management of proliferative diabetic retinopathy. Ophthalmic Surgery, Lasers and Imaging Retina. 2014;**45**:188-193. DOI: 10.3928/23258160-20140505-01

[5] Centers for Disease Control and Prevention (CDC). Blindness caused by diabetes--Massachusetts, 1987-1994. MMWR Morbidity and Mortality Weekly Report. 1996;**45**:937-941

[6] Salam A, Mathew R, Sivaprasad S. Treatment of proliferative diabetic retinopathy with anti-VEGF agents. Acta Ophthalmologica. 2011;**89**:405-411. DOI: 10.1111/j.1755-3768.2010.02079.x

[7] Barzideh N, Johnson TM. Subfoveal fluid resolves slowly after pars plana vitrectomy for tractional retinal detachment secondary to proliferative diabetic retinopathy. Retina. 2007;**27**:740-743. DOI: 10.1097/iae.0b013e318030c663

[8] Sivaprasad S, Prevost AT, Bainbridge J, Edwards RT, Hopkins D, Kelly J, et al. Clinical efficacy and mechanistic evaluation of aflibercept for proliferative diabetic retinopathy (acronym CLARITY): A multicenter phase IIb randomized active-controlled clinical trial. BMJ Open. 2015;**5**:e008405. DOI: 10.1136/bmjopen-2015-008405

[9] Fong DS, Strauber SF, Aiello LP, Beck RW, Callanan DG, Danis RP, et al. Comparison of the modified early treatment diabetic retinopathy study and mild macular grid laser photocoagulation strategies for diabetic macular edema. Archives of Ophthalmology. 2007;**125**:469-480. DOI: 10.1001/archopht.125.4.469

[10] Sivaprasad S, Prevost AT, Vasconcelos JC, Riddell A, Murphy C, Kelly J, et al. Clinical efficacy of intravitreal aflibercept versus panretinal photocoagulation for best corrected visual acuity in patients with proliferative diabetic retinopathy at 52 weeks (CLARITY): A multicenter, single-blinded, randomized, controlled, phase 2b, noninferiority trial. Lancet. 2017;**389**:2193-2203. DOI: 10.1016/S0140-6736(17)31193-5

[11] Mikhail M, Ali-Ridha A, Chorfi S, Kapusta MA. Long-term outcomes of sutureless 25-G+ pars-plana vitrectomy for the management of diabetic tractional retinal detachment. Graefe's Archive for Clinical and Experimental Ophthalmology. 2017;**255**:255-261. DOI: 10.1007/s00417-016-3442-7

[12] Sun JK, Lin MM, Lammer J, Prager S, Sarangi R, Silva PS, et al. Disorganization of the retinal inner layers as a predictor of visual acuity in eyes with center-involved diabetic macular edema. JAMA

Ophthalmology. 2014;**132**:1309-1316. DOI: 10.1001/jamaophthalmol.2014.2350

[13] Gorczynska I, Migacz JV, Zawadzki RJ, Capps AG, Werner JS. Comparison of amplitude-decorrelation, speckle-variance and phase-variance OCT angiography methods for imaging the human retina and choroid. Biomedical Optics Express. 2016;**7**:911-942. DOI: 10.1364/boe.7.000911

[14] Gill A, Cole ED, Novais EA, Louzada RN, de Carlo T, Duker JS, et al. Visualization of changes in the foveal avascular zone in both observed and treated diabetic macular edema using optical coherence tomography angiography. International Journal of Retina and Vitreous. 2017;**3**:19. DOI: 10.1186/s40942-017-0074-y

[15] Yannuzzi LA, Rohrer KT, Tindel LJ, Sobel RS, Costanza MA, Shields W, et al. Fluorescein angiography complication survey. Ophthalmology. 1986;**93**:611-617. DOI: 10.1016/s0161-6420(86)33697-2

[16] Ho AC, Yannuzzi LA, Guyer DR, Slakter JS, Sorenson JA, Orlock DA. Intraretinal leakage of indocyanine green dye. Ophthalmology. 1994;**101**:534-541. DOI: 10.1016/s0161-6420(94)31323-6

[17] Hwang TS, Zhang M, Bhavsar K, Zhang X, Campbell JP, Lin P, et al. Visualization of 3 distinct retinal plexuses by projection-resolved optical coherence tomography angiography in diabetic retinopathy. JAMA Ophthalmology. 2016;**134**:1411-1419. DOI: 10.1001/jamaophthalmol.2016.4272

[18] Spaide RF, Klancnik JM, Cooney MJ, Yannuzzi LA, Balaratnasingam C, Dansingani KK, et al. Volume-rendering optical coherence tomography angiography of macular telangiectasia type 2. Ophthalmology. 2015;**122**:2261-2269. DOI: 10.1016/j.ophtha.2015.07.025

[19] Matsunaga D, Yi J, Puliafito CA, Kashani AH. OCT angiography in healthy human subjects. Ophthalmic Surgery, Lasers and Imaging Retina. 2014;**45**:510-515. DOI: 10.3928/23258160-20141118-04

[20] Tan PEZ, Balaratnasingam C, Xu J, Mammo Z, Han SX, Mackenzie P, et al. Quantitative comparison of retinal capillary images derived by speckle variance optical coherence tomography with histology. Investigative Opthalmology & Visual Science. 2015;**56**:3989-3996. DOI: 10.1167/iovs.14-15879

[21] Huang D, Jia Y, Gao SS, Lumbroso B, Rispoli M. Optical coherence tomography angiography using the optovue device. Developments in Ophthalmology. 2016;**56**:6-12. DOI: 10.1159/000442770

[22] Kwiterovich KA, Maguire MG, Murphy RP, Schachat AP, Bressler NM, Bressler SB, et al. Frequency of adverse systemic reactions after fluorescein angiography. Ophthalmology. 1991;**98**:1139-1142. DOI: 10.1016/s0161-6420(91)32165-1

[23] Bhavsar AR, Torres K, Glassman AR, Jampol LM, Kinyoun JL. Evaluation of results 1 year following short-term use of ranibizumab for vitreous hemorrhage due to proliferative diabetic retinopathy. JAMA Ophthalmology. 2014;**132**:889-890. DOI: 10.1001/jamaophthalmol.2014.287

[24] de Carlo TE, Filho MAB, Baumal CR, Reichel E, Rogers A, Witkin AJ, et al. Evaluation of preretinal neovascularization in proliferative diabetic retinopathy using optical coherence tomography angiography. Ophthalmic Surgery, Lasers and Imaging Retina. 2016;**47**:115-119. DOI: 10.3928/23258160-20160126-03

[25] Matsunaga DR, Yi JJ, De Koo LO, Ameri H, Puliafito CA, Kashani AH.

Opticalcoherencetomographyangiography of diabetic retinopathy in human subjects. Ophthalmic Surgery, Lasers and Imaging Retina. 2015;**46**:796-805. DOI: 10.3928/23258160-20150909-03

[26] Ishibazawa A, Nagaoka T, Takahashi A, Omae T, Tani T, Sogawa K, et al. Optical coherence tomography angiography in diabetic retinopathy: A prospective pilot study. American Journal of Ophthalmology. 2015;**160**:35-44.e1. DOI: 10.1016/j.ajo.2015.04.021

[27] Quiroz-Reyes MA, Quiroz-Gonzalez EA, Esparza-Correa F, Kim-Lee J, Morales-Navarro J, Montano M, et al. Outcomes for successfully repaired macula-off diabetic tractional retinal detachment. International Journal of Ophthalmology and Clinical Research. 2021;**8**:131. DOI: 10.23937/2378-346x/1410131

[28] Quiroz-Reyes MA, Quiroz-Gonzalez EA, Quiroz-Gonzalez MA, Lima-Gomez V. Postoperative choroidal vascularity index after the management of macula-off rhegmatogenous retinal detachment. International Journal of Retina and Vitreous. 2023;**9**:19. DOI: 10.1186/s40942-023-00464-x

[29] Agrawal R, Gupta P, Tan KA, Cheung CMG, Wong TY, Cheng CY. Choroidal vascularity index as a measure of vascular status of the choroid: Measurements in healthy eyes from a population-based study. Scientific Reports. 2016;**6**:21090. DOI: 10.1038/srep21090

[30] Agrawal R, Salman M, Tan K-A, Karampelas M, Sim DA, Keane PA, et al. Choroidal vascularity index (CVI) - a novel optical coherence tomography parameter for monitoring patients with panuveitis? PLoS One. 2016;**11**:e0146344. DOI: 10.1371/journal.pone.0146344

[31] Bernabei F, Pellegrini M, Taroni L, Roda M, Toschi PG, Schiavi C, et al. Choroidal vascular changes after encircling scleral buckling for rhegmatogenous retinal detachment. Eye. 2021;**35**:2619-2623. DOI: 10.1038/s41433-020-01307-x

[32] Agrawal R, Ding J, Sen P, Rousselot A, Chan A, Nivison-Smith L, et al. Exploring choroidal angioarchitecture in health and disease using choroidal vascularity index. Progress in Retinal and Eye Research. 2020;**77**:100829. DOI: 10.1016/j.preteyeres.2020.100829

[33] Hayreh SS. Segmental nature of the choroidal vasculature. British Journal of Ophthalmology. 1975;**59**:631-648. DOI: 10.1136/bjo.59.11.631

[34] Aribas YK, Hondur AM, Tezel TH. Choroidal vascularity index and choriocapillary changes in retinal vein occlusions. Graefe's Archive for Clinical and Experimental Ophthalmology. 2020;**258**:2389-2397. DOI: 10.1007/s00417-020-04886-3

[35] Quiroz-Reyes MA, Quiroz-Gonzalez EA, Quiroz-Gonzalez MA, Lima-Gomez V. Long-term postoperative perfusion indices in surgically resolved myopic traction maculopathy. Open Journal of Ophthalmology. 2023;**13**:143-171. DOI: 10.4236/ojoph.2023.131014

[36] Koçak N, Subaşı M, Yeter V. Effects of age and binarising area on choroidal vascularity index in healthy eyes: An optical coherence tomography study. International Ophthalmology. 2021;**41**:825-834. DOI: 10.1007/s10792-020-01636-6

[37] Yazdani N, Ehsaei A, Hoseini-Yazdi H, Shoeibi N, Alonso-Caneiro D, Collins MJ. Wide-field choroidal thickness and vascularity index in myopes and emmetropes. Ophthalmic

and Physiological Optics. 2021;**41**:1308-1319. DOI: 10.1111/opo.12875

[38] Sakata K, Funatsu H, Harino S, Noma H, Hori S. Relationship between macular microcirculation and progression of diabetic macular edema. Ophthalmology. 2006;**113**:1385-1391. DOI: 10.1016/j.ophtha.2006.04.023

[39] Shimada N, Tanaka Y, Tokoro T, Ohno-Matsui K. Natural course of myopic traction maculopathy and factors associated with progression or resolution. American Journal of Ophthalmology. 2013;**156**:948-957.e1. DOI: 10.1016/j.ajo.2013.06.031

[40] Singh SR, Invernizzi A, Rasheed MA, Cagini C, Goud A, Vupparaboina KK, et al. Wide-field choroidal vascularity in healthy eyes. American Journal of Ophthalmology. 2018;**193**:100-105. DOI: 10.1016/j.ajo.2018.06.016

[41] Staurenghi G, Sadda S, Chakravarthy U, Spaide RF. Proposed lexicon for anatomic landmarks in normal posterior segment spectral-domain optical coherence tomography. Ophthalmology. 2014;**121**:1572-1578. DOI: 10.1016/j.ophtha.2014.02.023

[42] Sun JK, Glassman AR, Beaulieu WT, Stockdale CR, Bressler NM, Flaxel C, et al. Rationale and application of the protocol S anti–vascular endothelial growth factor algorithm for proliferative diabetic retinopathy. Ophthalmology. 2019;**126**:87-95. DOI: 10.1016/j.ophtha.2018.08.001

[43] Borrelli E, Sarraf D, Freund KB, Sadda SR. OCT angiography and evaluation of the choroid and choroidal vascular disorders. Progress in Retinal and Eye Research. 2018;**67**:30-55. DOI: 10.1016/j.preteyeres.2018.07.002

[44] Hsieh Y-T, Alam MN, Le D, Hsiao C-C, Yang C-H, Chao DL, et al. OCT angiography biomarkers for predicting visual outcomes after ranibizumab treatment for diabetic macular edema. Ophthalmology Retina. 2019;**3**:826-834. DOI: 10.1016/j.oret.2019.04.027

[45] Freiberg FJ, Pfau M, Wons J, Wirth MA, Becker MD, Michels S. Optical coherence tomography angiography of the foveal avascular zone in diabetic retinopathy. Graefe's Archive for Clinical and Experimental Ophthalmology. 2016;**254**:1051-1058. DOI: 10.1007/s00417-015-3148-2

[46] Ishibashi T, Sakimoto S, Shiraki N, Nishida K, Sakaguchi H, Nishida K. Association between disorganization of retinal inner layers and visual acuity after proliferative diabetic retinopathy surgery. Scientific Reports. 2019;**9**:12230. DOI: 10.1038/s41598-019-48679-z

[47] Hwang TS, Gao SS, Liu L, Lauer AK, Bailey ST, Flaxel CJ, et al. Automated quantification of capillary nonperfusion using optical coherence tomography angiography in diabetic retinopathy. JAMA Ophthalmology. 2016;**134**:367-373. DOI: 10.1001/jamaophthalmol.2015.5658

[48] Shin HJ, Lee SH, Chung H, Kim HC. Association between photoreceptor integrity and visual outcome in diabetic macular edema. Graefe's Archive for Clinical and Experimental Ophthalmology. 2011;**250**:61-70. DOI: 10.1007/s00417-011-1774-x

[49] Moein H-R, Novais EA, Rebhun CB, Cole ED, Louzada RN, Witkin AJ, et al. Optical coherence tomography angiography to detect macular capillary ischemia in patients with inner retinal changes after resolved diabetic macular edema. Retina. 2018;**38**:2277-2284. DOI: 10.1097/iae.0000000000001902

[50] Durbin MK, An L, Shemonski ND, Soares M, Santos T, Lopes M, et al.

Quantification of retinal microvascular density in optical coherence tomographic angiography images in diabetic retinopathy. JAMA Ophthalmology. 2017;**135**:370-376. DOI: 10.1001/jamaophthalmol.2017.0080

[51] Tortorella P, D'Ambrosio E, Iannetti L, De Marco F, La Cava M. Correlation between visual acuity, inner segment/outer segment junction, and cone outer segment tips line integrity in uveitic macular edema. BioMed Research International. 2015;**2015**:1-5. DOI: 10.1155/2015/853728

[52] Dou N, Yu S, Tsui C-K, Yang B, Lin J, Lu X, et al. Choroidal vascularity index as a biomarker for visual response to antivascular endothelial growth factor treatment in diabetic macular edema. Journal of Diabetes Research. 2021;**2021**:1-9. DOI: 10.1155/2021/3033219

[53] Betzler BK, Ding J, Wei X, Lee JM, Grewal DS, Fekrat S, et al. Choroidal vascularity index: A step toward software as a medical device. British Journal of Ophthalmology. 2022;**106**:149-155. DOI: 10.1136/bjophthalmol-2021-318782

[54] Singh RB, Perepelkina T, Testi I, Young BK, Mirza T, Invernizzi A, et al. Imaging-based assessment of choriocapillaris: A comprehensive review. Seminars in Ophthalmology. 2022;**38**:405-426.DOI:10.1080/08820538.2022.2109939

[55] Foo VHX, Gupta P, Nguyen QD, Chong CCY, Agrawal R, Cheng C-Y, et al. Decrease in choroidal vascularity index of Haller's layer in diabetic eyes precedes retinopathy. BMJ Open Diabetes Research & Care. 2020;**8**:e001295. DOI: 10.1136/bmjdrc-2020-001295

[56] Nicolini N, Tombolini B, Barresi C, Pignatelli F, Lattanzio R, Bandello F, et al. Assessment of diabetic choroidopathy using ultrawidefield optical coherence tomography. Translational Vision Science & Technology. 2022;**11**:35. DOI: 10.1167/tvst.11.3.35

[57] Rizzo S, Savastano A, Finocchio L, Savastano MC, Khandelwal N, Agrawal R. Choroidal vascularity index changes after vitreomacular surgery. Acta Ophthalmologica. 2018;**96**:e950-e955. DOI: 10.1111/aos.13776

[58] Chun H, Kim JY, Kwak JH, Kim RY, Kim M, Park Y-G, et al. The effect of phacoemulsification performed with vitrectomy on choroidal vascularity index in eyes with vitreomacular diseases. Scientific Reports. 2021;**11**:19898. DOI: 10.1038/s41598-021-99440-4

[59] Invernizzi A, Pellegrini M, Cornish E, Teo KYC, Cereda M, Chabblani J. Imaging the choroid: From indocyanine green angiography to optical coherence tomography angiography. Asia-Pacific Journal of Ophthalmology. 2020;**9**:335-348. DOI: 10.1097/apo.0000000000000307

[60] Dolz-Marco R, Gallego-Pinazo R, Dansingani KK, Yannuzzi LA. The History of the Choroid. Choroidal Disorders. The Macula Foundation. New York, NY, USA: Academic Press; 2017

[61] Kim M, Ha MJ, Choi SY, Park YH. Choroidal vascularity index in type-2 diabetes analyzed by swept-source optical coherence tomography. Scientific Reports. 2018;**8**:70. DOI: 10.1038/s41598-017-18511-7

[62] Agrawal R, Chhablani J, Tan K-A, Shah S, Sarvaiya C, Banker A. Choroidal vascularity index in central serous chorioretinopathy. Retina. 2016;**36**:1646-1651. DOI: 10.1097/iae.0000000000001040

[63] Quiroz-Reyes MA, Quiroz-Gonzalez EA, Quiroz- Gonzalez MA,

Lima-Gomez V. Choroidal perfusion changes after vitrectomy for myopic traction maculopathy. Seminars in Ophthalmology. 2023. pp. 261-270 DOI: 10.1080/08820538.2023.2283029

[64] Iovino C, Pellegrini M, Bernabei F, Borrelli E, Sacconi R, Govetto A, et al. Choroidal vascularity index: An in-depth analysis of this novel optical coherence tomography parameter. Journal of Clinical Medicine. 2020;**9**:595. DOI: 10.3390/jcm9020595

[65] Stem MS, Gardner TW. Neurodegeneration in the pathogenesis of diabetic retinopathy: Molecular mechanisms and therapeutic implications. Current Medicinal Chemistry. 2013;**20**:3241

[66] Chen X, Nie C, Gong Y, Zhang Y, Jin X, Wei S, et al. Peripapillary retinal nerve fiber layer changes in preclinical diabetic retinopathy: A meta-analysis. PLoS One. 2015;**10**:e0125919

[67] Dou N, Yu S, Tsui C-K, Yang B, Lin J, Lu X, et al. Choroidal vascularity index as a biomarker for visual response to antivascular endothelial growth factor treatment in diabetic macular edema. Journal of Diabetes Research. 2021;**26**:3033219. DOI: 10.1155/2021/3033219. PMID: 34869776; PMCID: PMC8642029

[68] Quiroz-Reyes MA, Quiroz-Gonzalez EA, Quiroz-Gonzalez MA, Lima-Gomez V. Postoperative choroidal vascular biomarkers in eyes with rhegmatogenous retinal detachment-related giant retinal tears. International Journal of Retina and Vitreous. 2023;**9**(1):45

[69] Keskin Ç, Dilekçi ENA, Üçgül AY, Üçgül RK, Toprak G, Cengiz D. Choroidal vascularity index as a predictor for the development of retinopathy in diabetic patients. Journal of Endocrinological Investigation. 2024;**47**(5):1175-1180. DOI: 10.1007/s40618-023-02236-8. Epub 2023 Nov 22

[70] Jing R, Sun X, Cheng J, Li X, Wang Z. Vascular changes of the choroid and their correlations with visual acuity in diabetic retinopathy. Frontiers in Endocrinology (Lausanne). 2024;**15**:1327325. DOI: 10.3389/fendo.2024.1327325

Chapter 6

The Role of Müller Cells in Diabetic Retinopathy

Durgul Acan

Abstract

Diabetic retinopathy (DR), the most common cause of vision loss in diabetes, is characterized by vascular and neuronal abnormalities of the retina. As the main glial cells of the retina, Müller cells (MCs) are essential to the homeostasis and functionality of the retina. According to recent studies, MCs exhibit morphological and functional alterations, triggering the disease's progression in DR. Retinal damage becomes exacerbated by their contribution in neurovascular unit disruption, pro-inflammatory cytokine release, and oxidative stress. Additionally, abnormal reactivity of these cells to high glucose circumstances compromises the health of neurons by causing glutamate accumulation and reducing potassium buffering. Comprehending the diverse functions of MCs in DR could facilitate the development of focused treatments aiming at slowing down the progression of the illness.

Keywords: diabetic retinopathy, glial fibrillary acidic protein, glutamate, Kir4.1 channel, Müller cell, retinal glial cell, inflammation

1. Introduction

Diabetic retinopathy (DR) is one of the microvascular complications of diabetes and a leading cause of visual impairment and blindness in adults worldwide. As a result of international differences in healthcare systems, diagnostic criteria, and population demographics, the prevalence of DR is worrisome and varies globally. The global rise in diabetes heralds an impending increase in DR and imposes a serious burden on society and healthcare systems. A significant increase is expected in the number of adults with DR by 2045, and it highlights the need for effective new public health solutions [1]. The pathogenesis of DR involves multiple interactions between inflammatory processes, vascular damage, and metabolic deteriorations that lead to structural and functional changes in the retina. And the term "neuro-vascular coupling" highlights the significance of retinal neurovascular dysfunction in the pathophysiology [2, 3].

As the major glial cell, MCs are essential to the unique multilayered cellular organization of the retina. These cells traverse the entire thickness of the retina and are positioned to support and connect the layers of it. Minimizing light scattering in retina, recycling neurotransmitters, controlling the blood-retinal barrier

(BRB), supporting neuronal metabolism, and preserving retinal homeostasis are some of their various functions. The overall health of the retina depends on the integrity of MCs, since injury or dysfunction of them can result in serious retinal disorders.

In DR, MCs undergo plenty of functional and structural alterations. Chronic hyperglycemia triggers reactivity, characterized by cellular hypertrophy, altered gene expression, and a shift in functional state. It contributes to the breakdown of the BRB, a characteristic component of DR, and exacerbates the progression of disease. Reactive MCs also emit growth factors and pro-inflammatory cytokines, which exacerbate retinal neovascularization and inflammation. The interaction between MCs and other retinal cells is complex and crucial to the development of DR. MCs play an active role in the pathogenesis of DR, rather than just being spectators.

The aim of this chapter is to provide a comprehensive review about the functions of the MCs in the development and progression of DR. Pathophysiological alterations in MCs caused by diabetes, their role in the development of the illness, and potential treatment approaches targeting these cells will be focused. Gaining insight into the role of MCs in DR is crucial to improve our knowledge of the pathophysiology of the disease and develop treatment strategies.

2. Basic anatomy and physiology of Müller cells

As the main glial cells within the retina, MCs are crucial for maintaining the retinal structure and functionality of it. Strategically positioned by extending radially across the retina from the inner limiting membrane to the outer limiting membrane, these cells interact with almost all types of retinal neurons as well as retinal blood vessels. Because of this special arrangement, MCs can provide vital support that keeps the structural integrity of the retina intact.

2.1 Structural characteristics

MCs, which constitute approximately 90% of the glial cell population in the retina, were first identified by Heinrich Müller in 1851 [4, 5]. Originating from a common progenitor cell with retinal neurons embryologically, they play a role in controlling neural differentiation and directing neuronal migration [6, 7]. Their nuclei are located in the inner nuclear layer, but they exhibit a bipolar morphology that extends through the entire thickness of the retina, from the inner limiting membrane to the outer limiting membrane. This broad reach facilitates interactions with the vitreous body, the subretinal region, and a variety of retinal neurons and arteries. This structure also serves as a critical scaffold supporting the neural components of the retina [8]. The outermost cell membrane of MCs forms the outer limiting membrane through tight junctions, while the innermost funnel-shaped endfeet contribute to the outer part of the inner limiting membrane without specialized junctions [9]. Outer limiting membrane demarcates the inner and outer segments of photoreceptors. Within the retinal architecture, MCs also form an intricate network that maintains contact with each other. Numerous apical microvilli at the cell surface facing the pigment epithelium and the subretinal space encapsulate the perikarya of rods and cones in the outer nuclear layer [10]. Each MC is central to a column of retinal neurons, encompassing one cone, up to 10 rods, 4–6 neurons from the inner nuclear layer, and 0.3–2.5 neurons from the ganglion cell layer, constituting the smallest functional unit for "advanced information processing" [10].

2.2 Functional features

2.2.1 Metabolic support

Providing metabolic support to neurons in retina is one of the primary functions of MCs. Because they mostly use glycolysis rather than oxidative phosphorylation to convert glucose to lactate, they are crucial to retinal glucose metabolism [11]. This strategy is essential because it retains oxygen for the use of retinal neurons, which rely on oxidative phosphorylation to produce ATP. Additionally, lactate, produced by MCs, serves as an alternative energy substrate for photoreceptors, under critic conditions [11–13]. In both favorable and unfavorable circumstances, the survival and function of retinal neurons depend on this metabolic support system [14].

2.2.2 Protection against oxidative stress

The retina requires strong antioxidant defenses due to its constant exposure to light, high rate of oxygen consumption, and abundance of polyunsaturated fatty acids in photoreceptors. In addition, the retina experiences oxidative stress as a result of cyclic variations in oxygen levels, going from extreme hypoxia in the dark to hyperoxia in the presence of light [15]. Retinal glutathione is a major antioxidant that is often present in large amounts in glial and horizontal cells [16–18]. In conditions of oxidative stress, such as ischemia, MCs swiftly release glutathione to neighboring neurons, where it acts as a crucial cofactor for the enzyme glutathione peroxidase [18]. Beyond its antioxidant role, released glutathione may function as a neuromodulator by interacting with ionotropic glutamate receptors and modulating the redox-sensitive domain of N-methyl-D-aspartate (NMDA) receptors, thereby enhancing receptor channel currents [19]. Glial release of antioxidants, including glutathione, as well as neuroprotective agents such as adenosine and basic fibroblast growth factor (bFGF), plays a part in protecting photoreceptors against the deleterious effects of daily light exposure [20]. Notably, the concentration of glutathione in MCs diminishes in aged animals, correlating with mitochondrial deterioration and membrane depolarization [21]. MCs also secrete other antioxidants such as pyruvate, α-ketoglutarate, metallothionein, lysozyme, ceruloplasmin, heme oxygenase, and ascorbate to support the survival of photoreceptor (especially cones) and neurons [22–27]. Secretion of neurotrophic factors, growth factors, and cytokines by MCs further underlines their vital role in neuronal maintanence [28]. Among these, the ciliary neurotrophic factor stands out for its neuroprotective properties, which include preventing apoptosis of photoreceptors and enhancing glial glutamate buffering [29, 30].

2.2.3 Recycling of photopigments

MCs phagocytose the shed outer segment discs of cones and play an auxiliary role in the regeneration of photoreceptor outer segments. Within the rod and cone visual cycles, which replenish the chromophores of photopigments, this mechanism is essential [31–33]. Whereas the pigment epithelium recycles rod-derived all-trans retinol back into 11-cis-retinal, cone-derived all-trans retinol is specifically processed by MCs. The efficient turnover of cone chromophore by MCs is vital for enhancing the dynamic response of cones under bright light conditions and facilitating their quick adaptation to darkness following light exposure [34].

2.2.4 Mechanical support

Because of their naturally vulnerable structure, MCs provide little mechanical support under normal circumstances. However, the overexpression of intermediate filaments, such as vimentin and glial fibrillary acidic protein (GFAP) during reactive gliosis, greatly enhances their ability to provide structural integrity [35–37]. In addition, MCs have calcium-permeable cation channels that open in response to retinal stretching, which causes calcium to mediate an increase in the activity of big-conductance potassium (BK) channels [38]. Growth factors, such as bFGF, and ATP are further released as a consequence of this activation [39, 40]. Therefore, MCs are crucial for inducing gliosis in response to mechanical stress as well as contribution to mechanical neuroprotection.

2.2.5 Maintenance of retinal homeostasis

MCs ensure the maintenance of retinal homeostasis by regulating the extracellular environment. This critical mission involves regulating ionic balance and promoting water transport across the retina, with a particular focus on potassium ions [41, 42]. Additionally, by controlling cellular swelling that influences retinal thickness and light transmission, MCs have an important role in regulating the response of retina to light [29].

Under normal physiological conditions, water and potassium ions (K+) produced by retinal neuronal activity are released into the interstitial fluid. As an essential potassium shuttle, MCs acquire K^+ via the inwardly rectifying potassium Kir2.1 channel, which is mainly expressed in regions nearby neurons and synapses. Kir4.1 channels are located on the perivascular glial membranes of MCs and responsible for shifting K+ toward retinal vessels [43, 44]. Maintaining the structural and functional integrity of the retina depends on the functionality of these channels. The efficiency of these homeostatic ways is primarily reliant on a very low membrane potential of approximately −80 mV, which is made possible by the extensive presence of Kir4.1 channels [42]. Additionally, Kir4.1 is implicated in regulation of intracellular water under varying osmotic conditions, collaborating closely with aquaporin-4 (AQP4) [44–46]. Interestingly, both AQP4 and Kir channels are co-localized on similar regions of the MC membrane, ensuring that ionic alterations linked with neuronal activity are promptly counterbalanced by swift water movement through glial barriers [44, 47]. After episodes of transient pressure-induced retinal ischemia, it has been observed that Kir4.1 expression is markedly downregulated, while Kir2.1 levels stay steady. As a result, K+ ion accumulation and an increase in osmotic pressure may develop in MCs [42, 48]. As a bidirectional water transporter, AQP4 helps to overcome the resistance of the synaptic barriers and promote fluid exchange between the extracellular space and the blood vessels or vitreous [49]. The synergistic function of Kir4.1 and AQP4 highlights a tightly coordinated process in which water transport is regulated by K+ currents managed by MCs [42].

Glutamate receptor activation causes a reduction in extracellular volume, swelling of synapses and retinal neurons during periods of intense neuronal activity [50]. The osmolarity of the extracellular fluid decreases due to significant decreases in extracellular calcium and sodium chloride levels after this activity [51]. Despite these hypoosmotic conditions, the ability of MCs to remain unswollen is important in preventing potential neuronal hyperexcitation. Noticeably, MCs can sustain their volume without swell for as long as 10–15 minutes, which is mainly due to the coordinated activities of AQP4 and Kir4.1 channels in the transport of potassium and water [10, 52].

2.2.6 Balancing extracellular pH

Photoreceptor cells, being the highest consumers of glucose and oxygen within the human body, inevitably generate considerable amounts of carbon dioxide and water as by-products of glycolysis. The efficient removal of carbon dioxide through its rapid conversion into bicarbonate and protons by carbonic anhydrases is termed "carbon dioxide siphoning" [53]. In this process, carbonic anhydrase II within Müller and amacrine cells, along with carbonic anhydrase XIV in other glial cells and the vascular endothelium, facilitates the transformation. The resulting bicarbonate is then transported to the blood and vitreous via sodium-bicarbonate cotransporters and anion exchangers present in the glial end-foot membranes [54].

Light-stimulated neuronal activity leads to extracellular alkalinization [55]. The release of potassium from active neurons induces depolarization of MCs and leads to bicarbonate influx into these cells [8]. On the other hand, protons produced by carbonic anhydrase activities remain extracellular, which causes acidification [8]. The acidification process can modulate synaptic transmission, suggesting that MC-mediated pH adjustments may protect neurons against potential overactivity [56].

2.2.7 Regulation of the blood-retinal barrier

Another important mission of MCs is the management of BRB, which controls the exchange of substances between the retina and the blood vessels. MCs establish tight junctions with retinal blood vessels, maintaining the structural integrity of the BRB and the unique retinal environment necessary for neuronal activity [42]. Synthesis of thrombospondin-1, glial cell line-derived neurotrophic factor (GDNF), and pigment epithelium-derived factor (PEDF), which are strongly linked to MC functionality, enhances the barrier efficiency of the vascular endothelium [57–60]. On the other hand, MCs may release substances that increase vascular permeability, such as tumor necrosis factor (TNF) and vascular endothelial growth factor (VEGF), in response to adverse conditions such as hypoxia, inflammation, or glucose deficiency [61]. MCs can also influence the permeability of the barrier by modifying the tight junction protein occludin via their matrix metalloproteinases [62]. It's interesting to note that by releasing soluble antiangiogenic factors like PEDF, MCs have been related to the suppression of retinal neovascularization under ischemia conditions [63]. The release has a continuous antiangiogenic effect on retinal vascular endothelial cells, which may explain why, in diabetic retinopathy, new blood vessels tend to form on the vitreous surface instead of in the ischemic retinal areas.

2.2.8 Regulation of retinal blood flow

In the healthy retina, increased light exposure causes an increase in retinal blood flow, which is crucial for the delivery of oxygen and nutrients to the relevant neurons. Because they release metabolites that affect the dilatation and constriction of retinal blood vessels, MCs play a crucial role in this neurovascular coupling [64, 65]. The synthesis of ATP by retinal neurons in the inner plexiform layer, in response to light, initiates IP3-mediated calcium signaling in MCs [64]. This, in turn, triggers glial calcium waves that stimulate phospholipase A2, generating signals that modulate blood flow along the inner surface of the retina, where arterioles reside [64, 65]. The production of arachidonic acid metabolites from the process either dilates arterioles via epoxyeicosatrienoic acids or induces constriction through 20-hydroxyeicosatetraenoic acid [64].

2.2.9 Neurotransmitter recycling

MCs play a critical role in the recycling of neurotransmitters, especially glutamate and GABA, by utilizing high-affinity transporters such as the electrogenic glutamate-aspartate transporter (GLAST, also known as excitatory amino acid transporter-1, EAAT1) [10, 65, 66]. By absorbing these neurotransmitters from the synaptic gap, MCs ensure the precise resolution of neural signaling and transform them into glutamine through the action of the glia-specific enzyme, glutamine synthetase [67]. The glutamine then released back into the extracellular space is reabsorbed by retinal neurons, serving as a substrate for the synthesis of both glutamate and GABA. Notably, bipolar and ganglion cells source virtually all their glutamine from MCs, while photoreceptor cells derive a portion of their requirements from these glial cells as well [68]. Maintaining neurotransmitter balance in the retina and preventing excitotoxicity depend on this effective recycling process [69]. Studies show that blocking MC-mediated glutamate intake significantly reduces the amount of extracellular glutamate needed to trigger neurotoxicity, which can cause functional blindness in animals in only a few minutes [10, 69, 70].

2.2.10 Regulation of neuronal activity

MCs contribute to synaptic transmission by secreting "gliotransmitters" like glutamate and ATP, which activate nearby cells, as well as adenosine, which has an inhibitory effect [65]. They also release a variety of neuroactive signaling molecules, such as D-serine, acyl coenzyme A-binding protein (ACBP), GABA, retinoic acid, and nitric oxide [71]. Osmotic gradients, mechanical or electrical stimuli, and neurotransmitters can cause MCs to release ATP [72]. This ATP signaling is essential for the spread of calcium waves across the glial cell network in the retina, facilitating long-range communication [73, 74]. In rat studies, it has been observed that ATP-triggered calcium responses are limited to the ganglion cell and nerve fiber layers. Interestingly, the cell bodies and outer processes do not exhibit calcium responses to ATP [75]. The inhibition of light-induced spike activity might result from ATP and adenosine produced by the MCs [39].

2.2.11 Release of D-serine

The release of D-serine has an essential role in modulating the light sensitivity of retinal ganglion and amacrine cells [76]. This control is essential for the activation of NMDA receptors, which are found in numerous amacrine cells, retinal ganglion, and horizontal cells in some species [77, 78]. In retinal ganglion cells, D-serine acts as a potent endogenous ligand at the glycine modulator site of the NMDA receptor. It has a greater activation potency than glycine, demonstrating the complex chemical interactions that occur within the retinal environment [79, 80].

2.2.12 Light-guiding

MCs provide focused light transmission to the photoreceptors by significantly lowering the scattering of light across the neuroretina. Light is more likely to scatter before reaching the cones, outside the fovea [81]. MCs optimize visual resolution by mimicking the function of glass fiber optics and efficiently guiding light through the inner retinal layers toward the photoreceptors, like biological optical fibers [82].

However, some retinal diseases like macular edema can reduce the ability of MCs to guide light and increase light scattering.

2.2.13 Müller stem cells

Although the capacity varies by species and age, a subset of MCs in the mature retina contains latent neural progenitor/stem cell capabilities [83, 84]. Because MCs can develop into neural stem cells, the potential use of MCs in cell-based therapy for retinal diseases is extremely promising [83, 85]. Investigating the factors that inhibit the neuroregenerative abilities of MCs in damaged retinal tissue remains an important area of research.

3. Pathophysiological changes in Müller cells in diabetic retinopathy

3.1 Müller cell reactivity in diabetes

In diabetes, MCs are triggered by the high glucose levels that are characteristic of the disease and respond similarly to other retinal pathologies. Despite their resiliience and efforts to protect the retina from damage, sometimes they inadvertently contribute to the progression of the disease. Their activity is crucially modulated by factors like FGF-2 that are secreted in the diabetic retina [86]. The onset of glial reactivity heralds vascular and neurodegenerative alterations in the retina even before DR clinically manifests [87]. Evidence of early-stage neurodegeneration in DR, as indicated by Optical Coherence Tomography (OCT) studies, includes thinning of the inner nuclear, ganglion cell, and nerve fiber layers [88]. Diabetes-related experimental research has also demonstrated that these cells suffer apoptosis and mitochondrial malfunction in addition to evident alterations such as thicker basement membranes, lipid vacuole accumulation, cell nuclei disintegration, and organelle depletion [89]. These changes lead to damage to the BRB by impairing not only the structural integrity of MCs but also endothelial cell adhesion and pericyte stability [87]. **Figure 1** illustrates how diabetes mellitus affects MCs.

3.2 Structural and functional alterations

MCs maintain the "dry state" of the retina by manipulating the AQP4 and Kir4.1 channels, the function of which is impaired in conditions with high glucose levels. It has been shown in studies that MC depolarization results from decreased Kir4.1 channel activity in proliferative DR (PDR). This alteration inhibits the voltage-dependent assimilation of glutamate, GABA, and other neurotransmitters, resulting in decreased drainage efficiency, MC swelling, and disruption of retinal structure [90, 91]. Retinal injury is exacerbated by the increase in glutamate levels and a reduction in extracellular space caused by increased neuronal activity in the inner retinal layers [50, 92]. Due to the release of local factors, aging and partial vitreous detachment can exacerbate local MC traction, which can lead to chronic MC damage, gliosis, and vascular leakage.

Increase in extracellular potassium (K^+) depolarizes glial cells and neurons, leading to glutamate accumulation. The accumulation may lead to irreversible visual impairment by disrupting the function of neurons in the inner retina, which generates action potentials [93]. Interestingly, AQP4 levels in the aqueous humor of

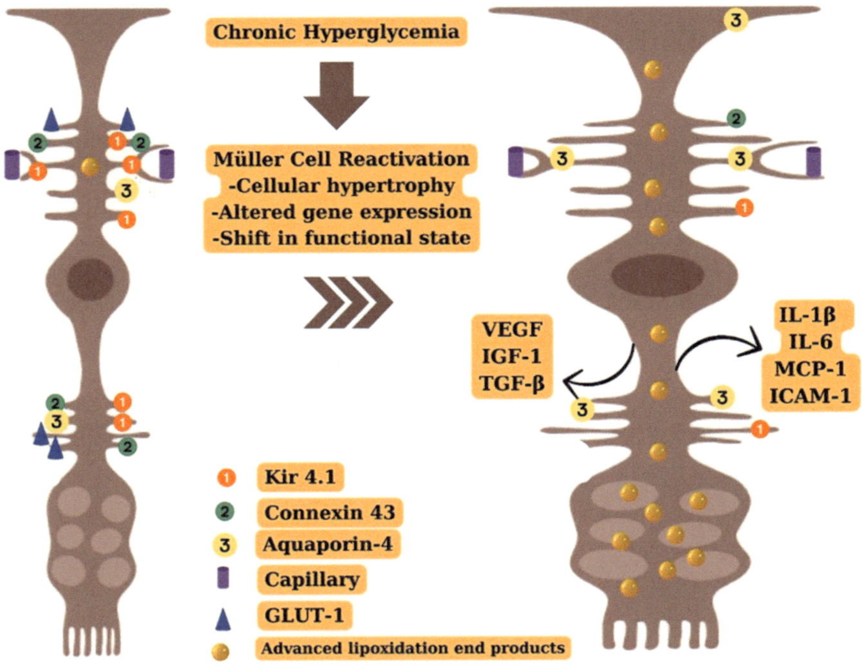

Figure 1.
Changes in Müller cell in diabetes. GLUT-1, Kir 4.1 receptors and connexin 43 are reduced, advanced lipoxidation end products increase. Müller cell becomes depolarized and edematous. It also contributes to the disruption of the blood-retina barrier by releasing inflammatory and angiogenic substances. GLUT-1; glucose transporter 1, ICAM-1; intercellular adhesion molecule-1, IGF-1; insülin-like growth factor 1, IL-1 β; interleukin 1 beta, MCP-1; Monocyte chemoattractant protein-1, TGF-β; transforming growth factor-beta, VEGF; vascular endothelial growth factor.

patients with diabetes (prior to DR onset) rise and are significantly elevated with the progression of DR, suggesting AQP4 as a potential early indicator of MC alterations in diabetes [94]. The amplification of AQP4 in DR facilitates the influx of fluid into retinal cells from the microvasculature, but this excess fluid is not efficiently reabsorbed into the bloodstream, resulting in retinal edema [95]. MC-originated exosomes, the nanosized vesicles between cells, contribute to the disruption of the BRB via damaging endothelial cells in hyperglycemic conditions [96].

Connexin 43 (Cx43) is a gap junction protein essential for cell-to-cell communication, and its translocation is regulated by a specific GTPase, Rab20. Rab20 expression increases noticeably in MCs under hyperglycemic circumstances, inhibiting localization of the Cx43 to the cell membrane and gap junction intercellular communication (GJIC), which results in protein kinase B inactivation and MC apoptosis [97]. The high-glucose-induced downregulation of Cx43 disrupts neurovascular homeostasis, contributing to the pathophysiology of DR. Rab20 siRNA treatments have demonstrated promise in reducing Rab20 overexpression and regaining GJIC activity, hence reducing the risk of neurovascular injury induced by elevated glucose levels [98].

3.3 Release of growth factors

The neovascularization that is frequently linked to PDR is mostly attributed to the growth factors produced by MCs. The interaction between these growth factors involves complex mechanisms. Critical growth factors such as VEGF [86], FGF [99], insulin-like growth factor-1 (IGF-1) [100], and transforming growth factor-beta (TGF-β) [101] are secreted in greater amounts in response to hyperglycemia. These factors have a major role in coordinating neovascularization processes, which can result in retinal fibrosis.

Elevated VEGF levels in MCs are linked to increased capillary permeability and neovascularization, which may cause irreversible visual impairment [102]. FGF, known as a neurotrophin and mitogen, supports neuronal differentiation, survival, and regeneration and fosters neovascularization via direct effects on vascular endothelial cells or indirectly by stimulating MCs to release a suite of pro-vascular growth factors and pro-inflammatory cytokines (including VEGF, IL-1β, IL-6, and interferon-γ) [86, 103]. Moreover, IGF-1 is noted for its ability to activate MCs under both normal and stress-induced conditions in the retina. It facilitates their migration to the stroma and enhances glucose transport to the retinal vascular endothelium through glucose transporter 1 (GLUT 1) [100, 104]. In PDR, MCs are associated with increased fibrosis and epithelial-mesenchymal transition (which results in the production of myofibroblasts). This is because they secrete a substantial amount of TGF-β and upregulate matrix proteins in the extracellular matrix [105, 106].

3.4 Role in inflammation and oxidative stress

Inflammation is a critical factor at all stages of DR and diabetic macular edema (DME) [107]. The receptor for advanced glycation end products (RAGE), belonging to the immunoglobulin superfamily, was initially identified for its role in recognizing advanced glycation end products (AGEs) [108]. RAGE is present in MCs, nerve cells, endothelial cells, pericytes, and retinal pigment epithelium and interacts with several ligands [109]. Activation of it contributes to neurodegeneration by increasing the release of growth factors, pro-inflammatory cytokines, cell adhesion molecules, and reactive oxygen species. Through the activation of NF-κB and the upregulation of VEGF, RAGE plays a significant role in the pathogenesis of DR [110].

Prolonged hyperglycemia induces an intense inflammatory response in MCs, leading to chronic inflammation, retinal vascular damage, neovascularization, fibrosis, and a decline in retinal function. The cytokine and chemokine release facilitates neutrophil and macrophage infiltration in the retina and vascular endothelial adhesion and compromises the BRB, further exacerbating neovascularization and fibrosis [111]. RAGE–ligand interactions also upregulate the mitogen-activated protein kinase (MAPK)-signaling pathway, enhancing pro-inflammatory cytokine expression [112].

Experiments in diabetic rats have revealed the upregulation of 78 genes, a majority of which are associated with cytokines such as IL-1β and IL-6, indicating their function in the acute-phase response of the retina [113, 114]. Interestingly, a moderate level of IL-6 secretion may provide partial protection against glucose toxicity through VEGF-A signaling, which is reversed by chronic hyperglycemia [115]. IL-6-signaling dynamics vary, with trans-signaling through the soluble IL-6 receptor being pro-inflammatory, whereas cis-signaling via membrane-bound IL-6R exhibits anti-inflammatory effects. Moreover, IL-6 cis-signaling in MCs supports the maintenance of bipolar neurons in the inner nuclear layer under diabetic conditions [116]. IL-1β amplifies leukocyte activation by stimulating IL-8 expression primarily through p38 MAPK and ERK1/2 pathways in MCs [117].

Research by Qiu et al. revealed that IL-17A levels rise in the plasma of diabetic patients, worsening retinal vascular leukostasis, vascular leakage, and ganglion cell apoptosis by inducing dysfunction through Act1 signaling in MCs [118, 119].

Additionally, IL-17A has been shown to increase retinal neovascularization in models of oxygen-induced retinopathy [120]. Monocyte chemoattractant protein-1 (MCP-1), a potent monocyte and macrophage attractant regulated by NF-κB, is also released by MCs, enhancing leukocytosis [121, 122].

Cluster of differentiation 40 (CD40) is part of the TNF receptor superfamily and expressed at low levels under normal conditions, while upregulated in a variety of cells, including MCs, in the diabetic retina [123, 124]. CD40 activation triggers leukocytosis by upregulating intercellular adhesion molecule-1 (ICAM-1) and MCP-1 in MCs of diabetic mice, and blocking this pathway reduces retinal inflammation [125, 126]. The chemokine axis CXCL16/CXCR6 and metalloproteinases ADAM10 and ADAM17 may play roles in the onset and progression of PDR, with CXCL16 inducing the upregulation of inflammatory pathways in MCs [127]. By focusing on these inflammatory pathways in MCs, new approaches for treating DR may become possible.

Advanced lipoxidation end products, such as Nε-(3-formyl-3,4-dehydropiperidino) lysine (FDP-lysine), an acrolein derivative, accumulate on MC proteins and impair their functionality. An effective acrolein scavenger, 2-hydrazino-4,6dimethylpyrimidine (2-HDP), has been linked to decreased oxidative stress marker expression and MC gliosis and partial normalization of Kir4.1 channel expression [128].

Physiological function of the Müller cells	Changes in Müller cells in diabetes
Metabolic support Converting glucose into lactate via glycolysis Reserve oxygen for retinal neurons	Alteration in glucose metabolism
Participate in the structure of limiting membranes	No data
Regulating the blood-retinal barrier	Disruption of the blood-retinal barrier Increased secretion of VEGF, FGF, IGF-1, and TGF-β
Recycling neurotransmitters	Decrease in GLUT-1 and glutamine synthetase expression Glutamate neurotoxicity
Minimizing light scattering in the retina	Impaired light guiding and visual resolution
Maintaining retinal homeostasis By Kir4.1, Kir2.1 and AQ4 channels	Diminished activity of Kir4.1 channels and AQ4 amplification Müller cell swelling
Protection against oxidative stress Releasing glutathione	Overexpression of inflammatory cytokines
Recycling of photopigments	Alteration in visual cycle-related proteins [88]
Mechanical support	Upregulation of intermediate filaments
Balancing extracellular pH	Müller cell depolarisation
Regulation of retinal blood flow	Changes in neurovascular coupling [133]
Regulation of neuronal activity	No data
Regulation of neuronal activity	No data
Release of D-serin	No data
Differentiation into neuronal stem cells	

Table 1.
The role of Müller cells physiologically and diabetic retinopathy associated pathological changes.

3.5 Retinal neurotoxicity

In DR, the capability of MCs to reduce glutamate excitotoxicity and to secrete neurotrophic factors, both vital for the survival of retinal neurons, becomes compromised. MCs typically try to preserve retinal equilibrium through reactive gliosis in response to retinal disorders. However, an overreaction in gliosis can eventually damage retinal cells [129]. In the early phases of DR, activation of Müller glia can promote neuroprotection by stimulating survival signals via the phosphorylation of ERK1/2. Yet, prolonged hyperglycemia can lead to a decrease in ERK1/2 activation [130].

Furthermore, the expression of the GLAST, crucial for the absorption of glutamate, is found to be diminished in the retinas of diabetic subjects, leading to neuronal cell death. Nonetheless, the introduction of GDNF within the eye has been identified to enhance GLAST expression and thus protect retinal cells from deterioration [131]. Furthermore, it is thought that VEGFR2-mediated signaling in diabetic MCs contributes significantly to neuroprotection, either directly or indirectly, by secreting substances such as brain-derived neurotrophic factor (BDNF) and GDNF [132]. **Table 1** summarizes the functions of MCs under physiological conditions, and the alterations occur due to diabetes.

4. Future therapeutic approaches

The following summarizes the most frequently discussed and promising MC-mediated treatment approaches in the litarature:

- A crucial metabolic regulator, 5′ adenosine monophosphate-activated protein kinase (AMPK), is activated by metformin, a drug that is frequently used for managing diabetes [90]. Studies have shown that metformin increases Kir4.1 channel proteins in mice, suggesting that it could be used as a therapy to compensate for DR-associated MC dysfunction [90].

- The interaction of AQP4, ROS, and VEGFR in the retina has been suggested by Oosuka et al. as a critical factor in the pathophysiology of DME and DR. Similar to the effect of bevacizumab, they discovered that intravitreal treatment of 2-(nicotinamide)-1,3,4-thiadiazole (TGN-020), a strong AQP4 inhibitor, significantly reduced VEGF, AQP4, and GFAP levels in diabetic animals and limited leakage and intracellular edema [134, 135].

- ATP-sensitive potassium (KATP) channels in the retinal microvasculature regulate retinal blood flow [136]. Pinacidil, a non-selective opener of these channels, has been used to treat hypertension by relaxing cardiovascular smooth muscles. It may also mitigate microglial-induced MC gliosis in diabetes by upregulating Kir6.1 expression, thereby indirectly reducing retinal inflammation and gliosis [137].

- Despite the effectiveness of intravitreal anti-VEGF agents in managing DME and preventing vascular permeability and neovascularization, their application in DR treatment remains under debate [138]. Wang et al. in 2021 demonstrated that ranibizumab, an anti-VEGF agent, safeguards MCs against diabetic intracellular edema by upregulating Kir4.1 and AQP4, thereby reducing intracellular osmotic pressure [139].

- Through numerous mechanisms, including gliosis, neurotoxicity, and neovascularization, the interaction between low-density lipoprotein receptor-related protein 1 (LRP1) and its ligand α2-macroglobulin (α2M) in MCs has been associated with proliferative retinopathies. Innovations targeting LRP1 present promising avenues for the treatment of DR [140].

- Glucagon-like peptide-1 (GLP-1), which has been shown to have neuroprotective effects, was topically administered to diabetic rats and prevented retinal malfunction and apoptosis and reversed reactive gliosis and vascular leakage. This protective impact is linked to the downregulation of VEGF, inflammatory markers, and NF-κB in addition to the activation of the Akt/GSK3b/β-catenin-signaling pathway, which promotes cell survival [141].

- The dysregulation of fatty acids, such as palmitic acid, may trigger DR progression via inflammatory cytokine release from MCs. Enhancing cytochrome P450 epoxygenase (CYP)-derived epoxygenated fatty acids in experimental settings reduced inflammation induced by palmitic acid and IL-1β in MCs, suggesting a therapeutic strategy for early DR inflammation [142].

- Moreover, by reducing the inflammatory response of the MCs, topical administration of suppressor of cytokine signaling-1 (SOCS1)-derived peptides has demonstrated reduction in retinal neuroinflammation and early microvascular damage [143].

- It has been reported that intravitreal delivery of peptides that impair CD40-TRAF2,3 signaling can reduce retinal inflammation in diabetic animals, providing a potential approach to treatment [144, 145].

- The elevated synthesis of Rho-associated protein kinase-1 (ROCK-1), VEGF, and MCP-1/CCL2 in MCs exposed to high glucose was normalized by fasudil, a Rho kinase inhibitor, highlighting its therapeutic potential [146].

- The fact that Oncostatin M reduces retinal neovascularization by 65.2% by influencing the secretome of MCs in the animal model of oxygen-induced retinopathy holds promise for the treatment of DR [147]

These various agents that can be used in the treatment of DR via Müller cells are schematized and shown in **Figure 2**.

Particularly in the last two decades, the significance of MCs in the retinopathies has attracted an extensive amount of attention. Several studies have highlighted the pivotal role that MCs play in the pathophysiology of DR. In diabetic patients, mitigating MC activation may provide protection against retinal neuronal damage and visual impairment. Even though much of the research is based on animal models and may not directly indicate human retinal physiology, their findings offer intriguing insights into possible treatments.

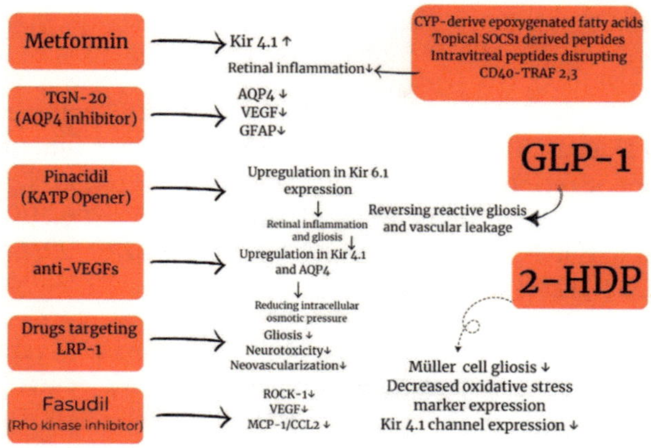

Figure 2.
Various agents that may act through Müller cells in the treatment of DR have been schematized. 2-HDP, 2-hydrazino-4,6dimethylpyrimidine; AQP4, aquaporin −4; GFAP, glial fibrillary acidic protein; GLP-1, glucagon-like peptide-1; KATP, ATP-sensitive potassium; LRP-1, low-density lipoprotein receptor-related protein 1; MCP-1/CCL2, monocyte chemoattractant protein-1; ROCK-1, Rho-associated protein kinase-1; SOCS1, suppressor of cytokine signaling-1; TGN-20, 2-(nicotinamide)-1,3,4-thiadiazole; VEGF, vascular endothelial growth factor.

5. Conclusion

In a hyperglycemic milieu associated with diabetes, the primary glial cells of the retina, MCs experience many alterations. Reactive MCs serve their functions initially, but they also play a role in the vascular and neurodegenerative alterations associated with DR. These pathways are explained in great detail in this paper. These cells are at the center of numerous intriguing therapy modalities that are presently being studied.

Author details

Durgul Acan
Department of Ophthalmology, School of Medicine, Balikesir University, Balikesir, Turkey

*Address all correspondence to: durgul2029@hotmail.com

References

[1] Teo ZL, Tham YC, Yu M, Chee ML, Rim TH, Cheung N, et al. Global prevalence of diabetic retinopathy and projection of burden through 2045. Systematic review and meta-analysis. Ophthalmology. 2021;**128**(11):1580-1591. DOI: 10.1016/j.ophtha.2021.04.027

[2] Moran EP, Wang Z, Chen J, Sapieha P, Smith LE, Ma JX. Neurovascular cross talk in diabetic retinopathy: Pathophysiological roles and therapeutic implications. American Journal of Physiology. Heart and Circulatory Physiology. 2016;**311**(3):H738-H749. DOI: 10.1152/ajpheart.00005.2016

[3] Sinclair SH, Schwartz SS. Diabetic retinopathy-an underdiagnosed and undertreated inflammatory, neuro-vascular complication of diabetes. Frontiers in Endocrinology. 2019;**10**:843. DOI: 10.3389/fendo.2019.00843

[4] Müller H. Zur Histologie der Netzhaut. [article in Germany]. Z Wissenschaft Zool. 1851;**3**:234-237

[5] Subirada PV, Paz MC, Ridano ME, Lorenc VE, Vaglienti MV, Barcelona PF, et al. A journey into the retina: Müller glia commanding survival and death. The European Journal of Neuroscience. 2018;**47**(12):1429-1443. DOI: 10.1111/ejn.13965

[6] Turner DL, Cepko CL. A common progenitor for neurons and glia persists in rat retina late in development. Nature. 1987;**328**:131-136. DOI: 10.1038/328131a0

[7] Kolb H. Glial cells of the retina. In: Kolb H, Fernandez E, Nelson R, editors. Webvision: The Organization of the Retina and Visual System [Internet]. Salt Lake City (UT): University of Utah Health Sciences Center; 2021. pp. 255-263

[8] Newman E, Reichenbach A. The Müller cell: A functional element of the retina. Trends in Neurosciences. 1996;**19**(8):307-312. DOI: 10.1016/0166-2236(96)10040-0

[9] Gao HLA, Huang X, Chen X. Müller glia-mediated retinal regeneration. Molecular Neurobiology. 2021;**58**(5):2342-2361. DOI: 10.1007/s12035-020-02274-w

[10] Reichenbach A, Bringmann A. New functions of Müller cells. Glia. 2013;**61**(5):651-678. DOI: 10.1002/glia.22477

[11] Winkler BS, Arnold MJ, Brassell MA, Puro DG. Energy metabolism in human retinal Müller cells. Investigative Ophthalmology & Visual Science. 2000;**41**(10):3183-3190

[12] Poitry-Yamate CL, Tsacopoulos M. Glucose metabolism in freshly isolated Müller glial cells from a mammalian retina. The Journal of Comparative Neurology. 1992;**320**(2):257-266. DOI: 10.1002/cne.903200209

[13] Poitry-Yamate CL, Poitry S, Tsacopoulos M. Lactate released by Müller glial cells is metabolized by photoreceptors from mammalian retina. Journal of Neuroscience. 1995;**15**(7 Pt 2):5179-5191. DOI: 10.1523/JNEUROSCI.15-07-05179.1995

[14] García VC, Chen Y, Cádiz B, Wang L, Paquet-Durand F, Schmachtenberg O. Imaging of lactate metabolism in retinal Müller cells with a FRET nanosensor. Experimental Eye Research. 2023;**226**:109352. DOI: 10.1016/j.exer.2022.109352

[15] Linsenmeier RA. Effects of light and darkness on oxygen distribution

and consumption in the cat retina. The Journal of General Physiology. 1986;**88**(4):521-542. DOI: 10.1085/jgp.88.4.521

[16] Huster D, Hjelle OP, Haug FM, Nagelhus EA, Reichelt W, Ottersen OP. Subcellular compartmentation of glutathione and glutathione precursors. A high resolution immunogold analysis of the outer retina of Guinea pig. Anatomy and Embryology (Berl). 1998;**198**(4):277-287. DOI: 10.1007/s004290050184

[17] Pow DV, Crook DK. Immunocytochemical evidence for the presence of high levels of reduced glutathione in radial glial cells and horizontal cells in the rabbit retina. Neuroscience Letters. 1995;**193**(1):25-28. DOI: 10.1016/0304-3940(95)11657-i

[18] Schütte M, Werner P. Redistribution of glutathione in the ischemic rat retina. Neuroscience Letters. 1998;**246**(1):53-56. DOI: 10.1016/s0304-3940(98)00229-8

[19] Janáky R, Ogita K, Pasqualotto BA, Bains JS, Oja SS, Yoneda Y, et al. Glutathione and signal transduction in the mammalian CNS. Journal of Neurochemistry. 1999;**73**(3):889-902. DOI: 10.1046/j.1471-4159.1999.0730889.x

[20] Ribelayga C, Mangel SC. A circadian clock and light/dark adaptation differentially regulate adenosine in the mammalian retina. The Journal of Neuroscience. 2005;**25**(1):215-222. DOI: 10.1523/JNEUROSCI.3138-04.2005

[21] Paasche G, Gärtner U, Germer A, Grosche J, Reichenbach A. Mitochondria of retinal Müller (glial) cells: The effects of aging and of application of free radical scavengers. Ophthalmic Research. 2000;**32**(5):229-236. DOI: 10.1159/000055618

[22] Arai-Gaun S, Katai N, Kikuchi T, Kurokawa T, Ohta K, Yoshimura N. Heme oxygenase-1 induced in muller cells plays a protective role in retinal ischemia-reperfusion injury in rats. Investigative Ophthalmology & Visual Science. 2004;**45**(11):4226-4232. DOI: 10.1167/iovs.04-0450

[23] Chen L, Dentchev T, Wong R, Hahn P, Wen R, Bennett J, et al. Increased expression of ceruloplasmin in the retina following photic injury. Molecular Vision. 2003;**9**:151-158

[24] Hollborn M, Francke M, Iandiev I, Bühner E, Foja C, Kohen L, et al. Early activation of inflammation- and immune response-related genes after experimental detachment of the porcine retina. Investigative Ophthalmology & Visual Science. 2008;**49**(3):1262-1273. DOI: 10.1167/iovs.07-0879

[25] Miyahara T, Kikuchi T, Akimoto M, Kurokawa T, Shibuki H, Yoshimura N. Gene microarray analysis of experimental glaucomatous retina from cynomologous monkey. Investigative Ophthalmology & Visual Science. 2003;**44**(10):4347-4356. DOI: 10.1167/iovs.02-1032

[26] Ulyanova T, Szél A, Kutty RK, Wiggert B, Caffé AR, Chader GJ, et al. Oxidative stress induces heme oxygenase-1 immunoreactivity in Müller cells of mouse retina in organ culture. Investigative Ophthalmology & Visual Science. 2001;**42**(6):1370-1374

[27] Woodford BJ, Tso MO, Lam KW. Reduced and oxidized ascorbates in Guinea pig retina under normal and light-exposed conditions. Investigative Ophthalmology & Visual Science. 1983;**24**(7):862-867

[28] Bringmann A, Iandiev I, Pannicke T, Wurm A, Hollborn M,

Wiedemann P, et al. Cellular signaling and factors involved in Müller cell gliosis: Neuroprotective and detrimental effects. Progress in Retinal and Eye Research. 2009;**28**(6):423-451. DOI: 10.1016/j.preteyeres.2009.07.001

[29] Shen W, Fruttiger M, Zhu L, Chung SH, Barnett NL, Kirk JK, et al. Conditional Müllercell ablation causes independent neuronal and vascular pathologies in a novel transgenic model. The Journal of Neuroscience. 2012;**32**(45):15715-15727. DOI: 10.1523/JNEUROSCI.2841-12.2012

[30] van Adel BA, Arnold JM, Phipps J, Doering JC, Ball AK. Ciliary neurotrophic factor protects retinal ganglion cells from axotomy-induced apoptosis via modulation of retinal glia *in vivo*. Journal of Neurobiology. 2005;**63**(3):215-234. DOI: 10.1002/neu.20117

[31] Fleisch VC, Neuhauss SCF. Parallel visual cycles in the zebrafish retina. Progress in Retinal and Eye Research. 2010;**29**(6):476-486. DOI: 10.1016/j.preteyeres.2010.05.001

[32] Muniz A, Villazana-Espinoza ET, Hatch AL, Trevino SG, Allen DM, Tsin ATC. A novel cone visual cycle in the cone-dominated retina. Experimental Eye Research. 2007;**85**(2):175-184. DOI: 10.1016/j.exer.2007.05.003

[33] Wang JS, Kefalov VJ. The cone-specific visual cycle. Progress in Retinal and Eye Research. 2011;**30**(2):115-128. DOI: 10.1016/j.preteyeres.2010.11.001

[34] Wang JS, Estevez ME, Cornwall MC, Kefalov VJ. Intra-retinal visual cycle required for rapid and complete cone dark adaptation. Nature Neuroscience. 2009;**12**(3):295-302. DOI: 10.1038/nn.2258

[35] Lu Y-B, Franze K, Seifert G, Steinhauser C, Kirchhoff F, Wolburg H, et al. Viscoelastic properties of individual glial cells and neurons in the CNS. Proceedings of the National Academy of Sciences of the United States of America. 2006;**103**:17759-17764. DOI: 10.1073/pnas.0606150103

[36] Lu YB, Iandiev I, Hollborn M, Korber N, Ulbricht E, Hirrlinger PG, et al. Reactive glial cells: Increased stiffness correlates with increased intermediate filament expression. The FASEB Journal. 2011;**25**:624-631. DOI: 10.1096/fj.10-163790

[37] Kobat SG, Turgut B. Importance of Müller cells. Beyoglu Eye Journal. 2020;**5**(2):59-63. DOI: 10.14744/bej.2020.28290

[38] Puro DG. Stretch-activated channels in human retinal Müller cells. Glia. 1991;**4**:456-460. DOI: 10.1002/glia.440040505

[39] Newman EA. Glial cell inhibition of neurons by release of ATP. The Journal of Neuroscience. 2003;**23**:1659-1666. DOI: 10.1523/JNEUROSCI.23-05-01659.2003

[40] Lindqvist N, Liu Q, Zajadacz J, Franze K, Reichenbach A. Retinal glial (Muller) cells: Sensing and responding to tissue stretch. Investigative Ophthalmology & Visual Science. 2010;**51**:1683-1690. DOI: 10.1167/iovs.09-4159

[41] Beverley KM, Pattnaik BR. Inward rectifier potassium (Kir) channels in the retina: Living our vision. American Journal of Physiology. Cell Physiology. 2022;**323**(3):C772-C782. DOI: 10.1152/ajpcell.00112.2022

[42] Bringmann A, Pannicke T, Grosche J, Francke M, Wiedemann P, Skatchkov SN, et al. Müller cells in the healthy and diseased retina. Progress in Retinal

and Eye Research. 2006;**25**:397-424. DOI: 10.1016/j.preteyeres.2006.05.003

[43] Bringmann A, Reichenbach A, Wiedemann P. Pathomechanisms of cystoid macular edema. Ophthalmic Research. 2004;**36**(5):241-249. DOI: 10.1159/000081203

[44] Nagelhus EA, Horio Y, Inanobe A, Fujita A, Haug FM, Nielsen S, et al. Immunogold evidence suggests that coupling of K^+ siphoning and water transport in rat retinal Müller cells is mediated by a coenrichment of Kir4.1 and AQP4 in specific membrane domains. Glia. 1999;**26**(1):47-54. DOI: 10.1002/(sici)1098-1136(199903)26:1<47::aid-glia5>3.0.co;2-5

[45] Iandiev I, Pannicke T, Reichel MB, Wiedemann P, Reichenbach A, Bringmann A. Expression of aquaporin-1 immunoreactivity by photoreceptor cells in the mouse retina. Neuroscience Letters. 2005;**388**(2):96-99. DOI: 10.1016/j.neulet.2005.06.046

[46] Nagelhus EA, Veruki ML, Torp R, Haug FM, Laake JH, Nielsen S, et al. Aquaporin-4 water channel protein in the rat retina and optic nerve: Polarized expression in Müller cells and fibrous astrocytes. The Journal of Neuroscience. 1998;**18**(7):2506-2519. DOI: 10.1523/JNEUROSCI.18-07-02506.1998

[47] Binder DK, Nagelhus EA, Ottersen OP. Aquaporin-4 and epilepsy. Glia. 2012;**60**:1203-1214. DOI: 10.1002/glia.22317

[48] Pannicke T, Iandiev I, Uckermann O, Biedermann B, Kutzera F, Wiedemann P, et al. A potassium channel-linked mechanism of glial cell swelling in the postischemic retina. Molecular and Cellular Neurosciences. 2004;**26**:493-502. DOI: 10.1016/j.mcn.2004.04.005

[49] Antcliff RJ, Hussain AA, Marshall J. Hydraulic conductivity of fixed retinal tissue after sequential excimer laser ablation: Barriers limiting fluid distribution and implications for cystoid macular edema. Archives of Ophthalmology. 2001;**119**:539-544. DOI: 10.1001/archopht.119.4.539

[50] Uckermann O, Vargova L, Ulbricht E, Klaus C, Weick M, Rillich K, et al. Glutamate-evoked alterations of glial and neuronal cell morphology in the Guinea-pig retina. The Journal of Neuroscience. 2004;**24**:10149-10158. DOI: 10.1523/JNEUROSCI.3203-04.2004

[51] Dmitriev AV, Govardovskii VI, Schwahn HN, Steinberg RH. Light-induced changes of extracellular ions and volume in the isolated chick retina-pigment epithelium preparation. Visual Neuroscience. 1999;**16**:1157-1167. DOI: 10.1017/s095252389916615x

[52] Lipp S, Wurm A, Pannicke T, Wiedemann P, Reichenbach A, Chen J, et al. Calcium responses mediated by type 2 IP3-receptors are required for osmotic volume regulation of retinal glial cells in mice. Neuroscience Letters. 2009;**457**:85-88. DOI: 10.1016/j.neulet.2009.04.001

[53] Oakley B, Wen R. Extracellular pH in the isolated retina of the toad in darkness and during illumination. The Journal of Physiology. 1989;**419**:353-378. DOI: 10.1113/jphysiol.1989.sp017876

[54] Newman EA. A physiological measure of carbonic anhydrase in muller cells. Glia. 1994;**11**:291-299. DOI: 10.1002/glia.440110402

[55] Borgula GA, Karwoski CJ, Steinberg RH. Light-evoked changes in extracellular pH in frog retina. Vision Research. 1989;**29**(9):1069-1077. DOI: 10.1016/0042-6989(89)90054-0

[56] Warren TJ, Van Hook MJ, Supuran CT, Thoreson WB. Sources of protons and a role for bicarbonate in inhibitory feedback from horizontal cells to cones in Ambystoma tigrinum retina. The Journal of Physiology. 2016;**594**(22):6661-6677. DOI: 10.1113/JP272533

[57] Yang XM, Yafai Y, Wiedemann P, Kuhrt H, Wang YS, Reichenbach A, et al. Hypoxia-induced upregulation of pigment epithelium-derived factor by retinal glial (Müller) cells. Journal of Neuroscience Research. 2012;**90**(1):257-266. DOI: 10.1002/jnr.22732

[58] Yafai Y, Eichler W, Iandiev I, Unterlauft JD, Jochmann C, Wiedemann P, et al. Thrombospondin-1 is produced by retinal glial cells and inhibits the growth of vascular endothelial cells. Ophthalmic Research. 2014;**52**(2):81-88. DOI: 10.1159/000362371

[59] Harada C, Harada QHMA, Maekawa F, Yoshida K, Ohno S, Wada K, et al. Potential role of glial cell line-derived neurotrophic factor receptors in Müller glial cells during light-induced retinal degeneration. Neuroscience. 2003;**122**(1):229-235. DOI: 10.1016/s0306-4522(03)00599-2

[60] Nishikiori N, Osanai M, Chiba H, Kojima T, Mitamura Y, Ohguro H, et al. Glial cell-derived cytokines attenuate the breakdown of vascular integrityin diabetic retinopathy. Diabetes. 2007;**56**:1333-1340. DOI: 10.2337/db06-1431

[61] Abu El-Asrar AM, Nawaz MI, Ahmad A, Siddiquei MM, Allegaert E, Gikandi PW, et al. CD146/soluble CD146 pathway is a novel biomarker of angiogenesis and inflammation in proliferative diabetic retinopathy. Investigative Ophthalmology & Visual Science. 2021;**62**(9):32. DOI: 10.1167/iovs.62.9.32

[62] Behzadian MA, Wang XL, Windsor LJ, Ghaly N, Caldwell RB. TGF-beta increases retinal endothelial cell permeability by increasing MMP-9: Possible role of glial cells in endothelial barrier function. Investigative Ophthalmology & Visual Science. 2001;**42**(3):853-859

[63] Eichler W, Yafai Y, Wiedemann P, Reichenbach A. Angiogenesis-related factors derived from retinal glial (Müller) cells in hypoxia. Neuroreport. 2004;**15**:1633-1637. DOI: 10.1097/01.wnr.0000133071.00786.a4

[64] Metea MR, Newman EA. Glial cells dilate and constrict blood vessels: A mechanism of neurovascular coupling. Journal of Neuroscience. 2006;**26**(11):2862-2870. DOI: 10.1523/JNEUROSCI.4048-05.2006

[65] Newman EA. Glial cell regulation of neuronal activity and blood flow in the retina by release of gliotransmitters. Philosophical Transactions of the Royal Society B. 2015;**370**(1672):20140195. DOI: 10.1098/rstb.2014.0195

[66] Sarthy VP, Pignataro L, Pannicke T, Weick M, Reichenbach A, Harada T, et al. Glutamate transport by retinal Muller cells in glutamate/aspartate transporter-knockout mice. Glia. 2005;**49**(2):184-196. DOI: 10.1002/glia.20097

[67] Bringmann A, Pannicke T, Biedermann B, Francke M, Iandiev I, Grosche J, et al. Role of retinal glial cells in neurotransmitter uptake and metabolism. Neurochemistry International. 2009;**54**:143-160. DOI: 10.1016/j.neuint.2008.10.014

[68] Pow DV, Robinson SR. Glutamate in some retinal neurons is derived solely

from glia. Neuroscience. 1994;**60**:355-366. DOI: 10.1016/0306-4522(94)90249-6

[69] Goldman D. Müller glial cell reprogramming and retina regeneration. Nature Reviews. Neuroscience. 2014;**15**(7):431-442. DOI: 10.1038/nrn3723

[70] Izumi Y, Shimamoto K, Benz AM, Hammerman SB, Olney JW, Zorumski CF. Glutamate transporters and retinal excitotoxicity. Glia. 2002;**39**(1):58-68. DOI: 10.1002/glia.10082

[71] Reichenbach A, Bringmann A. Müller Cells in the Healthy and Diseased Retina. New York, Dordrecht, Heidelberg, London: Springer; 2010

[72] Linnertz R, Wurm A, Pannicke T, Krugel K, Hollborn M, Hartig W, et al. Activation of voltage-gated Naþ and Ca2þ channels is required for vesicular release of glutamate from retinal glial cells implicated in cell volume regulation. Neuroscience. 2011;**188**:23-34. DOI: 10.1016/j.neuroscience.2011.04.058

[73] Lim D, Semyanov A, Genazzani A, Verkhratsky A. Calcium signaling in neuroglia. International Review of Cell and Molecular Biology. 2021;**362**:1-53. DOI: 10.1016/bs.ircmb.2021.01.003

[74] Newman EA, Zahs KR. Calcium waves in retinal glial cells. Science. 1997;**275**:844-847. DOI: 10.1126/science.275.5301.844

[75] Newman EA. Calcium increases in retinal glial cells evoked by light-induced neuronal activity. The Journal of Neuroscience. 2005;**25**:5502-5510. DOI: 10.1523/JNEUROSCI.1354-05.2005

[76] Sinha T, Ikelle L, Naash MI, Al-Ubaidi MR. The intersection of serine metabolism and cellular dysfunction in retinal degeneration. Cells. 2020;**9**(3):674. DOI: 10.3390/cells9030674

[77] Dixon DB, Copenhagen DR. Two types of glutamate receptors differentially excite amacrine cells in the tiger salamander retina. Journal of Physiology (London). 1992;**449**:589-606. DOI: 10.1113/jphysiol.1992.sp019103

[78] O'Dell TJ, Christensen BN. Horizontal cells isolated from catfish retina contain two types of excitatory amino acid receptors. Journal of Neurophysiology. 1989;**61**:1097-1109. DOI: 10.1152/jn.1989.61.6.1097

[79] Stevens ER, Esguerra M, Kim PM, Newman EA, Snyder SH, Zahs KR, et al. D-serine and serine racemase are present in the vertebrate retina and contribute to the physiological activation of NMDA receptors. Proceedings of the National Academy of Sciences of the United States of America. 2003;**100**:6789-6794. DOI: 10.1073/pnas.1237052100

[80] Pollegioni L, Sacchi S. Metabolism of the neuromodulator D-serine. Cellular and Molecular Life Sciences. 2010;**67**(14):2387-2404. DOI: 10.1007/s00018-010-0307-9

[81] Agte S, Junek S, Matthias S, Ulbricht E, Erdmann I, Wurm A, et al. Müller glial cell-provided cellular light guidance through the vital Guinea-pig retina. Biophysical Journal. 2011;**101**(11):2611-2619. DOI: 10.1016/j.bpj.2011.09.062

[82] Franze K, Grosche J, Skatchkov SN, Schinkinger S, Foja C, Schild D, et al. Müller cells are living optical fibers in the vertebrate retina. Proceedings of the National Academy of Sciences of the United States of America. 2007;**104**:8287-8292. DOI: 10.1073/pnas.0611180104

[83] Roesch K, Jadhav AP, Trimarchi JM, Stadler MB, Roska B, Sun BB, et al. The transcriptome of retinal Müller glial cells. The Journal of Comparative Neurology. 2008;**509**:225-238. DOI: 10.1002/cne.21730

[84] Jadhav AP, Roesch K, Cepko CL. Development and neurogenic potential of Müller glial cells in the vertebrate retina. Progress in Retinal and Eye Research. 2009;**28**(4):249-262. DOI: 10.1016/j.preteyeres.2009.05.002

[85] Eastlake K, Lamb WDB, Luis J, Khaw PT, Jayaram H, Limb GA. Prospects for the application of Müller glia and their derivatives in retinal regenerative therapies. Progress in Retinal and Eye Research. 2021;**85**:100970. DOI: 10.1016/j.preteyeres.2021.100970

[86] Rezzola S, Guerra J, Chandran AMK, Loda A, Cancarini A, Sacristani P, et al. Vegf-independent activation of Müller cells by the vitreous from proliferative diabetic retinopathy patients. International Journal of Molecular Sciences. 2021;**22**(4):2179. DOI: 10.3390/ijms22042179

[87] Carpi-Santos R, de Melo Reis RA, Gomes FCA, Calaza KC. Contribution of Müller cells in the diabetic retinopathy development: Focus on oxidative stress and inflammation. Antioxidants (Basel). 2022;**11**(4):617. DOI: 10.3390/antiox11040617

[88] Carpineto P, Toto L, Aloia R, Ciciarelli V, Borrelli E, Vitacolonna E, et al. Neuroretinal alterations in the early stages of diabetic retinopathy in patients with type 2 diabetes mellitus. Eye. 2016;**30**:673-679. DOI: 10.1038/eye.2016

[89] Yang S, Qi S, Wang C. The role of retinal Müller cells in diabetic retinopathy and related therapeutic advances. Frontiers in Cell and Development Biology. 2022;**10**:1047487. DOI: 10.3389/fcell.2022.1047487

[90] Alex A, Luo Q, Mathew D, Di R, Bhatwadekar AD. Metformin corrects abnormal circadian rhythm and Kir4.1 channels in diabetes. Investigative Ophthalmology & Visual Science. 2020;**61**(6):46. DOI: 10.1167/iovs.61.6.46

[91] Hassan I, Luo Q, Majumdar S, Dominguez JM 2nd, Busik JV. Tumor necrosis factor alpha (TNF-α) disrupts Kir4.1 channel expression resulting in Müller cell dysfunction in the retina. Investigative Ophthalmology & Visual Science. 2017;**58**(5):2473-2482. DOI: 10.1167/iovs.16-20712

[92] Wurm A, Pannicke T, Wiedemann P, Reichenbach A, Bringmann A. Glial cellderived glutamate mediates autocrine cell volume regulation in the retina: Activation by VEGF. Journal of Neurochemistry. 2008a;**104**:386-399. DOI: 10.1111/j.1471-4159. 2007.04992.x

[93] Gao F, Xu LJ, Zhao Y, Sun XH, Wang Z. K^+ channels of Müller glial cells in retinal disorders. CNS & Neurological Disorders Drug Targets. 2018;**17**(4):255-260. DOI: 10.2174/187152731 7666180202114233

[94] Vujosevic S, Micera A, Bini S, Berton M, Esposito G, Midena E. Aqueous humor biomarkers of Müller cell activation in diabetic eyes. Investigative Ophthalmology & Visual Science. 2015;**56**(6):3913-3918. DOI: 10.1167/iovs.15-16554

[95] Kida T, Oku H, Horie T, Fukumoto M, Okuda Y, Morishita S. Implication of VEGF and aquaporin 4 mediating Müller cell swelling to diabetic retinal edema. Graefe's Archive for Clinical and Experimental

Ophthalmology. 2017;**255**(6):1149-1157. DOI: 10. 1007/s00417-017-3631-z

[96] Gad MS, Elsherbiny NM, Refat D, Omar N, Ali S, Al-Shabrawey M, et al. Exploring the role of Müller cells-derived exosomes in diabetic retinopathy. Microvascular Research. 2024;7:104695. DOI: 10.1016/j.mvr.2024.104695

[97] Muto T, Tien T, Kim D, Sarthy VP, Roy S. High glucose alters Cx43 expression and gap junction intercellular communication in retinal müller cells: Promotes Müller cell and pericyte apoptosis. Investigative Ophthalmology & Visual Science. 2014;**55**(7):4327-4337. DOI: 10.1167/iovs.14-14606

[98] Kim D, Lewis CS, Sarthy VP. High-glucose-induced Rab20 upregulation disrupts gap junction intercellular communication and promotes apoptosis in retinal endothelial and Müller cells: Implications for diabetic retinopathy. Journal of Clinical Medicine. 2020;**9**(11):3710. DOI: 10.3390/jcm9113710

[99] Li X, Liu J, Hoh J, Liu J. Müller cells in pathological retinal angiogenesis. Translational Research. 2019;**207**:96-106. DOI: 10.1016/j.trsl.2018.12.006

[100] Actis Dato V, Sánchez MC, Chiabrando GA. LRP1 mediates the IGF-1-induced GLUT1 expression on the cell surface and glucose uptake in Müller glial cells. Scientific Reports. 2021;**11**(1):4742. DOI: 10.1038/s41598-021-84090-3

[101] Schmalen A, Lorenz L, Grosche A, Pauly D, Deeg CA, Hauck SM. Proteomic phenotyping of stimulated Müller cells uncovers profound proinflammatory signaling and antigen-presenting capacity. Frontiers in Pharmacology. 2021;**12**:771571. DOI: 10.3389/fphar.2021.771571

[102] Capozzi ME, McCollum GW, Cousins DB, Penn JS. Linoleic acid is a diabetes-relevant stimulator of retinal inflammation in human retinal muller cells and microvascular endothelial cells. Journal of Diabetes & Metabolism. 2016;7(12):718. DOI: 10.4172/2155-6156.1000718

[103] Xie Y, Su N, Yang J, Tan Q, Huang S, Jin M, et al. FGF/FGFR signaling in health and disease. Signal Transduction and Targeted Therapy. 2020;**5**(1):181. DOI: 10.1038/s41392-020-00222-7

[104] Xi G, Wai C, Clemmons D. Inhibition of aberrant IGF-I signaling in diabetic male rat retina prevents and reverses changes of diabetic retinopathy. Journal Diabetes Research. 2019;**2019**:6456032. DOI: 10.1155/2019/6456032

[105] Peng D, Fu M, Wang M, Wei Y. Targeting TGF-β signaltransd uction for fibrosis and cancer therapy. Molecular Cancer. 2022;**21**(1):104. DOI: 10. 1186/s12943-022-01569-x

[106] Wu D, Kanda A, Liu Y, Noda K, Murata M, Ishida S. Choroidal thickness in diabetes and diabetic retinopathy: A swept source oct study. Investigative Ophthalmology & Visual Science. 2020;**61**(14):29. DOI: 10.1167/iovs.61.4.29

[107] Buyuktepe TC, Demirel S, Batıoğlu F, Özmert E. The correlation of inflammation and microvascular changes with diabetic retinal neurodegeneration. Current Eye Research. 2021;**46**(10):1559-1566. DOI: 10.1080/02713683.2021.1908567

[108] Kim HJ, Jeong MS, Jang SB. Molecular characteristics of RAGE and advances in small-molecule inhibitors. International Journal of Molecular Sciences. 2021;**22**(13):6904. DOI: 10.3390/ijms22136904

[109] Barile GR, Schmidt AM. RAGE and its ligands in retinal disease. Current Molecular Medicine. 2007;**7**(8):758-765. DOI: 10.2174/156652407783220778

[110] Dvoriantchikova G, Hernandez E, Grant J, Santos AR, Yang H, Ivanov D. The high-mobility group box-1 nuclear factor mediates retinal injury after ischemia reperfusion. Investigative Ophthalmology & Visual Science. 2011;**52**(10):7187-7194. DOI: 10.1167/iovs.11-7793

[111] Forrester JV, Kuffova L, Delibegovic M. The role of inflammation in diabetic retinopathy. Frontiers in Immunology. 2020;**11**:583687. DOI: 10.3389/fimmu.2020.583687

[112] Rübsam A, Parikh S, Fort PE. Role of inflammation in diabetic retinopathy. International Journal of Molecular Sciences. 2018;**19**(4):942. DOI: 10.3390/ijms19040942

[113] Gerhardinger C, Costa MB, Coulombe MC, Toth I, Hoehn T. Expression of acute-phase response proteins in retinal Müller cells in diabetes. Investigative Ophthalmology & Visual Science. 2005;**46**(1):349-357. DOI: 10.1167/iovs.04-0860

[114] Wang Y, Zhai WL, Yang YW. Association between NDRG2/IL-6/STAT3 signaling pathway and diabetic retinopathy in rats. European Review for Medical and Pharmacological Sciences. 2020;**24**(7):3476-3484. DOI: 10.26355/eurrev_202004_20806

[115] Coughlin BA, Trombley BT. Interleukin-6 (IL-6) mediates protection against glucose toxicity in human Müller cells via activation of VEGF-A signaling. Biochemical and Biophysical Research Communications. 2019;**517**(2):227-232. DOI: 10. 1016/j.bbrc.2019.07.044

[116] Glass J, Robinson RL, Greenway G, Jones G, Sharma S. Diabetic Müller-glial-cell-specific Il6ra knockout mice exhibit accelerated retinal functional decline and thinning of the inner nuclear layer. Investigative Ophthalmology & Visual Science. 2023;**64**(15):1. DOI: 10.1167/iovs.64.15.1

[117] Liu X, Ye F, Xiong H, Hu D, Limb GA, Xie T, et al. IL-1β upregulates IL-8 production in human Müller cells through activation of the p38 MAPK and ERK1/2 signaling pathways. Inflammation. 2014;**37**(5):1486-1495. DOI: 10.1007/s10753-014-9874-5

[118] Qiu AW, Bian Z, Mao PA. IL-17A exacerbates diabetic retinopathy by impairing Müller cell function via Act1 signaling. Experimental & Molecular Medicine. 2016;**48**(12):e280. DOI: 10.1038/emm.2016.117

[119] Qiu AW, Liu QH. Blocking IL-17a alleviates diabetic retinopathy in rodents. Cellular Physiology and Biochemistry. 2017;**41**(3):960-972. DOI: 10.1159/000460514

[120] Taylor BE, Lee CA, Zapadka TE, Zhou AY, Barber KG, Taylor ZRR, et al. IL-17A enhances retinal neovascularization. International Journal of Molecular Sciences. 2023;**24**(2):1747. DOI: 10.3390/ijms24021747

[121] Ueda A, Okuda K, Ohno S, Shirai A, Igarashi T, Matsunaga K, et al. NF-kappa B and Sp1 regulate transcription of the human monocyte chemoattractant protein-1 gene. Journal of Immunology. 1994;**153**(5):2052-2063

[122] Taghavi Y, Hassanshahi G, Kounis NG, Koniari I, Khorramdelazad H. Monocyte chemoattractant protein-1 (MCP-1/CCL2) in diabetic retinopathy: Latest evidence and clinical considerations.

Journal of Cell Communication. 2019;**13**(4):451-462. DOI: 10.1007/s12079-018-00500-8

[123] Portillo J-AC, Greene JA, Okenka G, Miao Y, Sheibani N, Kern TS, et al. CD40 promotes the development of early diabetic retinopathy in mice. Diabetologia. 2014;**57**:2222-2231. DOI: 10.1007/s00125-014-3321-x

[124] Portillo JC, Pfaff A, Vos S, Weng M, Nagaraj RH, Subauste CS. Advanced glycation end products upregulate CD40 in human retinal endothelial and Müller cells: Relevance to diabetic retinopathy. Cells. 2024;**13**(5):429. DOI: 10.3390/cells13050429

[125] Portillo JC, Lopez Corcino Y, Miao Y, Tang J, Sheibani N, Kern TS, et al. CD40 in retinal müller cells induces P2X7-dependent cytokine expression in macrophages/microglia in diabetic mice and development of early experimental diabetic retinopathy. Diabetes. 2017;**66**(2):483-493. DOI: 10.2337/db16-0051

[126] Vos S, Aaron R, Weng M, Daw J, Rodriguez-Rivera E, Subauste CS. CD40 upregulation in the retina of patients with diabetic retinopathy: Association with TRAF2/TRAF6 upregulation and inflammatory molecule expression. Investigative Ophthalmology & Visual Science. 2023;**64**(7):17. DOI: 10.1167/iovs.64.7.17

[127] Abu El-Asrar AM, Nawaz MI, Ahmad A, De Zutter A, Siddiquei MM, Blanter M, et al. Evaluation of proteoforms of the transmembrane chemokines CXCL16 and CX3CL1, their receptors, and their processing metalloproteinases ADAM10 and ADAM17 in proliferative diabetic retinopathy. Frontiers in Immunology. 2021;**11**:601639. DOI: 10.3389/fimmu.2020.601639

[128] McDowell RE, Barabas P, Augustine J, Chevallier O, McCarron P, Chen M, et al. Müller glial dysfunction during diabetic retinopathy in rats is reduced by the acrolein-scavenging drug, 2-hydrazino-4, 6-dimethylpyrimidine. Diabetologia. 2018;**61**(12):2654-2667. DOI: 10.1007/s00125-018-4707-y

[129] de Hoz R, Rojas B, Ramírez AI, Salazar JJ, Gallego BI, Triviño A. Retinal macroglial responses in health and disease. BioMed Research International. 2016;**2016**:2954721. DOI: 10.1155/2016/2954721), 10.1155/2016/2954721)

[130] Matteucci A, Gaddini L, Villa M, Varano M, Parravano M, Monteleone V, et al. Neuroprotection by rat Müller glia against high glucose-induced neurodegeneration through a mechanism involving ERK1/2 activation. Experimental Eye Research. 2014;**125**:20-29. DOI: 10.1016/j.exer.2014.05.011

[131] Wang L, Deng QQ, Wu XH, Yu J, Yang XL, Zhong YM. Upregulation of glutamate-aspartate transporter by glial cell line-derived neurotrophic factor ameliorates cell apoptosis in neural retina in streptozotocininduced diabetic rats. CNS Neuroscience & Therapeutics. 2013;**19**(12):945-953. DOI: 10.1111/cns.12150

[132] Fu S, Dong S, Zhu M, Sherry DM, Wang C, You Z, et al. Müllerglia are a major cellular source of survival signals for retinal neurons in diabetes. Diabetes. 2015;**64**(10):3554-3563. DOI: 10.2337/db15-0180

[133] Nipper AR, Newman EA. Regulation of blood flow in diabetic retinopathy. Visual Neuroscience. 2020;**20**(37):E004. DOI: 10.1017/S0952523820000036

[134] Huber VJ, Tsujita M, Nakada T. Identification of aquaporin 4 inhibitors

using *in vitro* and in silico methods. Bioorganic & Medicinal Chemistry. 2009;**17**:411-417. DOI: 10.1016/j.bmc.2007.12.040

[135] Oosuka S, Kida T, Oku H, Horie T, Morishita S, Fukumoto M, et al. Effects of an aquaporin 4 inhibitor, TGN-020, on murine diabetic retina. International Journal of Molecular Sciences. 2020;**21**(7):2324. DOI: 10.3390/ijms21072324

[136] Ishizaki E, Fukumoto M, Puro DG. Functional K(ATP) channels in the rat retinal microvasculature: Topographical distribution, redox regulation, spermine modulation and diabetic alteration. The Journal of Physiology. 2009;**587**:2233-2253. DOI: 10.1113/jphysiol.2009.169003

[137] Li H, Chen D, Sun W, Chen J, Luo C, Xu H, et al. KATP opener attenuates diabetic-induced müller gliosis and inflammation by modulating Kir6.1 in microglia. Investigative Ophthalmology & Visual Science. 2021;**62**(2):3. DOI: 10.1167/iovs.62.2.3

[138] Chatziralli I, Loewenstein A. Intravitreal anti-vascular endothelial growth factor agents for the treatment of diabetic retinopathy: A review of the literature. Pharmaceutics. 2021;**13**(8):1137. DOI: 10.3390/pharmaceutics13081137

[139] Wang T, Zhang C, Xie H, Jiang M, Tian H, Lu L, et al. Anti-VEGF therapy prevents Müller intracellular edema by decreasing VEGF-A in diabetic retinopathy. Eye and Vision. 2021;**8**(1):13. DOI: 10.1186/s40662-021-00237-3

[140] Sanchez MC, Chiabrando GA. Multitarget activities of Müller glial cells and low-density lipoprotein receptor-related protein 1 in proliferative retinopathies. ASN Neuro. 2022;**14**:17590914221136365. DOI: 10.1177/17590914221136365

[141] Sampedro J, Bogdanov P, Ramos H, Solà-Adell C, Turch M, Valeri M, et al. New insights into the mechanisms of action of topical administration of GLP-1 in an experimental model of diabetic retinopathy. Journal of Clinical Medicine. 2019;**8**(3):339. DOI: 10.3390/jcm8030339)

[142] Ontko CD, Capozzi M, Kim MJ, McCollum GW. Cytochrome P450-epoxygenated fatty acids inhibit Müller glial inflammation. Scientific Reports. 2021;**11**(1):9677. DOI: 10.1038/s41598-021-89000-1

[143] Hernández C, Bogdanov P, Gómez-Guerrero C, Sampedro J, Solà-Adell C, Espejo C, et al. SOCS1-derived peptide administered by eye drops prevents retinal neuroinflammation and vascular leakage in experimental diabetes. International Journal of Molecular Sciences. 2019;**20**(15):3615. DOI: 10.3390/ijms20153615

[144] Bishop GA, Hostager BS, Brown KD. Mechanisms of TNF receptor-associated factor (TRAF) regulation in B lymphocytes. Journal of Leukocyte Biology. 2002;**72**(1):19-23. DOI: 10.1189/jlb.72.1.19

[145] Portillo JC, Yu JS, Vos S, Bapputty R, Lopez Corcino Y, Hubal A, et al. Disruption of retinal inflammation and the development of diabetic retinopathy in mice by a CD40-derived peptide or mutation of CD40 in Müller cells. Diabetologia. 2022;**65**(12):2157-2171. DOI: 10.1007/s00125-022-05775-6

[146] Mohammad G, AlSharif HM, Siddiquei MM, Ahmad A, Alam K, Abu El-Asrar AM. Rho-associated protein Kinase-1 mediates the regulation of

inflammatory markers in diabetic retina and in retinal Müller cells. Annals of Clinical and Laboratory Science. 2018;**48**(2):137-145

[147] Rapp J, Hospach A, Liang P, Schwämmle M, Renz L, Agostini H, et al. Oncostatin M reduces pathological neovascularization in the retina through Müller cell activation. Investigative Ophthalmology & Visual Science. 2024;**65**(1):22. DOI: 10.1167/iovs.65.1.22

Section 3

Therapies in the Management of Diabetic Retinopathy: Limitation and Future Prospects

Chapter 7

Extracellular Vesicles and Diabetic Retinopathy: Nano-Sized Vesicles with Mega-Sized Hopes

Samar Habib, Alaa M. Mansour, Babak Baban and Khaled Elmasry

Abstract

Diabetic retinopathy (DR) is a major health problem, being the leading cause of vision loss in the working-age group. Novel discoveries facilitating the early diagnosis and curative treatment of DR are still greatly needed. Extracellular vesicles (EVs) are nano-sized vesicles released from different kinds of body cells including various retinal cells for intercellular communication. EVs recently attracted attention because of their non-immunogenic, biocompatible, and biodegradable characteristics. Recent studies investigated EV cargoes in DR patient samples, animal models, and *in vitro* models of DR. Although a thorough understanding of the trafficking of EVs in the retina still needs extensive investigations, these studies will pave the way for the discovery of novel biomarkers for early diagnosis of DR. Furthermore, EVs-based therapeutics could be of great interest in the treatment of DR. They are presented as promising delivery tools for both pharmacological and genetic therapies. Here, we highlighted the studies that discussed the role of EVs in both inflammation and angiogenesis as two main pathophysiological events occurring in DR. We also tried to portray what we know so far about the role of EVs in DR as a diagnostic, prognostic, and therapeutic tool.

Keywords: diabetic retinopathy, extracellular vesicles, exosomes, microvesicles, inflammation, angiogenesis, retina

1. Introduction

Diabetic retinopathy (DR) is a diabetes-related complication characterized by various molecular, metabolic, functional, and structural changes in the retina. It is considered the leading cause of acquired preventable sight loss in the working-age population worldwide. It causes visual impairment that negatively impacts the individual's quality of life [1–5]. DR has several risk factors such as the duration of diabetes mellitus (DM), poor glycemic control, hypertension, hyperlipidemia, obesity, smoking, alcohol intake, and pregnancy [6–8]. Moreover, genetic determinants have a role in the development and progression of DR [9].

Regular DR screening is recommended for diabetic patients to recognize high-risk DR characteristics. Therefore, it is essential to detect cases that require timely full ophthalmic examination and treatment for permanent visual loss prevention and to reduce the new cases of blindness. Additionally, screening is useful for identifying cases at the risk of cardiovascular disease, which expands their role beyond the prevention of sight-threatening disease. Screening is done using diagnostic modalities for DR which are important for the detection and classification of DR. Current diagnostic modalities include ophthalmoscopy and retinal photography, standard color fundus photography, multicolor fundus photography, fundus fluorescein angiography, optical coherence tomography, optical coherence tomography angiography, ultrawide-field imaging systems, swept-source wide-field optical coherence tomography angiography, smartphone-based imaging, and artificial intelligence systems [10].

There are several stages for DR. The reduction in visual acuity (VA), distortion of visual images, and sight loss can occur at any stage of the disease. In the early stages, the disease may remain asymptomatic, but later on, retinal examination reveals progressive retinal damage. This retinal damage appears firstly as microaneurysms, followed by the appearance of cotton wool spots, retinal hemorrhages, and intraretinal microvascular abnormalities. Eventually, this may lead to neovascularization with fragile new blood vessels, so they can be easily damaged, causing vision obstruction. Neovascularization can also detach the retina, resulting in blindness [4].

Regarding the pathophysiology of DR, oxidative stress and inflammation occupy a major role in the development and progression of DR. Sustained high-circulating glucose level activates several inflammatory pathways such as the protein kinase C pathway, the hexosamine biosynthetic pathway, and advanced glycation end-products accumulation (**Figure 1**). This chronic hyperglycemia increases reactive oxygen species

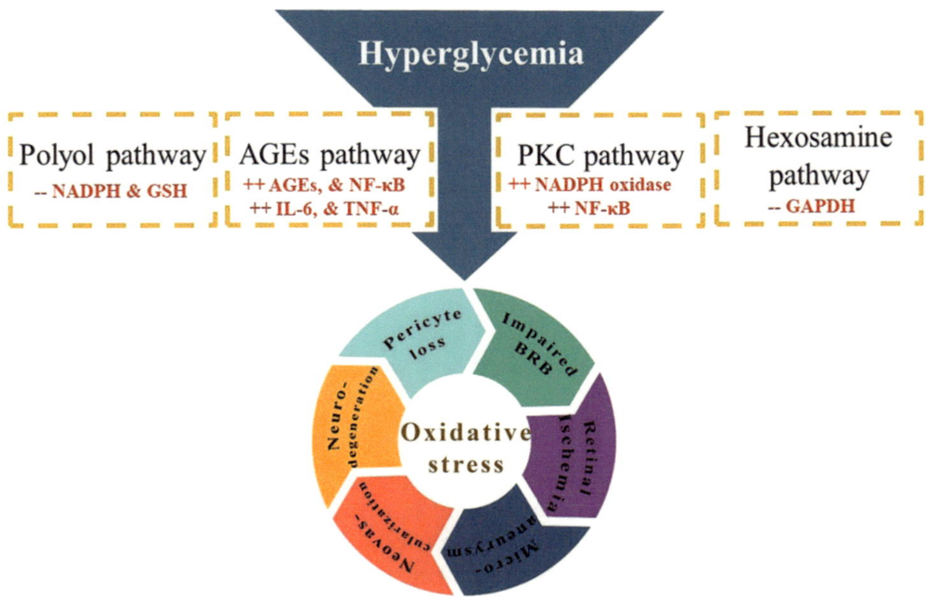

Figure 1.
Schematic diagram showing different pathways involved in DR pathogenesis. These pathways induce oxidative stress and inflammation that lead to diabetic retinopathy. NADPH; Polyol pathway downregulates the nicotinamide adenine dinucleotide phosphate, AGEs; advanced glycation end products, NF-κB; nuclear factor κappa-B, IL; interleukin, TNF- α; tumor necrosis factor-α, GAPDH; glyceraldehyde 3-phosphate dehydrogenase.

(ROS) exacerbating retinal oxidative stress and inflammation [2, 11]. This leads to a vicious circle of ROS inducing an increase of the inflammatory factors, and then, inflammation induces ROS generation. The nuclear factor κappa-B (NF-κB) is activated also in DM. It is a transcription factor regulating many cytokines, for example, interleukin (IL)-1β, IL-8, tumor necrosis factor (TNF)-α, and several chemokines [4, 12, 13]. Moreover, oxidative stress and inflammation can cause epigenetic modifications. These epigenetic modifications are rapid and transmissible to the next generation [4, 14].

The upregulation of inflammatory mediators in DM, together with growth factors such as vascular endothelial growth factor (VEGF), cause blood-retinal barrier (BRB) breakdown, vascular damage, and neuro-inflammation, as well as pathological neovascularization (NV) noticed in DR [15, 16]. VEGF is a major pathogenic factor in DR. Upregulated VEGF induces the expression of more inflammatory cytokines, inducing endothelial dysfunction and breakdown of the BRB. The sub- and intraretinal fluid accumulation causes macular thickening, known as diabetic macular edema (DME), and is considered a complication of DR [2, 17]. As DR is a neurovascular complication of diabetes, non-vascular cells, including retinal neurons and glial cells, are also affected, showing many abnormalities or accelerated apoptosis. Retinal microglia and astrocytes are two main sources of ROS causing oxidative stress in chronic neurodegeneration [4, 18, 19]. Diabetic retinal neurodegeneration is shown as a significant thinning of the inner retinal layers, including the retinal nerve fiber layer, and ganglion cell layer [20–22].

The current therapies available for DR aim to stop the inflammatory response, prevent retinal NV, and stabilize the BRB [23]. There is a wide range of therapies for DR which are always under development. The selection of the treatment modality depends on several factors. For instance, vitrectomy, where the blood and scar tissue is removed along with vitreous removal, is important in the management of certain cases in DR, for example, non-clearing vitreous hemorrhages. Laser photocoagulation of the abnormal leaky blood vessels is also used to treat pathological NV [24].

Pharmacotherapy has also been used and it produces more progress in the treatment of DR than laser or surgical therapy, but its cost is still a challenge [24]. Corticosteroids, such as dexamethasone, triamcinolone, and fluocinolone, are potent anti-inflammatory agents. They antagonize various pathologic inflammatory mediators such as TNF-α, IL-1β, and IL-6 [25]. As VEGF plays a major role in the pathogenesis of DR, it is considered a critical therapeutic target. Intravitreal injection of anti-VEGF therapy such as bevacizumab, brolucizumab, ranibizumab, and aflibercept can improve non-proliferative DR (NPDR) and prevent the onset of angiogenesis and DME [20, 26–29]. Unfortunately, not all patients respond properly to anti-VEGF such as in the case of DME with subretinal fluid [2]. Another treatment modality, depending on the integration of laser therapy with pharmacotherapy, may provide a more durable and effective response [24]. It can also result in optimum clinical efficacy with reduced treatment burden for the patient. In proliferative DR (PDR), the combination treatment between anti-VEGF and pan-retinal photocoagulation may be superior to monotherapy [30].

As DR is a polygenetic disease influenced by both environmental and genetic factors, gene therapy is considered a potential alternative therapy for DR. Generally, gene therapy is proposed to introduce genetic material into the cells to compensate for defective genes or deliver therapeutic transgenes. It has several benefits, such as prolonged effect with less frequency of intravitreal injection [31, 32]. One of the methods used for gene delivery is extracellular vesicles (EVs), as it is considered an immune-friendly gene therapy-delivering approach.

Generally, EVs are lipid-bound structures released by cells into the extracellular space carrying bioactive components that interact with target cells, causing subsequent modification. They can be detected in different biological fluids. EVs represent important tools of intercellular communication that allow the exchange of various messages including proteins, lipids, and nucleic acids between adjacent and/or distant cells. These intercellular messages have critical rules in normal homeostasis and disease development [33]. Therefore, EVs are considered novel diagnostic/prognostic biomarkers, promising drug delivery vehicles, and unique tools for targeted therapy [34, 35]. EVs can effectively deliver their cargo, including drugs or nucleic acids, to targeted tissues or organs as they possess several natural advantages, such as stability in circulation, transportation capability, and natural barriers-traversing capacity [36].

According to the pathways involved in their biogenesis and release, size, contents, and functions, EVs are classified into exosomes, microvesicles (MVs), and apoptotic bodies [37]. Exosomes are generated via the inward budding of the limiting membrane of early endosomes during maturation into multivesicular bodies (MVBs). They vary in size from 50 to 150 nm [38]. Their formation and release are regulated by endosomal sorting complexes required for transport (ESCRT) [39]. Nonetheless, ESCRT-independent pathways have also been identified, where sphingomyelinase converts sphingomyelin into ceramides, which allows the sorting of the cargoes in the exosomes and enhances the formation of curvatures in the membrane [40]. Exosomes were shown to have higher levels of transmembrane proteins and glycoproteins compared to whole-cell lysate [41]. Based on the cholesterol contents, MVBs are degraded by lysosomes, or they merge with the plasma membrane and liberate their exosome contents into the extracellular space [42, 43]. Exosomes interact with the target cells by micropinocytosis, endocytosis, or they fuse with the cell membrane and deliver their contents into the cell [44]. **Figure 2** describes the biogenesis and uptake of exosomes.

Microvesicles are formed by external budding and then scission from the plasma membrane of both healthy and damaged cells. Their size ranges between 50 and 500 nm, and up to 10 μm in cases of cancer-derived EVs, known as oncosomes. Cytoskeletal components, molecular motors, and fusion machinery were shown to contribute to MVs formation [45]. In comparison to exosomes, MVs tend to contain higher levels of proteins with post-translational modifications [41]. Different mechanisms are adopted to mediate MVs-cellular communications such as receptor-ligand interaction, fusion of MVs membrane with that of the recipient cell, endocytic-mediated internalization of MVs contents, and membrane protease cleavage resulting in the release of MVs soluble proteins, which interact with specific receptors on the target cells [46].

Regarding apoptotic bodies, they are typically larger, ranging from 50 to 5000 nm. They are generated during the process of programmed cell death (apoptosis) as blebbing from the plasma membrane of cells [47]. They enclose intact organelles, chromatin, and proteins [48]. In contrast to exosomes and MVs, the proteomic analysis of apoptotic bodies is similar to that of cell lysate [49]. The features of different subtypes of EVs were summarized by Hu et al. [50].

The basics of uptake and intercellular trafficking of different subtypes of EVs are thought to be shared despite different sizes and components [36]. Inside the recipient cell, endocytosed EVs either follow the degradation pathway or release their contents into the cytoplasm [35]. Van der Pol et al. [51] and Lv et al. [52] have reviewed the functions of exosomes and MVs and highlighted their crucial roles in cell-to-cell communication and signaling, particularly in the immune response, tumorigenesis,

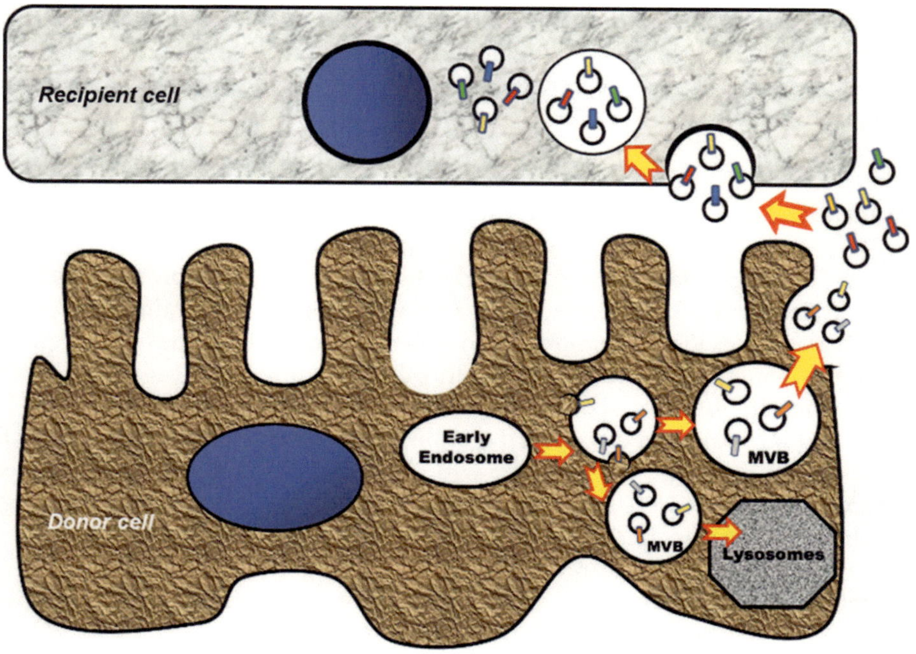

Figure 2.
A schematic diagram illustrating different steps of EVs biogenesis and release from donor cells. EVs uptake by the recipient cells can occur via endocytosis, pinocytosis, or membrane fusion.

thrombus formation, and waste removal. **Figure 3** portrays retinal intercellular communication via EVs [51, 52].

In this book chapter, we briefly discuss the EVs' isolation. We emphasize EVs originating from various sources, either intraocular or extraocular sources, and explain

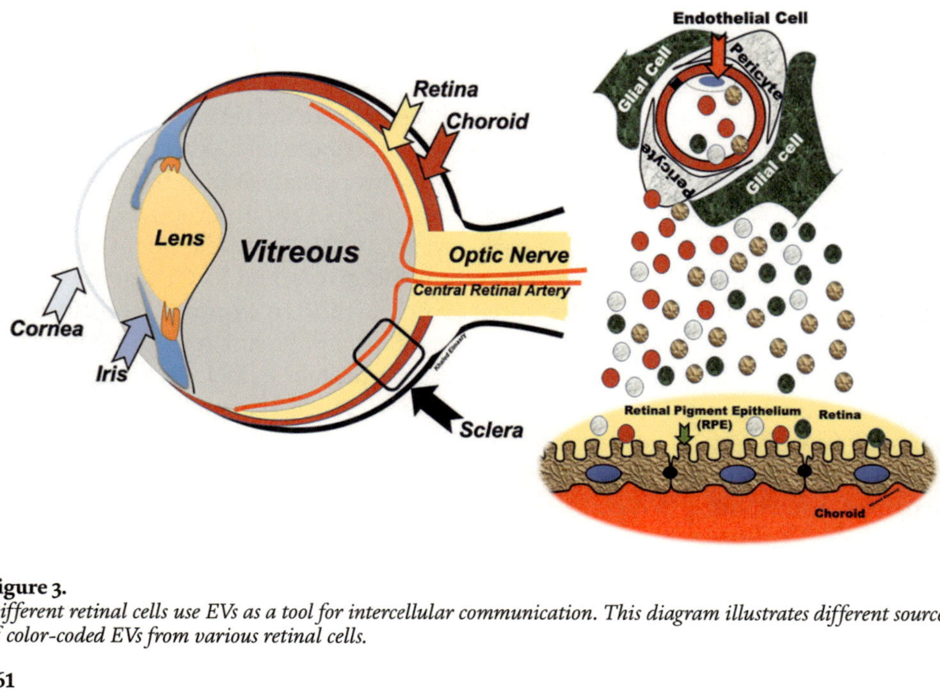

Figure 3.
Different retinal cells use EVs as a tool for intercellular communication. This diagram illustrates different sources of color-coded EVs from various retinal cells.

how they contribute to inflammation and angiogenesis, as two major arms of DR pathophysiology. Additionally, we highlight the EVs as promising diagnostic biomarkers and therapeutic tools in the field of DR. Finally, we list the related challenges and future recommendations.

2. Isolation and characterization of EVs

As most isolation methods depend on the distinction of EVs according to the size, and due to size overlap between exosomes and MVs, it is hard to obtain a pure population of EVs subtypes [53]. Commonly used isolation methods include immunoprecipitation, polymer-based precipitation, ultrafiltration, ultracentrifugation, density gradient, microfluidics, and size exclusion chromatography. An interesting study by Helwa et al. [54] compared ultracentrifugation versus commercially available kits for exosome isolation and showed that even with limited volumes of biological samples, commercially available isolation kits were feasible alternatives to the ultracentrifugation technique. The principle of the techniques, advantages, disadvantages, yield, and purity are neatly tabled by Massoumi et al. [55]. Regarding identification and characterization, tetraspanins, such as CD9, CD63, and CD81, are generally used as markers for exosomes. CD40, selectins, integrins, and annexin 1 are used for MVs characterization. As far as apoptotic bodies, DNA, histone, and phosphatidylserine are commonly used [55–57]. Electron microscopy (EM) studies including transmission EM, scanning EM, or immune-gold labeling using different EVs markers are generally used as an additional confirmatory step for EVs characterization [58, 59]. Nanoparticle tracking analysis is commonly used to report the concentration and the size range of EVs in isolated samples [54].

3. Role of EVs in inflammation

Inflammation and immune dysfunction result from chronic hyperglycemia and hyperlipidemia, are believed to be key mechanisms in the development of DR. Increased levels of inflammatory cytokines and angiogenic factors were noticed in plasma EVs from diabetic patients, which find their way to the retina because of increased permeability of BRB and are known to contribute to the pathophysiology of DR [60]. Our previous work highlighted the pathway analysis of retinal pigment epithelium (RPE)-derived exosomal microRNAs (miRNAs or miRs) that showed their involvement in different cellular pathways related to the development of DR such as oxidative stress, endoplasmic reticulum (ER) stress, and VEGF signaling [61]. Our ongoing research noticed a differential exosomal miRNA expression profile of retinal endothelial cells treated with proinflammatory lipid mediators. Inflammatory mediators such as TNF-α, thrombin, and C-reactive protein (CRP) were found to enhance endothelial cells (ECs) to form MVs *in vitro*. These MVs promote inflammation by triggering target cells to produce ROS, leading to oxidative stress [62–64]. High glucose causes increased NADPH oxidase activity in endothelium-derived microparticles, contributing to disturbed retinal barrier functions [65]. EVs derived from RPE under oxidative stress promoted apoptosis and inflammation through Apaf1/caspase-9 axis [66]. Additionally, Tokarz et al. [67] found a correlation between chemokine receptor (CCR)-5 positive MVs with NPDR progression.

Platelet-derived MVs from patients with DR enhanced the interaction between monocytes and endothelial cells [68]. Also, in diabetic patients, high levels of CXCL-10 in platelet-derived EVs stimulated the Toll-like receptor (TLR)-4 pathway, triggered ROS production, inhibited superoxide dismutase (SOD) activity, and lessened tight junction proteins, with the net result of increased BRB permeability [69]. Additionally, exosomes derived from platelet-rich plasma from diabetic rats enhanced the proliferation and fibrogenic activity of human retinal Müller cells (hMCs) through PI3K/AKT signaling [70].

Microglia are the principal immune cells in the retina which respond to paracrine signals carried by EVs. DM promotes a chronic inflammatory status in the body, which causes polarization of the microglia to the proinflammatory M1 phenotype [71]. Furthermore, M1-polarized microglia accumulate around the capillaries and release EVs, which heighten neuro-inflammation and increase vascular permeability [72, 73]. Beltramo et al. [74] reported a significant increase in inflammatory markers, including chemokine ligand (CCL)-2, matrix metalloproteinase (MMP)-2, and MMP-9, in M1-polarized microglia-derived EVs. A significant increase in the miRNAs related to inflammation and angiogenesis (miR-21 and miR-155) was also marked. Interestingly, exposure of human retinal pericytes (HRPs) and Human retinal endothelial cells (HRECs) to EVs derived from M1-polarized microglia caused a significant increase in their proliferation, apoptosis, migration, and ROS production. In addition, HRPs displayed significant production of IL-1β, IL-6, MMP-9, CCL-2, and VEGF, while HRECs exhibited significant release of TNF-α, angiopoietin (Ang)-2, VEGF, and platelet-derived growth factor (PDGF)-B, when exposed to M1-polarized microglia-derived EVs. Of note, Müller glia cells-derived exosomes were found to aggravate vascular dysfunction under high glucose through exosomal miR-9-3p, which is transferred to retinal endothelial cells and binds to the sphingosine-1-phosphate receptor S1P1 coding sequence, which subsequently activates VEGFR2 phosphorylation [75].

The complement system is a key mechanism deployed by the innate and adaptive immune responses and causes damage to opsonized pathogens and cells via deposition of the membrane attack complex (MAC) on the plasma membrane, resulting in osmotic disturbance and lysis of the target cell [76, 77]. The expression of MAC was marked in the chorio-capillaries and around larger choroidal vessels in patients with DR [78]. This complement-mediated damage is attributed to continuous complement activation, in addition to the lack of complement regulatory proteins on the retinal endothelium [79]. Interestingly, Huang et al. [80, 81] reported robust complement activation in the plasma of diabetic rats by immunoglobulin (Ig) G-enriched EVs. Further, these IgG-laden EVs caused MAC deposition and lysis of HRECs *in vitro*, which was abrogated by the depletion of EVs from the plasma.

4. Role of EVs in angiogenesis

The involvement of EVs in the pathogenesis of DR, particularly in establishing microvascular dysfunction and angiogenesis, has been investigated in numerous studies. Although RPE-derived EVs are believed to induce protective effects in physiological states and during the early stages of DR, EVs originated from stressed ARPE-19 cells enhanced angiogenesis, through upregulation of VEGF receptors on HUVEC cells [82]. A longitudinal cohort study conducted by Wu et al. [83] reported the significant link between EVs levels of VEGF-A, the diabetes situation, and parameters of insulin resistance, in diabetic patients when compared to euglycemic controls. Moreover, when endothelial cells were treated with EVs from diabetic patients, the formation of lamellipodia increased and led to enhanced migration of endothelial cells.

Plasma-derived EVs from patients with DR were capable of inducing retinopathy indices in retinal microvascular *in vitro* models in the form of detachment and migration of pericytes, increased permeability, and new vessel-like structure formation [84]. TNF-α-induced protein 8 (TNFAIP8) was demonstrated in the small EVs (sEVs) isolated from DR patients' plasma and was linked to increased viability, proliferation, migration, and tube formation of HRECs [85].

Circulating EVs were reported to increase in diabetic patients and to induce phenotypic changes similar to those of DR in different study models owing to their bioactive cargoes, especially miRNAs [86]. Free miRNAs in the plasma are liable to degradation by enzymes; however, EVs' lipid membrane protects them [74]. Plasma-derived EVs from patients with DR did not display differences in the surface markers when compared to diabetic patients with no DR or healthy controls; however, microarray analysis revealed significant changes in several miRNAs [84]. One of the important miRNAs reported to promote angiogenesis is miR-30b, which was found to be prominently enriched in plasma-derived EVs and was the most differentially expressed miRNA in the retinal tissues of mice with PDR, compared to control mice. miR-30b exerts its pro-angiogenic effect on retinal microvascular endothelial cells (RMECs) through repression of sirtuin (SIRT)-1; the latter was stated to preserve vascular integrity of the retina and protect against the development of DR in the early phases [87, 88]. Besides, upregulation of miR-30a-5p was recognized in the vitreous specimens of patients diagnosed with PDR [89]. It promotes angiogenesis by enhancing endothelial cells' motility and tube formation [90]. miR-21 was also found to enhance angiogenesis through repression of peroxisome proliferator-activated receptor-α (PPARα) [91]. In addition, the expression of miR-30b-5p, miR-21-3p, and hypoxia-inducible factor (HIF)-1α increased, and that of miR-150-5p decreased in EVs derived from DR patients, compared to healthy controls and diabetic patients with no DR [92]. Noteworthy, miR-150 was stated to inhibit the migration of endothelial cells (ECs) through inhibition of numerous angiogenic factors [93].

Pericytes regulate the blood capillaries tone, control the interchange of molecules between the blood and the neuroretina, and limit the proliferation and motility of ECs; thus, their loss leads to the development of angiogenesis, which is a key mechanism in the early stages of DR [94]. EVs control the interplay between pericytes and ECs in DR, where circular RNA (circRNA) cPWWP2A is shuttled from pericytes to ECs by EVs, inducing retinal vascular malformations through enhanced expression of Ang-1, occludin, and SIRT-1 [95]; however, a protective role of Ang-1 in DR has been described [96]. EVs derived from microglia and photoreceptors were reported to increase in the vitreous of PDR patients and were found to promote ECs proliferation and angiogenesis [97]. Maisto et al. [98, 99] demonstrated a decrease in the anti-angiogenic miRNAs (miR-20a-3p, miR-20a-5p, miR-20b, and miR-106a-5p), together with increased expression of VEGF in retinal photoreceptors/ARPE-19 cells and their derived EVs, when challenged with high glucose.

The role of MVs in the development of DR was summarized by Zhang et al. [46], where the diabetic milieu causes MVs of platelet origin to activate MMPs, which cause mitochondrial damage and release of cytochrome c, which in turn enhances apoptosis of capillary endothelial cells and consequently, capillary hypoxia, which

Source of EVs		Method of isolation and/or purification	Role of EVs in DR	Refs.
Extraocular cell-derived EVs	Plasma	Isolated by ultracentrifugation and purified by OptiPrep Density Gradient	Circulating IgG-laden exosomes are responsible for the activation of the complement cascade that subsequently upregulates proinflammatory cytokines and chemokines and causes MAC deposition and lysis of HRECs *in vitro*.	[80, 81]
		Isolated using total exosome isolation reagent for cell culture media	Plasma-EVs transferred miR-30b to retinal microvascular endothelial cells (RMECs), where miR-30b increases VEGF expression by downregulating SIRT1. This enhances angiogenesis and proliferative DR.	[87]
	Platelet-rich plasma (PRP)	Isolated by ultracentrifugation	Hyperglycemia elevates the level of circulating PRP-Exos which activates the TLR4 pathway through the release of CXCL10. This led to endothelial injury and dysfunction in early DR.	[69]
		Isolated by ultracentrifugation	Platelet rich plasma derived exosomes in hyperglycemia enhance both the proliferation and fibrogenic activity of Müller cells through PI3K/AKT signaling.	[70]
	Pancreatic β cells	Isolated using total exosome isolation reagent for cell culture media	Exposing Müller cells to exosomes derived from pancreatic β-cells under high-glucose conditions caused miR-15a overexpression in Müller cells and increased the oxidative stress and apoptotic cell death.	[103]

Source of EVs		Method of isolation and/or purification	Role of EVs in DR	Refs.
Intraocular cell-derived EVs	Retinal pigment epithelial (RPE) cells	Isolated by multi-step differential centrifugation	Exosomes derived from RPE cells under oxidative stress increased Apaf1 expression, so oxidative injury and cell apoptosis increased.	[66]
		Isolated using total exosome isolation reagent for cell culture media	RPE cells cultured in a high glucose level led to ROS formation and release of VEGF containing exosomes.	[99]
	Retinal Astrocytes (RACs)	Isolated by ultra centrifugation	Apoptosis and autophagy levels in RACs were positively correlated with the oxidative stress level, and the exosomes generated from RACs under oxidative stress condition. These exosomes can promote endothelial cell proliferation, migration, and tube formation.	[57]
	Retinal Photoreceptor	Isolated using total exosomes isolation reagent	High glucose increased VEGF levels and decreased anti-angiogenic miR-20a-3p, miR-20a-5p, miR-106a-5p, and miR-20b expression in retinal photoreceptor-derived EVs due to ROS-induced NF-κB signaling.	[98]
	Müller glia cells	Isolated using ultracentrifugation	Müller glia-derived exosomes aggravate vascular dysfunction under high glucose, through exosomal miRNA-9-3p which is transferred to retinal endothelial cells and binds to the sphingosine-1-phosphate receptor S1P1 coding sequence, with subsequent activation of VEGFR2 phosphorylation.	[75]
	Retinal Pericytes	Not mentioned	Pericytes transferred cPWWP2A, miR-579, and angiopoietin 1/occludin/SIRT1 to endothelial cells by exosomes. These transferred materials induced retinal vascular dysfunction.	[95]

Table 1.
Role of EVs in the initiation and progression of the pathogenesis of DR.

leads to NV over time. MVs of monocyte origin were claimed to cause damage to RPE, compromising the barrier function and increasing the permeability. Noteworthy, monocyte-derived MVs were the most prominent during the transition of DR from the non-proliferative to the proliferative stage, where abnormal leaky blood vessels are formed [100].

Significantly, mesenchymal stem cells (MSCs) were established to contribute to the homeostasis and the pathology of different tissues, including the retina, through the paracrine effect of EVs [101]. Beltramo et al. [102] reported that HRPs display enhanced detachment when exposed to EVs isolated from MSCs, which were grown in high glucose and/or hypoxia to mimic diabetic conditions, regardless of the origin of MSCs. The detached cells were viable and were able to re-attach again, suggesting that these cells tend to localize in the walls of the newly formed vessels for stabilization. They also described increased permeability of the blood barrier, and enhanced formation of vessel-like structures in HRP/EC co-cultures on Matrigels when treated with the same EVs. Moreover, they attributed the effect of MSCs-derived EVs on HRPs and ECs to the active form of MMP-2, which causes degradation of the proteins in the extracellular matrix, facilitating pericyte loss and angiogenesis. Interestingly, pancreatic β cells were proved to release EVs rich in miR-15a, which spread to distant sites and promote DR through induction of oxidative stress and apoptosis in Müller cells [103].

It is worth mentioning that procoagulant MVs in patients with DR correlate with the duration of diabetes [104]. Phosphatidyl serine (PS)-positive MVs are linked to enhanced coagulant activity in patients with PDR and NPDR [105]. Additionally, endothelial-derived MVs are considered a risk factor for the development of thromboembolic DR [106]. The roles of EVs in the initiation and progression of DR are summarized in **Table 1**.

5. How can EVs help in the diagnosis of DR?

The clinical diagnosis of DR is challenging since the disease is asymptomatic during the early stages. Development of symptoms in the form of blurred vision may occur with more progressive pathology [86]. Given that EVs reflect the molecular profile of the parent cells and the important role played by EVs, particularly the miRNAs shuttled by EVs in the pathophysiology of DR [107], it appeared valuable to use them as diagnostic biomarkers. Several studies aimed at the detection of EVs-miRNAs exclusive to DR.

As mentioned before, cPWWP2A circRNA is shuttled by EVs derived from pericytes in DR, and it is thought to have a protective role in refining pericytes-endothelial cells communication and amelioration of vascular pathology. This circRNA can be used as a diagnostic biomarker [95]. Likewise, EVs positive for miR-15a [103], IgG [108], or TNFAIP8 [85], all can be used for the diagnosis of DR. EVs with increased expression of miR-30b-5p, miR-21-3p, miR-26b-5p, or decreased expression of miR-150-5p were identified in the sera of DR patients [92, 109]. Additionally, EVs carrying CCR-5 can be used to detect NPDR progression [67]. Remarkably, Mighty et al. [110] confirmed the expression of junction plakoglobin protein (JUP) in the EVs isolated from retinal tissue explants and urine of DR patients but not in healthy controls. This was the first study to provide a novel non-invasive diagnosis for DR through urinary specimens. **Table 2** shows examples of EV-derived cargoes that could be used as biomarkers for DR.

EVs marker	Origin	Role	Reference
cPWWP2A	Pericytes	Refining pericytes-endothelial cells communication and amelioration of vascular pathology	[95]
miR-15a	Pancreatic β cells	Induction of oxidative stress and apoptosis in Müller cells	[103]
IgG	Plasma of diabetic rats	Robust complement activation MAC deposition and lysis of HRECs *in vitro*	[80]
TNFAIP8	Plasma of DR patients	Increased viability, proliferation, migration, and tube formation of HRECs	[85]
CCR-5	Plasma of DR patients	Regulates trafficking and effector functions of immune cells NPDR progression	[67]
JUP	Retinal tissue explants and urine of DR patients	Early screening biomarker for DR diagnosis	[110]

Table 2.
Examples of EVs cargoes that could serve as potential biomarkers for DR.

Interestingly, some studies have proved the effectiveness of certain miRNAs as diagnostic markers; however, these studies did not consider their expression in EVs. For instance, miR-181c, miR-21, and miR-1179 were reported to increase significantly in the sera of PDR patients when compared to NPDR patients [111]. Detection of such miRNAs in serum EVs may provide higher diagnostic values. Similarly, Friedrich et al. [112] found higher levels of six miRNAs in the vitreous of PDR patients when compared to non-diabetic patients namely, hsa-miR-23b-3p, hsa-miR-20a-5p, hsa-miR-142-3p, hsa-miR-185-5p, hsa-miR-362-5p, and has-miR-326. The first one, hsa-miR-23b-3p, was found to be downregulated in anti-VEGF-treated patients in comparison to non-treated PDR patients. On the other hand, miR-126 decreased in DR patients and could serve as a diagnostic biomarker for PDR [113]. We recommend conducting future studies to verify the expression of these miRNAs in circulating EVs, which might spot the time of alteration in their levels and allow their use as diagnostic and prognostic markers through non-invasive sampling procedures.

6. Are EVs a promising new therapeutic tool for DR?

Impairment and loss of vision are unavoidable if DR is left untreated. During the initial stages, proper control of blood glucose levels may prevent the deterioration of the disease. Treatment of hypertension and hyperlipidemia is also important; however, medical intervention is necessary in the late stages. Anti-VEGF, corticosteroids, lipid-lowering drugs, argon laser photocoagulation, and vitrectomy are commonly used, as reviewed by Martins et al. [86]. Immunotherapy such as anti-TNF-α and anti-IL-1β are being tested [114, 115]. Although current interventions may help prevent or delay the sequelae of the disease, lack of curative treatment, adverse reactions, and ineffectiveness of these regimens in some patients are still considerable challenges [116]. Therefore, it is important to seek novel and more tolerable therapies, such as EVs, which can deliver many factors including miRNAs and medications to the retina, in addition to enhancing the efficacy of certain drugs (**Figure 4**) [117].

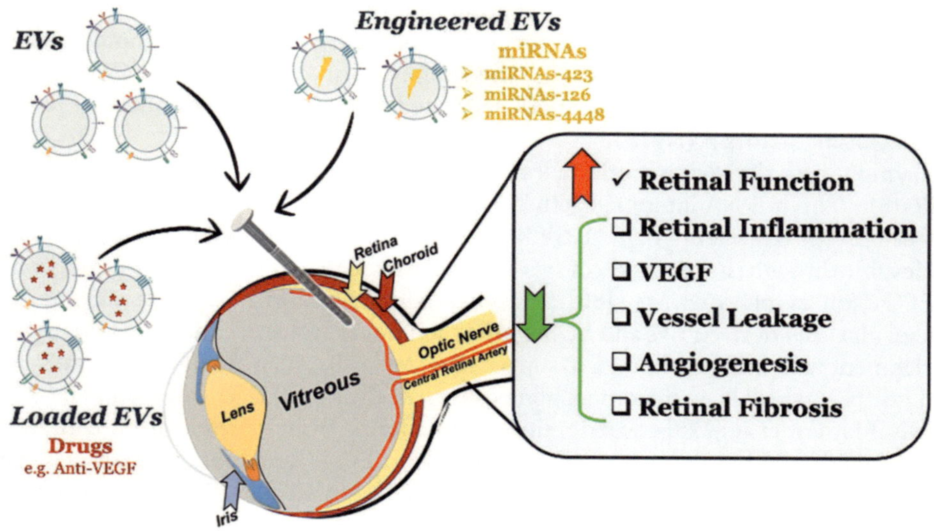

Figure 4.
EVs derived from intra- or extra-ocular sources can be used as a therapy for DR directly, as a drug delivery nanocarrier, or engineered EVs with elevated levels of targeted miRNAs.

Intriguingly, intraocular injection of exosomes derived from rabbit adipose tissue MSCs in diabetic rabbits resulted in well-organized retinal layers. The link between increased miR-222 in MSCs-derived exosomes and the regenerative events in the retina was highlighted [118]. In addition, Zhang and colleagues [119], used umbilical cord MSCs-derived exosomes as a vehicle for miR-126. Intravitreal injection of these exosomes in diabetic rats suppressed retinal inflammation. The authors confirmed the role of miR-126-over expression in MSCs-derived exosomes in the reduction of high-mobility group box (HMGB)-1 and inflammasome, which resulted in amelioration of retinal inflammation. Gu et al. [120] reported that MSCs-derived EVs, which shuttle miR-192, ameliorated retinal inflammation and angiogenesis. Reddy et al. [121] reported that intravitreal injection of MSCs-derived sEVs loaded with anti-VEGF caused prolonged inhibition of VEGF and leukostasis and decreased exudates in diabetic rats for more than 2 months following injection, supporting the value of sEVs as drug delivery system. Furthermore, the anti-oxidant and anti-apoptotic effect of MSCs-derived EVs was reported in an animal model of DR. The *in vitro* experiments attributed this therapeutic effect to neuronal precursor cell-expressed developmentally downregulated 4 (NEDD4), which regulates PTEN/AKT/NRF2 pathway [122]. On the other hand, EVs derived from MSCs, which were grown in high glucose, were claimed to accelerate vascular dysfunction [102]; therefore, the use of MSCs-derived EVs in the treatment of DR needs more extensive studies.

Interestingly, exosomes derived from retinal astroglial cells (RACs), but not from RPE, inhibited vessel leakage and choroidal neovascularization (CNV) in a laser-induced CNV model. These anti-angiogenic properties may be useful when applied in DR models [123]. RPE-derived exosomes were found to inhibit endothelial-to-mesenchymal transition (EMT) and retinal fibrosis due to their miR-202-5p content, which inhibits transforming growth factor/Smad signaling [124]. Of note, our study showed that RPE-treated with homocysteine, which is reported as a risk factor for retinopathies, released exosomes with micro-RNA cargo close to the miRs profile noticed in the diabetic mouse retina, such as miR-17, let-7, and miR-122 [61]. Recently, Huang et al. [125] analyzed sEVs derived from human embryonic stem cell-derived retinal organoids (hERO-RPCs) and found them to delay the degeneration of photoreceptors, inhibit gliosis of Müller glia cells, and support retinal functions in RCS rats. They attributed these effects to miRNA-mediated downregulation of nuclear factor I transcription factors B (NFIB).

Lymphocyte-derived microparticles (LMPs) were found to contain high levels of miR-181a. This miRNA interferes with VEGF signaling in HREC; therefore, it could be used for the treatment of DR [126]. Besides, control of complement activation was achievable through the exclusion of IgG-laden plasma EVs, which led to the protection of the ECs from cytolytic damage [80]. A recent study by Lamb et al. [127] investigated the Müller glia cells-derived EVs and highlighted their neuroprotective functions through enrichment with miRNAs known to support the stem cells, such as miR-21 and miR-16, and miRNAs which keep the retinal homeostasis; such as miR-125b, miR-9, and let-7 family. Mathew et al. [128] treated retinal cells suffering from ischemic insult with functionally engineered EVs overexpressing miR-424 (FEE424), and found them to achieve anti-inflammatory and neuroprotective functions. They also used FEE424 in an animal model of retinal ischemia and reported that retinal functions were restored.

Other miRNAs were confirmed to have a protective effect on the retinal tissue. For instance, Shaker et al. [129] found that miR-20b and miR-17-3p decrease significantly in the sera of both PDR and NPDR patients, in comparison to healthy controls. miR-20b and miR-17-3p are believed to regulate the expression of HIF-1α and VEGF-A genes. Another study reported downregulation of four miRNAs in the sera of DR patients namely, miR-338-3p, miR-4448, miR-9-5p, and miR-485-5p [130]. These miRNAs regulate inflammation, oxidative stress, and angiogenesis through the regulation of dozens of genes. miR-200b expression in different DR animal models revealed controversial results; nevertheless, McArthur et al. [131] reported its decrease in the retinas and endothelial cells of diabetic rats and linked this decrease to enhanced VEGF expression. Blum et al. [132] confirmed the link between decreased levels of miRNA-423 and increased levels of VEGF in the sera of DR patients. Also, Qin et al. [113] highlighted miR-126 lower levels in DR patients. While EVs were not included in these studies, it is possible to establish a drug delivery system using those EVs to deliver such deficient miRNAs.

In contrast, some studies reported higher values of certain miRNAs in DR patients without the inclusion of EVs in these studies. For example, miR-181c, miR-21, and miR-1179 were proven to increase the sera of DR patients and were known to play important roles in ischemia and angiogenesis [111]. Using EVs as vehicles to deliver such deficient miRNAs may be a valuable drug delivery tool in DR. Sun et al. [133] developed engineered MSCs-EVs with increased levels of miR-5068 and miR-10228 as therapeutic molecules. They used both MSCs-EVs and engineered ones to treat two diabetic animal models, including db/db mice and STZ-induced diabetic rats. The presence of miR-5068 and miR-10228 in both EVs targeted the HIF-1α/EZH2/PGC-1α pathway. However, the engineered MSCs-EVs showed more enhanced retinal repair efficiency than MSCs-EVs.

7. Challenges and future recommendations

The therapeutic potential of EVs requires the construction of clinical-grade EVs, where enormous quantities, in addition to preserved phenotypes, are necessary. As different cell culture procedures aim at increasing the harvest, such as using different stimuli to expand the production or using 3D culture technology, the phenotype of the cultured cells and, consequently, their EVs may change [134]. Passage of the cultured cells, media composition, and oxygen levels could affect the cells/EVs number and quality [135]. The use of the third to fifth passage was recommended to preserve consistency in MSCs [136]. Regarding media composition, while fetal bovine serum was found to influence the behavior of cells, serum-free media changed the protein content of EVs [137]. Platelet lysate with an EV-depleted medium was reported to preserve the phenotype of MSCs and the RNA profile of their EVs [138].

Another challenge is the isolation of EVs. Although several techniques are available, there is no standardized technique for isolation of clinical-grade EVs. Low yield in ultracentrifugation, low purity, or chemical contamination in the other techniques interfere with their use in such settings [50]. Ultrafiltration followed by size exclusion chromatography was confirmed to obtain a higher yield of EVs and preserve their phenotype [139, 140]. Cryopreservation using glycerol and dimethyl sulfoxide (DMSO) was found to disintegrate EVs [141]. Using phosphate-buffered saline (PBS) was reported to form calcium nanoparticles, which intervene with quantification of EVs [142]. Concerning the temperature of storage, different studies reported different results, such as −20 or −80° C [141, 143]. To extend the shelf life and decrease the cost, lyophilization was proposed, with a storage temperature of 4°C [144].

Directing EVs to specific cells is another challenge. While the factors that control the targeting of EVs to certain cells are not fully described, surface molecules, the physiological status of the target cells, and the route of administration play important roles in the process [50, 118]. Using certain labels to track EVs was confirmed to enhance their targeting of certain cells [145, 146]. Improving the therapeutic properties of EVs to reach the target cells is required to decrease the dose or the frequency of administration. Priming, loading, engineering, artificial EVs, and bio nanotechnology were developed for that purpose [147].

Finally, the safety of EV-based therapy is crucial. Although cell therapy may induce tumorigenesis, EVs have been shown to be well tolerated in several animal models. Immunogenicity and toxicity monitoring in humans must be extensively studied [53].

8. Conclusion

DR is a neurovascular disease where different retinal cells may be involved in pathophysiological changes occurring throughout the disease course. Retinal endothelial cells exposed to high glucose levels during diabetes may send early warning messages to other retinal cells, initiating various signaling pathways via endothelial-derived EVs. Retinal Müller glia cells, as important master regulators of retinal homeostasis, may talk to other retinal cells via EVs, trying to fight against the high-glucose-induced retinal injury. Other retinal cells may use this salient method of communication to synergize their actions during the disease. Understanding these EVs-carried messages may help in understanding a more detailed picture of the process of DR development. That is why EVs are promising new tools that could carry novel biomarkers for early diagnosis and prognosis of DR. EVs have been used recently as an encouraging drug delivery method in cases of DR. The field of EVs is an emerging area of research that still needs more extensive studies to portray a thorough understanding of EVs' retinal trafficking, various cargoes, isolation purity, proper characterization, and therapeutic safety.

Acknowledgements

Dr. Khaled Elmasry would like to thank Augusta University, Augusta, GA, USA, for the start-up fund.

Conflict of interest

The authors have no conflict of interest to declare.

Author details

Samar Habib[1,2,3], Alaa M. Mansour[1,4], Babak Baban[1,2] and Khaled Elmasry[1,2,5,6]*

1 Department of Oral Biology and Diagnostic Sciences, The Dental College of Georgia, Augusta University, Augusta, GA, USA

2 DCG Center for Excellence in Research, Scholarship, and Innovation (CERSI), Augusta University, Augusta, GA, USA

3 Mansoura Faculty of Medicine, Department of Medical Parasitology, Mansoura University, Mansoura, Egypt

4 Faculty of Dentistry, Department of Oral Biology, Mansoura University, Mansoura, Egypt

5 Department of Cellular Biology and Anatomy, The Medical College of Georgia, Augusta University, Augusta, GA, USA

6 Mansoura Faculty of Medicine, Department of Human Anatomy and Embryology, Mansoura University, Mansoura, Egypt

*Address all correspondence to: khelmasry@augusta.edu; elmasryretina@gmail.com

References

[1] Frank RN. Diabetic retinopathy. New England Journal of Medicine. 2004;**350**(1):48-58

[2] Gomulka K, Ruta M. The role of inflammation and therapeutic concepts in diabetic retinopathy-a short review. International Journal of Molecular Sciences. 2023;**24**(2):1024

[3] Altmann C, Schmidt MHH. The role of microglia in diabetic retinopathy: Inflammation, microvasculature defects and neurodegeneration. International Journal of Molecular Sciences. 2018;**19**(1):110

[4] Kowluru RA. Cross talks between oxidative stress, inflammation and epigenetics in diabetic retinopathy. Cells. 2023;**12**(2):300

[5] Ola MS, Nawaz MI, Khan HA, Alhomida AS. Neurodegeneration and neuroprotection in diabetic retinopathy. International Journal of Molecular Sciences. 2013;**14**(2):2559-2572

[6] Chew EY, Davis MD, Danis RP, Lovato JF, Perdue LH, Greven C, et al. The effects of medical management on the progression of diabetic retinopathy in persons with type 2 diabetes: The action to control cardiovascular risk in diabetes (ACCORD) eye study. Ophthalmology. 2014;**121**(12):2443-2451

[7] Lachin JM, Genuth S, Nathan DM, Zinman B, Rutledge BN. Effect of glycemic exposure on the risk of microvascular complications in the diabetes control and complications trial--revisited. Diabetes. 2008;**57**(4):995-1001

[8] Yau JW, Rogers SL, Kawasaki R, Lamoureux EL, Kowalski JW, Bek T, et al. Global prevalence and major risk factors of diabetic retinopathy. Diabetes Care. 2012;**35**(3):556-564

[9] Arar NH, Freedman BI, Adler SG, Iyengar SK, Chew EY, Davis MD, et al. Heritability of the severity of diabetic retinopathy: The FIND-eye study. Investigative Ophthalmology & Visual Science. 2008;**49**(9):3839-3845

[10] Vujosevic S, Aldington SJ, Silva P, Hernandez C, Scanlon P, Peto T, et al. Screening for diabetic retinopathy: New perspectives and challenges. The Lancet Diabetes and Endocrinology. 2020;**8**(4):337-347

[11] Whitehead M, Wickremasinghe S, Osborne A, Van Wijngaarden P, Martin KR. Diabetic retinopathy: A complex pathophysiology requiring novel therapeutic strategies. Expert Opinion on Biological Therapy. 2018;**18**(12):1257-1270

[12] Yuuki T, Kanda T, Kimura Y, Kotajima N, Ji T, Kobayashi I, et al. Inflammatory cytokines in vitreous fluid and serum of patients with diabetic vitreoretinopathy. Journal of Diabetes and its Complications. 2001;**15**(5):257-259

[13] Rübsam A, Parikh S, Fort PE. Role of inflammation in diabetic retinopathy. International Journal of Molecular Sciences. 2018;**19**(4):942

[14] Kowluru RA, Kowluru A, Mishra M, Kumar B. Oxidative stress and epigenetic modifications in the pathogenesis of diabetic retinopathy. Progress in Retinal and Eye Research. 2015;**48**:40-61

[15] Tang L, Xu GT, Zhang JF. Inflammation in diabetic retinopathy: Possible roles in pathogenesis and

potential implications for therapy. Neural Regeneration Research. 2023;**18**(5):976-982

[16] Wang W, Lo ACY. Diabetic retinopathy: Pathophysiology and treatments. International Journal of Molecular Sciences. 2018;**19**(6):1816

[17] Tang L, Zhang C, Lu L, Tian H, Liu K, Luo D, et al. Melatonin maintains inner blood-retinal barrier by regulating microglia via inhibition of PI3K/Akt/Stat3/NF-κB signaling pathways in experimental diabetic retinopathy. Frontiers in Immunology. 2022;**13**:831660

[18] Tan TE, Finkelstein MT, Tan GSW, Tan ACS, Chan CM, Mathur R, et al. Retinal neural dysfunction in diabetes revealed with handheld chromatic pupillometry. Clinical & Experimental Ophthalmology. 2022;**50**(7):745-756

[19] Kowluru RA, Mishra M. Chapter three—Regulation of matrix metalloproteinase in the pathogenesis of diabetic retinopathy. In: Khalil RA, editor. Progress in Molecular Biology and Translational Science. 148: Academic Press; 2017. pp. 67-85

[20] Tan TE, Wong TY. Diabetic retinopathy: Looking forward to 2030. Frontiers in Endocrinology (Lausanne). 2022;**13**:1077669

[21] Chen X, Nie C, Gong Y, Zhang Y, Jin X, Wei S, et al. Peripapillary retinal nerve fiber layer changes in preclinical diabetic retinopathy: A meta-analysis. PLoS One. 2015;**10**(5):e0125919

[22] Sohn EH, van Dijk HW, Jiao C, Kok PH, Jeong W, Demirkaya N, et al. Retinal neurodegeneration may precede microvascular changes characteristic of diabetic retinopathy in diabetes mellitus. Proceedings of the National Academy of Sciences of the United States of America. 2016;**113**(19):E2655-E2664

[23] Elmasry K, Habib S, Moustafa M, Al-Shabrawey M. Bone morphogenetic proteins and diabetic retinopathy. Biomolecules. 2021;**11**(4):593

[24] Mansour SE, Browning DJ, Wong K, Flynn HW Jr, Bhavsar AR. The evolving treatment of diabetic retinopathy. Clinical Ophthalmology. 2020;**14**:653-678

[25] Jeong S, Ku SK, Bae JS. Anti-inflammatory effects of pelargonidin on TGFBIp-induced responses. Canadian Journal of Physiology and Pharmacology. 2017;**95**(4):372-381

[26] Wells JA, Glassman AR, Ayala AR, Jampol LM, Bressler NM, Bressler SB, et al. Aflibercept, bevacizumab, or ranibizumab for diabetic macular edema: Two-year results from a comparative effectiveness randomized clinical trial. Ophthalmology. 2016;**123**(6):1351-1359

[27] Brown DM, Wykoff CC, Boyer D, Heier JS, Clark WL, Emanuelli A, et al. Evaluation of intravitreal aflibercept for the treatment of severe nonproliferative diabetic retinopathy: Results from the PANORAMA randomized clinical trial. JAMA Ophthalmology. 2021;**139**(9):946-955

[28] Wykoff CC, Eichenbaum DA, Roth DB, Hill L, Fung AE, Haskova Z. Ranibizumab induces regression of diabetic retinopathy in Most patients at high risk of progression to proliferative diabetic retinopathy. Ophthalmology Retina. 2018;**2**(10):997-1009

[29] Maturi RK, Glassman AR, Josic K, Antoszyk AN, Blodi BA, Jampol LM, et al. Effect of intravitreous anti-vascular endothelial growth factor vs sham treatment for prevention of vision-threatening complications of diabetic retinopathy: The protocol W randomized clinical trial. JAMA Ophthalmology. 2021;**139**(7):701-712

[30] Filho JA, Messias A, Almeida FP, Ribeiro JA, Costa RA, Scott IU, et al. Panretinal photocoagulation (PRP) versus PRP plus intravitreal ranibizumab for high-risk proliferative diabetic retinopathy. Acta Ophthalmologica. 2011;**89**(7):e567-e572

[31] Raman R, Swathipriya N, Sripriya S. Gene therapy in diabetic retinopathy. In: Genetics of Ocular Diseases. Singapore: Springer; 2022. pp. 187-194

[32] Han J, Lando L, Skowronska-Krawczyk D, Chao DL. Genetics of diabetic retinopathy. Current Diabetes Reports. 2019;**19**:1-8

[33] Raposo G, Stoorvogel W. Extracellular vesicles: Exosomes, microvesicles, and friends. The Journal of Cell Biology. 2013;**200**(4):373-383

[34] Bettio V, Mazzucco E, Antona A, Cracas S, Varalda M, Venetucci J, et al. Extracellular vesicles from human plasma for biomarkers discovery: Impact of anticoagulants and isolation techniques. PLoS One. 2023;**18**(5):e0285440

[35] Liu YJ, Wang C. A review of the regulatory mechanisms of extracellular vesicles-mediated intercellular communication. Cell Communication and Signaling: CCS. 2023;**21**(1):77

[36] Van Niel G, d'Angelo G, Raposo G. Shedding light on the cell biology of extracellular vesicles. Nature Reviews Molecular Cell Biology. 2018;**19**(4):213-228

[37] Zaborowski MP, Balaj L, Breakefield XO, Lai CP. Extracellular vesicles: Composition, biological relevance, and methods of study. Bioscience. 2015;**65**(8):783-797

[38] Chaudhary PK, Kim S, Kim S. Shedding light on the cell biology of platelet-derived extracellular vesicles and their biomedical applications. Life (Basel). 2023;**13**(6):1403

[39] Wollert T, Hurley JH. Molecular mechanism of multivesicular body biogenesis by ESCRT complexes. Nature. 2010;**464**(7290):864-869

[40] Trajkovic K, Hsu C, Chiantia S, Rajendran L, Wenzel D, Wieland F, et al. Ceramide triggers budding of exosome vesicles into multivesicular endosomes. Science. 2008;**319**(5867):1244-1247

[41] Sinha A, Ignatchenko V, Ignatchenko A, Mejia-Guerrero S, Kislinger T. In-depth proteomic analyses of ovarian cancer cell line exosomes reveals differential enrichment of functional categories compared to the NCI 60 proteome. Biochemical and Biophysical Research Communications. 2014;**445**(4):694-701

[42] Mobius W, Ohno-Iwashita Y, van Donselaar EG, Oorschot VM, Shimada Y, Fujimoto T, et al. Immunoelectron microscopic localization of cholesterol using biotinylated and non-cytolytic perfringolysin O. The Journal of Histochemistry and Cytochemistry. 2002;**50**(1):43-55

[43] Simons M, Raposo G. Exosomes--vesicular carriers for intercellular communication. Current Opinion in Cell Biology. 2009;**21**(4):575-581

[44] Chen H, Wang L, Zeng X, Schwarz H, Nanda HS, Peng X, et al. Exosomes, a new star for targeted delivery. Frontiers in Cell and Development Biology. 2021;**9**:751079

[45] Cai H, Reinisch K, Ferro-Novick S. Coats, tethers, rabs, and SNARES work together to mediate the intracellular destination of a transport vesicle. Developmental Cell. 2007;**12**(5):671-682

[46] Zhang W, Chen S, Liu ML. Pathogenic roles of microvesicles in diabetic retinopathy. Acta Pharmacologica Sinica. 2018;**39**(1):1-11

[47] Hristov M, Erl W, Linder S, Weber PC. Apoptotic bodies from endothelial cells enhance the number and initiate the differentiation of human endothelial progenitor cells in vitro. Blood. 2004;**104**(9):2761-2766

[48] Thery C, Boussac M, Veron P, Ricciardi-Castagnoli P, Raposo G, Garin J, et al. Proteomic analysis of dendritic cell-derived exosomes: A secreted subcellular compartment distinct from apoptotic vesicles. Journal of Immunology. 2001;**166**(12):7309-7318

[49] Doyle LM, Wang MZ. Overview of extracellular vesicles, their origin, composition, purpose, and methods for exosome isolation and analysis. Cells. 2019;**8**(7):727

[50] Hu W, Song X, Yu H, Sun J, Zhao Y. Therapeutic potentials of extracellular vesicles for the treatment of diabetes and diabetic complications. International Journal of Molecular Sciences. 2020;**21**(14):5163

[51] van der Pol E, Boing AN, Harrison P, Sturk A, Nieuwland R. Classification, functions, and clinical relevance of extracellular vesicles. Pharmacological Reviews. 2012;**64**(3):676-705

[52] Lv Y, Tan J, Miao Y, Zhang Q. The role of microvesicles and its active molecules in regulating cellular biology. Journal of Cellular and Molecular Medicine. 2019;**23**(12):7894-7904

[53] Sun F, Xu W, Qian H. The emerging role of extracellular vesicles in retinal diseases. American Journal of Translational Research. 2021;**13**(12):13227-13245

[54] Helwa I, Cai J, Drewry MD, Zimmerman A, Dinkins MB, Khaled ML, et al. A comparative study of serum exosome isolation using differential ultracentrifugation and three commercial reagents. PLoS One. 2017;**12**(1):e0170628

[55] Massoumi H, Amin S, Soleimani M, Momenaei B, Ashraf MJ, Guaiquil VH, et al. Extracellular-vesicle-based therapeutics in neuro-ophthalmic disorders. International Journal of Molecular Sciences. 2023;**24**(10):9006

[56] Zoller M. Tetraspanins: Push and pull in suppressing and promoting metastasis. Nature Reviews: Cancer. 2009;**9**(1):40-55

[57] Zhu L, Zang J, Liu B, Yu G, Hao L, Liu L, et al. Oxidative stress-induced RAC autophagy can improve the HUVEC functions by releasing exosomes. Journal of Cellular Physiology. 2020;**235**(10):7392-7409

[58] Jung MK, Mun JY. Sample preparation and imaging of exosomes by transmission electron microscopy. Journal of Visualized Experiments. 2018;**131**:56482

[59] Ibrahim SA, Khan YS. Histology, extracellular vesicles. In: StatPearls. Treasure Island (Florida) ineligible companies. Disclosure: Yusuf Khan declares no relevant financial relationships with ineligible companies; 2024

[60] Tokarz A, Szuscik I, Kusnierz-Cabala B, Kapusta M, Konkolewska M, Zurakowski A, et al. Extracellular vesicles participate in the transport of cytokines and angiogenic factors in diabetic patients with ocular complications. Folia Medica Cracoviensia. 2015;**55**(4):35-48

[61] Elmasry K, Mohamed R, Sharma I, Elsherbiny NM, Liu Y, Al-Shabrawey M, et al. Epigenetic modifications in

hyperhomocysteinemia: Potential role in diabetic retinopathy and age-related macular degeneration. Oncotarget. 2018;**9**(16):12562-12590

[62] Bastiaans J, van Meurs JC, Mulder VC, Nagtzaam NM, Smits-te Nijenhuis M, Dufour-van den Goorbergh DC, et al. The role of thrombin in proliferative vitreoretinopathy. Investigative Ophthalmology & Visual Science. 2014;**55**(7):4659-4666

[63] Vitkova V, Zivny J, Janota J. Endothelial cell-derived microvesicles: Potential mediators and biomarkers of pathologic processes. Biomarkers in Medicine. 2018;**12**(2):161-175

[64] Huang H, Gandhi JK, Zhong X, Wei Y, Gong J, Duh EJ, et al. TNFalpha is required for late BRB breakdown in diabetic retinopathy, and its inhibition prevents leukostasis and protects vessels and neurons from apoptosis. Investigative Ophthalmology & Visual Science. 2011;**52**(3):1336-1344

[65] Jansen F, Yang X, Franklin BS, Hoelscher M, Schmitz T, Bedorf J, et al. High glucose condition increases NADPH oxidase activity in endothelial microparticles that promote vascular inflammation. Cardiovascular Research. 2013;**98**(1):94-106

[66] Ke Y, Fan X, Rui H, Xinjun R, Dejia W, Chuanzhen Z, et al. Exosomes derived from RPE cells under oxidative stress mediate inflammation and apoptosis of normal RPE cells through Apaf1/caspase-9 axis. Journal of Cellular Biochemistry. 2020;**121**(12):4849-4861

[67] Tokarz A, Konkolewska M, Kusnierz-Cabala B, Maziarz B, Hanarz P, Zurakowski A, et al. Retinopathy severity correlates with RANTES concentrations and CCR 5-positive microvesicles in diabetes. Folia Medica Cracoviensia. 2019;**59**(3):95-112

[68] Jansen F, Wang H, Przybilla D, Franklin BS, Dolf A, Pfeifer P, et al. Vascular endothelial microparticles-incorporated microRNAs are altered in patients with diabetes mellitus. Cardiovascular Diabetology. 2016;**15**:49

[69] Zhang W, Dong X, Wang T, Kong Y. Exosomes derived from platelet-rich plasma mediate hyperglycemia-induced retinal endothelial injury via targeting the TLR4 signaling pathway. Experimental Eye Research. 2019;**189**:107813

[70] Zhang W, Jiang H, Kong Y. Exosomes derived from platelet-rich plasma activate YAP and promote the fibrogenic activity of muller cells via the PI3K/Akt pathway. Experimental Eye Research. 2020;**193**:107973

[71] Arroba AI, Valverde AM. Modulation of microglia in the retina: New insights into diabetic retinopathy. Acta Diabetologica. 2017;**54**(6):527-533

[72] Madeira MH, Boia R, Santos PF, Ambrosio AF, Santiago AR. Contribution of microglia-mediated neuroinflammation to retinal degenerative diseases. Mediators of Inflammation. 2015;**2015**:673090

[73] Aires ID, Ribeiro-Rodrigues T, Boia R, Catarino S, Girao H, Ambrosio AF, et al. Exosomes derived from microglia exposed to elevated pressure amplify the neuroinflammatory response in retinal cells. Glia. 2020;**68**(12):2705-2724

[74] Beltramo E, Mazzeo A, Porta M. Release of pro-inflammatory/angiogenic factors by retinal microvascular cells is mediated by extracellular vesicles derived from M1-activated microglia.

International Journal of Molecular Sciences. 2023;**25**(1):15

[75] Liu Y, Yang Q, Fu H, Wang J, Yuan S, Li X, et al. Muller glia-derived exosomal miR-9-3p promotes angiogenesis by restricting sphingosine-1-phosphate receptor S1P(1) in diabetic retinopathy. Molecular Therapy - Nucleic Acids. 2022;**27**:491-504

[76] Merle NS, Church SE, Fremeaux-Bacchi V, Roumenina LT. Complement system part I—Molecular mechanisms of activation and regulation. Frontiers in Immunology. 2015;**6**:262

[77] Merle NS, Noe R, Halbwachs-Mecarelli L, Fremeaux-Bacchi V, Roumenina LT. Complement system part II: Role in immunity. Frontiers in Immunology. 2015;**6**:257

[78] Gerl VB, Bohl J, Pitz S, Stoffelns B, Pfeiffer N, Bhakdi S. Extensive deposits of complement C3d and C5b-9 in the choriocapillaris of eyes of patients with diabetic retinopathy. Investigative Ophthalmology & Visual Science. 2002;**43**(4):1104-1108

[79] Zhang J, Gerhardinger C, Lorenzi M. Early complement activation and decreased levels of glycosylphosphatidylinositol-anchored complement inhibitors in human and experimental diabetic retinopathy. Diabetes. 2002;**51**(12):3499-3504

[80] Huang C, Fisher KP, Hammer SS, Busik JV. Extracellular vesicle-induced classical complement activation leads to retinal endothelial cell damage via MAC deposition. International Journal of Molecular Sciences. 2020;**21**(5):1693

[81] Huang C, Fisher KP, Hammer SS, Navitskaya S, Blanchard GJ, Busik JV. Plasma exosomes contribute to microvascular damage in diabetic retinopathy by activating the classical complement pathway. Diabetes. 2018;**67**(8):1639-1649

[82] Atienzar-Aroca S, Flores-Bellver M, Serrano-Heras G, Martinez-Gil N, Barcia JM, Aparicio S, et al. Oxidative stress in retinal pigment epithelium cells increases exosome secretion and promotes angiogenesis in endothelial cells. Journal of Cellular and Molecular Medicine. 2016;**20**(8):1457-1466

[83] Wu SF, Noren Hooten N, Freeman DW, Mode NA, Zonderman AB, Evans MK. Extracellular vesicles in diabetes mellitus induce alterations in endothelial cell morphology and migration. Journal of Translational Medicine. 2020;**18**(1):230

[84] Mazzeo A, Beltramo E, Lopatina T, Gai C, Trento M, Porta M. Molecular and functional characterization of circulating extracellular vesicles from diabetic patients with and without retinopathy and healthy subjects. Experimental Eye Research. 2018;**176**:69-77

[85] Xiao J, Zhang H, Yang F, Xiao M, Zhou L, Yu R, et al. Proteomic analysis of plasma sEVs reveals that TNFAIP8 is a new biomarker of cell proliferation in diabetic retinopathy. Journal of Proteome Research. 2021;**20**(3):1770-1782

[86] Martins B, Amorim M, Reis F, Ambrosio AF, Fernandes R. Extracellular vesicles and MicroRNA: Putative role in diagnosis and treatment of diabetic retinopathy. Antioxidants (Basel). 2020;**9**(8):705

[87] Wang P, Li C, Deng Y, Yu Q, Meng X, Jiang T, et al. Effect of plasma-derived extracellular vesicles on angiogenesis and the ensuing proliferative diabetic retinopathy through a miR-30b-dependent mechanism. Diabetology and Metabolic Syndrome. 2022;**14**(1):188

[88] Mishra M, Duraisamy AJ, Kowluru RA. Sirt1: A guardian of the development of diabetic retinopathy. Diabetes. 2018;**67**(4):745-754

[89] Murinello S, Usui Y, Sakimoto S, Kitano M, Aguilar E, Friedlander HM, et al. miR-30a-5p inhibition promotes interaction of Fas(+) endothelial cells and FasL(+) microglia to decrease pathological neovascularization and promote physiological angiogenesis. Glia. 2019;**67**(2):332-344

[90] Gong M, Yu B, Wang J, Wang Y, Liu M, Paul C, et al. Mesenchymal stem cells release exosomes that transfer miRNAs to endothelial cells and promote angiogenesis. Oncotarget. 2017;**8**(28):45200-45212

[91] Chen Q, Qiu F, Zhou K, Matlock HG, Takahashi Y, Rajala RVS, et al. Pathogenic role of microRNA-21 in diabetic retinopathy through downregulation of PPARalpha. Diabetes. 2017;**66**(6):1671-1682

[92] Mazzeo A, Lopatina T, Gai C, Trento M, Porta M, Beltramo E. Functional analysis of miR-21-3p, miR-30b-5p and miR-150-5p shuttled by extracellular vesicles from diabetic subjects reveals their association with diabetic retinopathy. Experimental Eye Research. 2019;**184**:56-63

[93] Liu CH, Sun Y, Li J, Gong Y, Tian KT, Evans LP, et al. Endothelial microRNA-150 is an intrinsic suppressor of pathologic ocular neovascularization. Proceedings of the National Academy of Sciences of the United States of America. 2015;**112**(39):12163-12168

[94] Beltramo E, Porta M. Pericyte loss in diabetic retinopathy: Mechanisms and consequences. Current Medicinal Chemistry. 2013;**20**(26):3218-3225

[95] Liu C, Ge HM, Liu BH, Dong R, Shan K, Chen X, et al. Targeting pericyte-endothelial cell crosstalk by circular RNA-cPWWP2A inhibition aggravates diabetes-induced microvascular dysfunction. Proceedings of the National Academy of Sciences of the United States of America. 2019;**116**(15):7455-7464

[96] Lee J, Kim KE, Choi DK, Jang JY, Jung JJ, Kiyonari H, et al. Angiopoietin-1 guides directional angiogenesis through integrin alphavbeta5 signaling for recovery of ischemic retinopathy. Science Translational Medicine. 2013;**5**(203):203ra127

[97] Chahed S, Leroyer AS, Benzerroug M, Gaucher D, Georgescu A, Picaud S, et al. Increased vitreous shedding of microparticles in proliferative diabetic retinopathy stimulates endothelial proliferation. Diabetes. 2010;**59**(3):694-701

[98] Maisto R, Trotta MC, Petrillo F, Izzo S, Cuomo G, Alfano R, et al. Resolvin D1 modulates the intracellular VEGF-related miRNAs of retinal photoreceptors challenged with high glucose. Frontiers in Pharmacology. 2020;**11**:235

[99] Maisto R, Oltra M, Vidal-Gil L, Martinez-Gil N, Sancho-Pelluz J, Filippo CD, et al. ARPE-19-derived VEGF-containing exosomes promote neovascularization in HUVEC: The role of the melanocortin receptor 5. Cell Cycle. 2019;**18**(4):413-424

[100] Stepien E, Kablak-Ziembicka A, Czyz J, Przewlocki T, Malecki M. Microparticles, not only markers but also a therapeutic target in the early stage of diabetic retinopathy and vascular aging. Expert Opinion on Therapeutic Targets. 2012;**16**(7):677-688

[101] Ratajczak MZ. The emerging role of microvesicles in cellular therapies

for organ/tissue regeneration. Nephrology, Dialysis, Transplantation. 2011;**26**(5):1453-1456

[102] Beltramo E, Lopatina T, Berrone E, Mazzeo A, Iavello A, Camussi G, et al. Extracellular vesicles derived from mesenchymal stem cells induce features of diabetic retinopathy in vitro. Acta Diabetologica. 2014;**51**(6):1055-1064

[103] Kamalden TA, Macgregor-Das AM, Kannan SM, Dunkerly-Eyring B, Khaliddin N, Xu Z, et al. Exosomal microRNA-15a transfer from the pancreas augments diabetic complications by inducing oxidative stress. Antioxidants & Redox Signaling. 2017;**27**(13):913-930

[104] Razmara M, Hjemdahl P, Ostenson CG, Li N. Platelet hyperprocoagulant activity in type 2 diabetes mellitus: Attenuation by glycoprotein IIb/IIIa inhibition. Journal of Thrombosis and Haemostasis. 2008;**6**(12):2186-2192

[105] Su Y, Chen J, Dong Z, Zhang Y, Ma R, Kou J, et al. Procoagulant activity of blood and endothelial cells via phosphatidylserine exposure and microparticle delivery in patients with diabetic retinopathy. Cellular Physiology and Biochemistry. 2018;**45**(6):2411-2420

[106] Zhang X, McGeoch SC, Johnstone AM, Holtrop G, Sneddon AA, MacRury SM, et al. Platelet-derived microparticle count and surface molecule expression differ between subjects with and without type 2 diabetes, independently of obesity status. Journal of Thrombosis and Thrombolysis. 2014;**37**(4):455-463

[107] Li X, Yu ZW, Wang Y, Fu YH, Gao XY. MicroRNAs: Potential targets in diabetic retinopathy. Hormone and Metabolic Research. 2020;**52**(3):142-148

[108] Zhuang X, Ji L, Jiang H, Liu Y, Liu X, Bi J, et al. Exosomes derived from stem cells from the apical papilla promote dentine-pulp complex regeneration by inducing specific dentinogenesis. Stem Cells International. 2020;**2020**:5816723

[109] Zhang Y, Wei J, Zhang L, Jiang G, Wang B, Jiang L. Extracellular vesicle-derived miR-26b-5p is up-regulated in the serum of patients with diabetic retinopathy. Combinatorial Chemistry & High Throughput Screening. 2022;**25**(5):877-882

[110] Mighty J, Rubio-Navarro A, Shi C, Zhou J, Flores-Bellver M, Heissel S, et al. Extracellular vesicles of human diabetic retinopathy retinal tissue and urine of diabetic retinopathy patients are enriched for the junction plakoglo bin protein. Frontiers in Endocrinology (Lausanne). 2022;**13**:1077644

[111] Qing S, Yuan S, Yun C, Hui H, Mao P, Wen F, et al. Serum miRNA biomarkers serve as a fingerprint for proliferative diabetic retinopathy. Cellular Physiology and Biochemistry. 2014;**34**(5):1733-1740

[112] Friedrich J, Steel DHW, Schlingemann RO, Koss MJ, Hammes HP, Krenning G, et al. microRNA expression profile in the vitreous of proliferative diabetic retinopathy patients and differences from patients treated with anti-VEGF therapy. Translational Vision Science & Technology. 2020;**9**(6):16

[113] Qin LL, An MX, Liu YL, Xu HC, Lu ZQ. MicroRNA-126: A promising novel biomarker in peripheral blood for diabetic retinopathy. International Journal of Ophthalmology. 2017;**10**(4):530-534

[114] Markomichelakis NN, Theodossiadis PG, Sfikakis PP. Regression of neovascular age-related

macular degeneration following infliximab therapy. American Journal of Ophthalmology 2005;139(3):537-540

[115] Stahel M, Becker M, Graf N, Michels S. Systemic interleukin 1beta inhibition in proliferative diabetic retinopathy: A prospective open-label study using canakinumab. Retina. 2016;**36**(2):385-391

[116] Rodriguez ML, Perez S, Mena-Molla S, Desco MC, Ortega AL. Oxidative stress and microvascular alterations in diabetic retinopathy: Future therapies. Oxidative Medicine and Cellular Longevity. 2019;**2019**:4940825

[117] Habibi A, Zarei-Behjani Z, Falamarzi K, Malekpour M, Ebrahimi F, Soleimani M, et al. Extracellular vesicles as a new horizon in the diagnosis and treatment of inflammatory eye diseases: A narrative review of the literature. Frontiers in Immunology. 2023;**14**:1097456

[118] Safwat A, Sabry D, Ragiae A, Amer E, Mahmoud RH, Shamardan RM. Adipose mesenchymal stem cells-derived exosomes attenuate retina degeneration of streptozotocin-induced diabetes in rabbits. Journal of Circulating Biomarkers. 2018;**7**:1849454418807827

[119] Zhang W, Wang Y, Kong Y. Exosomes derived from mesenchymal stem cells modulate miR-126 to ameliorate hyperglycemia-induced retinal inflammation via targeting HMGB1. Investigative Ophthalmology & Visual Science. 2019;**60**(1):294-303

[120] Gu C, Zhang H, Gao Y. Adipose mesenchymal stem cells-secreted extracellular vesicles containing microRNA-192 delays diabetic retinopathy by targeting ITGA1. Journal of Cellular Physiology. 2021;**236**(7):5036-5051

[121] Reddy SK, Ballal AR, Shailaja S, Seetharam RN, Raghu CH, Sankhe R, et al. Small extracellular vesicle-loaded bevacizumab reduces the frequency of intravitreal injection required for diabetic retinopathy. Theranostics. 2023;**13**(7):2241-2255

[122] Sun F, Sun Y, Zhu J, Wang X, Ji C, Zhang J, et al. Mesenchymal stem cells-derived small extracellular vesicles alleviate diabetic retinopathy by delivering NEDD4. Stem Cell Research & Therapy. 2022;**13**(1):293

[123] Hajrasouliha AR, Jiang G, Lu Q, Lu H, Kaplan HJ, Zhang HG, et al. Exosomes from retinal astrocytes contain antiangiogenic components that inhibit laser-induced choroidal neovascularization. The Journal of Biological Chemistry. 2013;**288**(39):28058-28067

[124] Gu S, Liu Y, Zou J, Wang W, Wei T, Wang X, et al. Retinal pigment epithelial cells secrete miR-202-5p-containing exosomes to protect against proliferative diabetic retinopathy. Experimental Eye Research. 2020;**201**:108271

[125] Huang S, Zeng Y, Guo Q, Zou T, Yin ZQ. Small extracellular vesicles of organoid-derived human retinal stem cells remodel Muller cell fate via miRNA: A novel remedy for retinal degeneration. Journal of Controlled Release. 2024;**370**:405-420

[126] Yang C, Xiong W, Qiu Q, Shao Z, Hamel D, Tahiri H, et al. Role of receptor-mediated endocytosis in the antiangiogenic effects of human T lymphoblastic cell-derived microparticles. American Journal of Physiology. Regulatory, Integrative and Comparative Physiology. 2012;**302**(8):R941-R949

[127] Lamb WDB, Eastlake K, Luis J, Sharif NA, Khaw PT, Limb GA.

MicroRNA profile of extracellular vesicles released by Muller glial cells. Frontiers in Cellular Neuroscience. 2023;**17**:1325114

[128] Mathew B, Acha LG, Torres LA, Huang CC, Liu A, Kalinin S, et al. MicroRNA-based engineering of mesenchymal stem cell extracellular vesicles for treatment of retinal ischemic disorders: Engineered extracellular vesiclesand retinal ischemia. Acta Biomaterialia. 2023;**158**:782-797

[129] Shaker OG, Abdelaleem OO, Mahmoud RH, Abdelghaffar NK, Ahmed TI, Said OM, et al. Diagnostic and prognostic role of serum miR-20b, miR-17-3p, HOTAIR, and MALAT1 in diabetic retinopathy. IUBMB Life. 2019;**71**(3):310-320

[130] Li Z, Dong Y, He C, Pan X, Liu D, Yang J, et al. RNA-Seq revealed novel non-proliferative retinopathy specific circulating MiRNAs in T2DM patients. Frontiers in Genetics. 2019;**10**:531

[131] McArthur K, Feng B, Wu Y, Chen S, Chakrabarti S. MicroRNA-200b regulates vascular endothelial growth factor-mediated alterations in diabetic retinopathy. Diabetes. 2011;**60**(4):1314-1323

[132] Blum A, Meerson A, Rohana H, Jabaly H, Nahul N, Celesh D, et al. MicroRNA-423 may regulate diabetic vasculopathy. Clinical and Experimental Medicine. 2019;**19**(4):469-477

[133] Sun F, Sun Y, Wang X, Zhu J, Chen S, Yu Y, et al. Engineered mesenchymal stem cell-derived small extracellular vesicles for diabetic retinopathy therapy through HIF-1α/EZH2/PGC-1α pathway. Bioactive Materials. 2024;**33**:444-459

[134] Haraszti RA, Miller R, Stoppato M, Sere YY, Coles A, Didiot MC, et al. Exosomes produced from 3D cultures of MSCs by tangential flow filtration show higher yield and improved activity. Molecular Therapy. 2018;**26**(12):2838-2847

[135] Lener T, Gimona M, Aigner L, Borger V, Buzas E, Camussi G, et al. Applying extracellular vesicles based therapeutics in clinical trials—An ISEV position paper. Journal of Extracellular Vesicles. 2015;**4**:30087

[136] Zhao K, Lou R, Huang F, Peng Y, Jiang Z, Huang K, et al. Immunomodulation effects of mesenchymal stromal cells on acute graft-versus-host disease after hematopoietic stem cell transplantation. Biology of Blood and Marrow Transplantation. 2015;**21**(1):97-104

[137] Shelke GV, Lasser C, Gho YS, Lotvall J. Importance of exosome depletion protocols to eliminate functional and RNA-containing extracellular vesicles from fetal bovine serum. Journal of Extracellular Vesicles. 2014:**3**(1):24783

[138] Pachler K, Lener T, Streif D, Dunai ZA, Desgeorges A, Feichtner M, et al. A good manufacturing practice-grade standard protocol for exclusively human mesenchymal stromal cell-derived extracellular vesicles. Cytotherapy. 2017;**19**(4):458-472

[139] Nordin JZ, Lee Y, Vader P, Mager I, Johansson HJ, Heusermann W, et al. Ultrafiltration with size-exclusion liquid chromatography for high yield isolation of extracellular vesicles preserving intact biophysical and functional properties. Nanomedicine. 2015;**11**(4):879-883

[140] Benedikter BJ, Bouwman FG, Vajen T, Heinzmann ACA, Grauls G, Mariman EC, et al. Ultrafiltration

combined with size exclusion chromatography efficiently isolates extracellular vesicles from cell culture media for compositional and functional studies. Scientific Reports. 2017;**7**(1):15297

[141] Lorincz AM, Timar CI, Marosvari KA, Veres DS, Otrokocsi L, Kittel A, et al. Effect of storage on physical and functional properties of extracellular vesicles derived from neutrophilic granulocytes. Journal of Extracellular Vesicles. 2014;**3**:25465

[142] Larson MC, Luthi MR, Hogg N, Hillery CA. Calcium-phosphate microprecipitates mimic microparticles when examined with flow cytometry. Cytometry. Part A. 2013;**83**(2):242-250

[143] Kalra H, Adda CG, Liem M, Ang CS, Mechler A, Simpson RJ, et al. Comparative proteomics evaluation of plasma exosome isolation techniques and assessment of the stability of exosomes in normal human blood plasma. Proteomics. 2013;**13**(22):3354-3364

[144] Kusuma GD, Barabadi M, Tan JL, Morton DAV, Frith JE, Lim R. To protect and to preserve: Novel preservation strategies for extracellular vesicles. Frontiers in Pharmacology. 2018;**9**:1199

[145] Yin H, Chen CY, Liu YW, Tan YJ, Deng ZL, Yang F, et al. Synechococcus elongatus PCC7942 secretes extracellular vesicles to accelerate cutaneous wound healing by promoting angiogenesis. Theranostics. 2019;**9**(9):2678-2693

[146] Hu W, Song X, Yu H, Sun J, Zhao Y. Released exosomes contribute to the immune modulation of cord blood-derived stem cells. Frontiers in Immunology. 2020;**11**:165

[147] Murphy DE, de Jong OG, Brouwer M, Wood MJ, Lavieu G, Schiffelers RM, et al. Extracellular vesicle-based therapeutics: Natural versus engineered targeting and trafficking. Experimental & Molecular Medicine. 2019;**51**(3):1-12

Chapter 8

Treating Diabetic Retinopathy: Challenges and the Way Forward

Nikita Dash

Abstract

Diabetic retinopathy is a well-known complication of long-standing diabetes and is frequently encountered by ophthalmologists. While early changes may not impact vision, it is important to understand the need to follow up these patients regularly to avoid sight-threatening vision loss with timely management. Timely referral by physicians and increasing awareness about diabetic retinopathy is crucial to achieve this goal. Moreover, the advent of newer pharmacotherapeutics and better machinery and instrumentation for safe vitreoretinal surgery has played a significant role in changing the dynamics of the treatment of diabetic retinopathy. This chapter focuses on the difficulties faced in managing patients with diabetic retinopathy, as well as treatment options in practice and areas of future research.

Keywords: diabetic retinopathy, diabetic macular edema, photocoagulation, anti-vascular endothelial growth factor (VEGF) injections, diabetic vitrectomy

1. Introduction

Diabetes is a well-known metabolic disorder with an estimated global prevalence of 536.6 million (10%) in 20 to 79-year-olds in 2021. This is expected to rise to 783.2 million (12.2%) in 2045 [1]. With the increasing disease burden, the prevalence of people with microvascular complications such as nephropathy, neuropathy and retinopathy is on the rise. Diabetic retinopathy (DR) is a major ocular complication of this disease with known visual repercussions. With a global prevalence of more than 100 million, DR is known to cause significant sight-threatening complications that lead to blindness and visual impairment [2]. This is projected to increase significantly to 161 million in 2045 [3].

The prevalence of diabetic retinopathy has been noted in both type 1 and type 2 diabetics. In the former variant, 13% develop retinopathy after 5 years, and it increases to 90% after 10 to 15 years. After 15 years, proliferative retinopathy may be seen in about 25% of patients with type 1 diabetes [4]. Forty percent of type 2 diabetics treated with insulin develop retinopathy after 5 years as compared to 24% when treated with oral hypoglycemic agents. The prevalence increases to 84 and 53%, respectively, after 15 to 19 years of diabetes. Proliferative retinopathy has been detected in 2% of type 2 diabetics within 5 years of diagnosis and 25% after 25 years or more [5].

Although DR is preventable and treatable with appropriate screening strategies, newer imaging modalities and advances in pharmacotherapy, there are still several challenges that need to be faced to decrease the burden of the disease. This chapter shall discuss the problems encountered, current treatment strategies and key areas of further research. It will not only improve our insight on DR but also help us tackle this public health problem in a better manner.

2. Challenges of treating diabetic retinopathy

Although diabetic retinopathy and its pathogenesis is well-understood now, its management is fraught with challenges. Since the burden of the disease is high, it is important to screen established diabetics properly to detect retinopathy before it gets sight-threatening. Unfortunately, the degree of awareness regarding diabetic retinopathy in the community is still low, which can pose a hindrance to the detection and further management of retinopathy. Even when it is diagnosed, compliance issues, lack of motivation for blood sugar control, and failure to treat other microvascular complications like nephropathy can further aggravate retinopathy and pose problems for the patient as well as the physician.

Treatment of diabetic retinopathy complications includes retinal laser, anti-VEGF injections and surgical management in those with established retinal detachment and vitreous hemorrhage. This has been explained lucidly in **Figure 1**. While intravitreal anti-VEGF injections can work wonders, economic issues involving affordability remain. The advent of microincision vitreoretinal surgery (MIVS) may have made the lives of vitreoretinal surgeons better, but diabetic vitrectomy is not without challenges.

In the subsequent sections, the management of diabetic retinopathy and the challenges faced thereof shall be discussed.

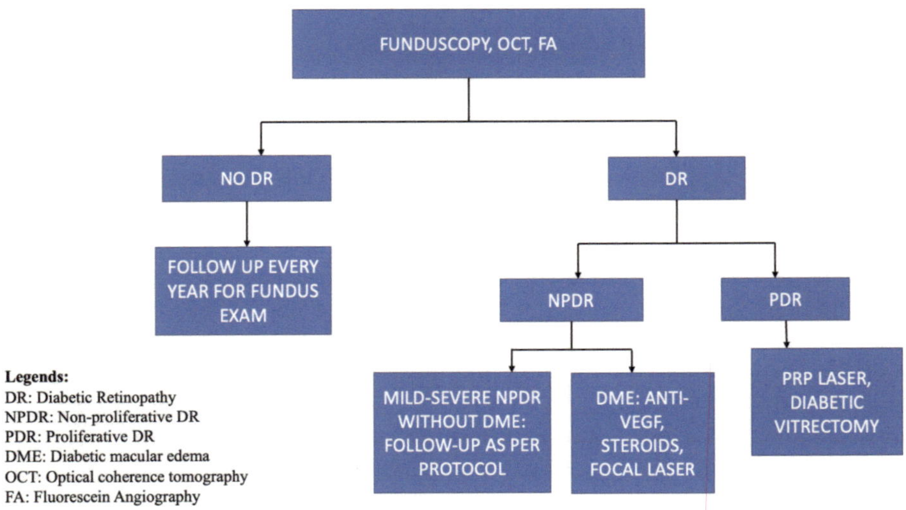

Figure 1.
A simplistic flowchart on approach to management in diabetic retinopathy.

3. Role of glycemic control

Glycemic control has an important role in the management of diabetic retinopathy. Several studies have highlighted the importance of glycated hemoglobin (HbA1c) in predicting the course of retinopathy. The Wisconsin Epidemiologic Study reported that HbA1c levels at baseline had a significant correlation with the incidence and progression of proliferative retinopathy in diabetic individuals younger than 30 years and in those who were older and treated with oral hypoglycemic agents and insulin [6].

The Diabetes Control and Complications Trial (DCCT) studied the effects of intensive glycemic control on the incidence and progression of retinopathy and its management in type 1 diabetes [7]. Participants treated with conventional therapy had a mean HbA1c of 9.2% at follow-up as compared to 7.2% in the intensive control group. There was a risk reduction of 70% for clinically important sustained retinopathy, 56% for laser photocoagulation and 60% for sustained microalbuminuria. Even after 4 years of completion of study, the intensive control group not only reported lower HbA1c but also a reduction in proliferative retinopathy, macular edema and need for laser therapy by 74, 77% and 77%, respectively [8].

The United Kingdom Prospective Diabetes Study (UKPDS) also achieved lower HbA1c levels in the intensive therapy group in type 2 diabetic individuals [9, 10]. A risk reduction of 27% for retinal photocoagulation was reported at 12 years in the intensive treatment group. In addition, the effects of blood pressure control in type 2 diabetics with hypertension were also studied. Those with tight blood pressure control experienced a 34% reduction in two-step deterioration of retinopathy, a 35% reduction in retinal photocoagulation, and a 47% risk reduction in three-line deterioration in Early Treatment of Diabetic Retinopathy Study (ETDRS) visual acuity over 7.5 years [11, 12].

Therefore, not only should one understand the need for strict glycemic control but also the requirement for blood pressure control in patients with coexisting hypertension.

4. Diabetic retinopathy study (DRS) and ETDRS studies: stepping stones in diabetic retinopathy treatment

Two major landmark trials made a huge impact on the classification and management of diabetic retinopathy. They were the Diabetic Retinopathy Study (DRS) and the Early Treatment of Diabetic Retinopathy Study (ETDRS).

4.1 Diabetic retinopathy study (DRS)

The DRS was a randomized, controlled clinical trial funded by the National Eye Institute (NEI) to evaluate photocoagulation for the treatment of proliferative diabetic retinopathy (PDR). The main aim of the DRS was to determine whether photocoagulation helps prevent severe vision loss (SVL) in PDR, with SVL being defined as visual acuity (VA) defined as less than 5/200 at two or more consecutively completed 4-month follow-up visits [13]. The results of DRS showed that the 2-year incidence of SVL was reduced by photocoagulation in more than half of eyes with PDR with or without high-risk characteristics (HRCs), which were described as follows:

- Moderate or severe new vessels on or within one disc diameter (DD) of the optic disc.
- Mild new vessels on or within one DD of the optic disc if fresh vitreous or pre-retinal hemorrhage is present.
- Moderate or severe new vessels elsewhere (NVE), if fresh vitreous or pre-retinal hemorrhage is present, and if the area of NVE was half DD or more.

On the contrary, in eyes with non-proliferative diabetic retinopathy (NPDR), photocoagulation reduced the risk of SVL to only 2.8% compared to 3.2% in the untreated NPDR subjects. Therefore, in NPDR, the risks of photocoagulation outweigh the benefits [13].

In conclusion, the DRS firmly established the benefits of laser photocoagulation in patients with PDR with HRCs and advised prompt treatment in such cases. It did not, however, include the effects of focal laser on macular edema [14].

4.2 The early treatment diabetic retinopathy study

The ETDRS was a multicenter, randomized clinical trial, funded by the NEI, to evaluate argon laser photocoagulation in the management of patients with non-proliferative or early PDR [15]. They not only studied the effects of scatter photocoagulation but also that of focal laser in patients with macular edema [16].

The ETDRS recommended that scatter photocoagulation should be considered without delay if the eye has already reached a high-risk proliferative stage. It is not recommended for mild to moderate NPDR cases as the side effects outweigh the benefits in those cases. It also showed that in eyes with macular edema, an immediate focal laser showed a statistically significant beneficial effect [17].

However, there were many gray areas that this study could not answer. Moreover, with the advent of modern pharmacotherapeutic agents for macular edema, many recommendations have changed over time.

5. Present role of laser photocoagulation

With the advent of anti-VEGF therapy in the management of PDR and diabetic macular edema (DME), several trials have been conducted to study the effect of pharmacologic therapy vis-à-vis laser therapy or combined therapy. Even corticosteroid agents have been the focus of certain clinical trials. The Diabetic Retinopathy Clinical Research Network (DRCR.net) has conducted many of these studies [18]. They establish the efficacy and benefits of intravitreal anti-VEGF therapy, either alone or in combination with laser, for the treatment of PDR and DME.

However, in the real-world scenario, various other factors also come into play. There might be several personal, social, financial or even medical constraints to seeking therapy by multiple intravitreal injections [19]. It is in these conditions that laser therapy emerges as the better option, considering that it not only reduces the number of injections required but also provides a lasting therapeutic effect [20].

Laser treatment in the form of Panretinal Photocoagulation (PRP) remains the gold standard for PDR as it offers a definitive and long-lasting therapeutic effect that prevents severe vision loss or complications of PDR. It also minimizes the number of intravitreal injections for treatment and reduces the number of follow-up visits.

Similarly, a focal laser can be done to treat leaking microaneurysms that cause persistent DME in patients with DR. However, it should be noted that only fovea-sparing microaneurysms can be lasered.

In addition, newer laser techniques and instrumentation are being introduced that can lead to better clinical efficacy and improvements in patient management. Examples include pattern scanning laser technology (PASCAL), which reduces the time taken to laser a patient as well as improves patient comfort levels. Selective Retinal Therapy (SRT) treats retinal pigment epithelial cells selectively, thus limiting damage to the neurosensory retina. Similarly, subthreshold laser induces a therapeutic effect without any visible tissue damage. Other innovations including End Point Management and Navigated Laser have improved the safety and efficacy of laser photocoagulation [21].

6. Anti-VEGF agents in diabetic retinopathy

Anti-VEGF agents were first developed in the 1990s and worked by blocking the vascular endothelial growth factor (VEGF) that is known to cause angiogenesis. Although they were majorly introduced as anti-cancer therapy, the beneficial effects of these agents were soon discovered in a range of eye conditions like diabetic macular edema and age-related macular degeneration [22]. Bevacizumab was the first anti-VEGF agent that was tried for treatment and is still used off-label [23]. Later, many anti-VEGF drugs were formulated that are FDA-approved and have been summarized in **Table 1**.

6.1 Mechanism of action

The major factor that drives angiogenesis in an eye with diabetic retinopathy is VEGF and its isoforms. Studies have shown that VEGF-A is the most significant of all in promoting vascular permeability and angiogenesis by interacting with the receptor

Name	Mechanism of action	FDA approval
Bevacizumab	149 KDa recombinant humanized monoclonal antibody targeting VEGF-A	Metastatic colorectal cancer (2004), Off-label use in Ophthalmology
Ranibizumab	48KDa recombinant monoclonal antibody fragment with one VEGF-A binding site	Wet AMD# (2006), DME* (2012), DR$ (2017)
Aflibercept	115 KDa soluble decoy receptor with two VEGF binding domains for VEGFR-1 and VEGFR-2	Wet AMD# (2011), DME* (2014), DR$ (2019)
Newer agents		
Brolucizumab	26KDa humanized monoclonal single-chain variable fragment that binds VEGF-A	Wet AMD# (2019), DME* (2022), not approved for DR$
Faricimab	149 KDa dual mechanism antibody that works against VEGF-A and Ang-2	Wet AMD# (2022), DME* (2022)

#Age-related macular degeneration.
**Diabetic macular edema.*
$Diabetic retinopathy.

Table 1.
List of anti-VEGF agents and their mechanism of action.

VEGFR-2 on vascular endothelial cells [24]. This leads to destruction of capillary endothelium tight junction that leads to endothelial cell fenestration and weakened blood vessels. It also stimulates endothelial proliferation and migration associated with the early stages of angiogenesis [25]. Different agents, however, differ in their specific actions.

6.2 Use of anti-VEGF agents

Anti-VEGF agents are popularly used to decrease the central macular thickness in cases of DME. Studies like the RISE and ranibizumab in diabetic macular edema studies (RIDE) evaluated ranibizumab as therapy for DME. Later Intravitreal Aflibercept injection in vision impairment due to DME (VIVID) and study of intravitreal aflibercept injection (IAI; EYLEA®; BAY86-5321) in patients with diabetic macular edema (VISTA) studied the effects of aflibercept [26, 27]. Both studies showed improvement in the eyes with injection. Comparison of anti-VEGF agents like bevacizumab, ranibizumab and aflibercept was done by the Protocol T. Post-hoc analysis after 2 years did not show any significant difference between the three groups [28]. At least a minimum of three injections every month is required following which the number of injections and duration of follow-up can be adjusted as per response.

In PDR, anti-VEGF agents can be used as an adjunct or as primary therapy. Protocol S demonstrated that ranibizumab was non-inferior to PRP laser therapy, with outcomes showing improvement in DME, reduction in rates of DME development and decrease in the need for rescue laser therapy [29]. Eyes with proliferative retinopathy that develop vitreous hemorrhage can also benefit from anti-VEGF therapy. They can be used to buy time for surgery or as therapy while waiting for media to clear up [30].

6.3 Safety and precautions of anti-VEGF agents

Ocular adverse events often associated anti-VEGF agents include cataracts, retinal detachment, endophthalmitis, elevated intraocular pressure, vitreous hemorrhage, uveitis, ocular inflammation, floaters, retinal vessel changes and risks of glaucomatous optic atrophy [31, 32]. Systemic side effects like thromboembolism, myocardial infarction, stroke, hypertension and bowel perforation [33]. Although most of the systemic adverse events have been associated with cancer trials, they have not been confirmed with low dose or intravitreal route of drug delivery. No difference has been noted between the anti-VEGF agents [34].

Another serious complication that can occur is the development of tractional detachment in cases of PDR with pre-existing membranes. It is hypothesized that when anti-VEGF medications are used, angiogenesis is suppressed, but connective tissue growth factor (CTGF) mediated fibrosis is not checked. This leads to the acceleration of fibrosis, which produces traction on the underlying retina [35, 36]. Long-standing diabetes and poorly controlled diabetic retinopathy are major risk factors [37].

7. Corticosteroid therapy in treatment of diabetic retinopathy

Corticosteroid therapy has mostly been used to treat diabetic macular edema, especially those refractory to anti-VEGF treatment. It has been found that apart from upregulation in VEGF, there is an increase in the levels of various growth factors and cytokines like interleukin-6, interleukin-8, interleukin-1β, monocyte chemotactic protein-1 and tumor necrosis factor α [38]. Sometimes, even after six consecutive monthly injections of anti-VEGF, 40-50% of the eyes can still have persistent DME, thus suggesting that in certain eyes, cytokines dominate over VEGF upregulation [39].

Triamcinolone acetonide (TA) was the first corticosteroid to be widely used for DME as an intravitreal pharmacotherapy [40]. Currently, apart from TA, the dexamethasone implant and the fluocinolone acetonide implant are in use.

Triamcinolone acetonide was first tried by Jonas et al. at a dose of 20 mg injected intravitreally in an eye with persistent DME following macular photocoagulation. The DME regressed visual gains were maintained for 5 months in the patient [40]. Thereafter, most retina specialists started using 4 mg for the dose of intravitreal TA as the commercial formulation was 40 mg/ml and it is readily available.

Dexamethasone implant was studied in the dexamethasone in macular edema (MEAD) trial that randomized patients to 0.7 mg dexamethasone (DEX) implant, 0.35 mg DEX implant and sham injections [41]. The DEX-treated eyes gained eight letters compared to two letters in the sham group. At around 15 months, development of cataract led to reduction in the visual improvement in the DEX-treated eyes. These were treated and cataract extraction and gained vision toward 3-year visit. About a third of patients who were treated with the DEX implant required medication for increased intraocular pressure (IOP) and 0.3% required incisional surgery for the same [42].

The fluocinolone acetonide implant is known to deliver drugs for 3 years and has the potential to reduce frequent injections and associated endophthalmitis [43]. The fluocinolone acetonide in macular edema (FAME) study assigned individuals with persistent DME to three groups: 0.2 μg Iluvien-fluorescein angiography (FA) per day, 0.5 μg Iluvien-FA per day, or sham injection. After 3 years, 28.7, 27.8, and 18.9% gained ≥15 letters, respectively [44]. Despite 0.2 μg Iluvien-FA per day implantation, rescue photocoagulation therapy was required in 40% of the eyes. Iluvien-FA has been approved for chronic DME in Europe. It was also found through a cost-effectiveness analysis in the United Kingdom that the Iluvien-FA implant provided good value for patients with persistent DME, specifically pseudophakic patients [45, 46].

Although several head-on trials with anti-VEGF have proved that corticosteroids are non-inferior, they are still associated with a number of side effects such as increased IOP and cataract that make them a less popular drug for the first line of treatment in phakic patients [47, 48].

8. Considerations in treating diabetic macular edema

While the efficacy of intravitreal anti-VEGF agents and corticosteroids is well established, there are certain factors that one must keep in mind while treating patients with DME. It is also advisable to obtain a fundus fluorescein angiogram (FFA) and optical coherence tomography (OCT) of the patient to tailor treatment as per individual needs. OCT further classifies DME into center-involving (CI) and non-center-involving (NCI), as discussed in **Table 2**, which can again lead to differences in therapeutic approach.

8.1 Non-center-involving DME

In a naïve case of NCI-DME, one can observe if the vision is good enough (6/6-6/9). However, if the vision is worse, one can consider lasering any leaking microaneurysm 500-3000 microns away from the fovea if it meets the Clinically significant

Clinically significant macular edema (CSME)	Retinal thickening at or within 500 microns from the center of fovea
	Hard exudates at or within 500 microns from the center of fovea with associated retinal thickening
	An area or areas of retinal thickening 1 disc area in size, a part of which is within 1 disc diameter of the center of macula
Center-involving DME (CI-DME)	Diagnosed on SD-OCT# when the central subfoveal thickness (CST) on the macular map is 305 microns or worse in women and 315 microns or worse in men on Heidelberg (or equivalent thickness on other SD-OCT machines)
Non-center-involving DME (NCI-DME)	Diagnosed on SD-OCT# when the central subfoveal thickness (CST) on the macular map is less than 305 microns in women and less than 315 microns in men on Heidelberg (or equivalent thickness on other SD-OCT machines) with increased thickness in inner and outer ETDRS subfields

#SD-OCT: Spectral domain optical coherence tomography.

Table 2.
Classification of Diabetic Macular Edema.

macular edema (CSME) criteria, as given in **Table 2** [49]. Sometimes, NCI-DME may result after treatment of CI-DME. In such cases, one can opt to observe every 2 months if the vision is more than equal to 6/9. If it is less than that, leaking microaneurysms may be lasered, as discussed above [50, 51]. However, it must be kept in mind that if there is a plaque of hard exudates near fovea, it often carries a poor prognosis and the patient must be counseled thusly [52].

8.2 Center-involving DME

Intravitreal anti-VEGF agents are often the first choice of treatment for center-involving DME. The drug doses commonly administered are – bevacizumab – 1.25 mg/0.05 ml, ranibizumab – 0.5 mg/0.05 ml and aflibercept – 2 mg/0.05 ml [51, 53].

Treatment usually involves monthly injections for 4-6 months initially followed by changing regimen as per response [54]. No further improvement has been described as a less than 10% decrease in the central subfield thickness on OCT and no more than a line improvement of visual acuity [49]. Treatment can be withdrawn and patients are observed if visual acuity improves to 6/7.5 despite persistent DME. Therapy can be reinstituted if there is worsening on follow-up [55].

In cases with sub-optimal response to anti-VEGF injections, focal macular laser or switch to corticosteroid therapy may be considered depending on the case [56, 57].

8.3 DME in special situations

DME in pregnancy has been reported to spontaneously regress. However, it is important to maintain a close follow-up [49, 58]. If vision is worsened, dexamethasone implants may be considered. Intravitreal anti-VEGF injections are not recommended owing to potential side effects on the developing embryo/fetus. It is also advised not to conceive immediately after the last intravitreal injection. A waiting time of 3 months is recommended in these cases [59].

In vitrectomized eyes, it has been reported that intravitreal anti-VEGF therapy may not be as effective. Instead, an intravitreal dexamethasone implant has been found to be effective in such a scenario. However, both these agents are preferred in vitrectomized eyes based on current evidence [60, 61].

Caution should also be practiced when dealing with DME patients with cardiovascular diseases. If there is a recent history of stroke or myocardial infarction (event less than 3 months), it is better to refrain from anti-VEGF agents; steroids or laser treatment should be used instead. If the event occurred more than 3 months ago, then anti-VEGF agents can be injected, although it is better to consult with the treating physician before proceeding if a high risk of thromboembolism is suspected [49].

9. Surgical treatment for diabetic retinopathy

Common indications for vitrectomy in diabetic retinopathy include vitreous hemorrhage, tractional retinal detachment involving or approaching fovea, combined rhegmatogenous and tractional detachment, pre-macular hemorrhage and diabetic macular edema due to vitreomacular traction [62].

The Diabetic Retinopathy Vitrectomy Study has shown a clear benefit of early vitrectomy in type 1 diabetics with vitreous hemorrhage. Since then, there has been a lower threshold for vitrectomy, with more and more ophthalmologists opting for early vitrectomy [63]. Current guidelines include managing conservatively for a month before proceeding for vitrectomy. The risk of intra-operative bleeding is usually reduced with the injection of anti-VEGF agent a week before surgery. However, care should be taken so that the gap between injection and surgery is not too long to avoid Crunch syndrome [64].

Tractional retinal detachment (TRD) is usually operated upon if it involves the fovea or if there is a risk of foveal involvement if not treated. Contraction of the TRD may also lead to breaks in the atrophic retina that can further result in a combined tractional and rhegmatogenous retinal detachment. Although better equipment and improvements in vitrectomy machinery have made these surgeries easier, they still have a variable prognosis. Older age, anterior segment neovascularization, poor preoperative visual acuity, greater extent of retinal detachment and macular heterotopia are the reasons for worse prognosis [65, 66].

Pars plana vitrectomy (PPV) with internal limiting membrane (ILM) peeling is considered if there is persistent macular edema with a taut posterior hyaloid or vitreomacular traction. However, there has been contrasting evidence in relation to this subject. While some studies show favorable outcomes, others do not show a clear benefit [67].

10. Challenges and the way forward

The major challenge with any disease with a long-term course is compliance issues. Even though the early treatment of DR can improve quality of life, a significant proportion fails to comply with follow-ups, thus leading to recommended screening exams in only 18 to 60% [68]. Therefore, awareness and outreach camps in diabetic screening should not only be organized but also should be compulsorily included in the national health policy. Moreover, various therapeutic options in diabetic retinopathy come with their own set of complications and limitations. This has been summarized in **Table 3**.

Treatment options	Limitations
Anti-VEGF Agents	Relative contraindication in patients with cerebrovascular accident and myocardial infarction. Cost prohibitive
Steroids	Can lead to increase in intraocular pressure, secondary glaucoma and cataract formation. Contraindicated in glaucoma patients. Implant migration can occur in patients with posterior capsular defect
Laser Photocoagulation	Precipitates macular edema. It can cause constriction of field of vision and consecutive optic atrophy
Diabetic Vitrectomy	Foveal contour may not return to normal even after the removal of tractional membranes. Not advocated in extramacular tractional retinal detachment

Table 3.
Limitations of treatment strategies for diabetic retinopathy.

Another major factor is the economic burden of the disease. While the advent of intravitreal injections has made treating DME a lot easier, at the same time, it has increased the cost burden by several notches [69]. Therefore, economically marginalized sections of society are deprived of treatment, which increases the burden of disease. To tackle this, progress is being made in formulating more long-acting preparations or drug delivery systems like the ranibizumab port delivery system and the verisome system. Both act as long-acting systems of drug delivery into the vitreous [70, 71].

The lack of skilled retina specialists for screening is also another challenge in treating diabetic retinopathy. Therefore, several training sessions need to be organized so that ophthalmologists can identify cases that require further evaluation and urgent attention. The use of teleophthalmology can also be helpful in such cases. Fundus photographs can be screened by experts, thus aiding management [72]. The use of artificial intelligence can also augment patient care with precision and reduce human errors [73].

11. Areas of future research

There are still many unanswered questions with regard to diabetic retinopathy and its future prospects. Certain areas that require clarification and provide scope for further research have been outlined below [74].

11.1 Diabetic retinal neurodegeneration

While the primary focus of research in DR was on its vascular pathophysiology, evidence of neuronal degeneration has been collected over the years [75]. OCT of retinal inner layers including nerve fiber layer (RNFL) and ganglion cell layer (GCL) has demonstrated significant thinning over a period of time that may even precede the appearance of microangiopathic lesions [76, 77]. This has been termed as "diabetic retinal neurodegeneration" and has been corroborated histologically [78]. However, it is yet to be known as to how it affects the quality of life in diabetics and what more this information can contribute. It remains to be seen if the knowledge of retinal neurodegeneration in diabetics will help in prognosis or play a role in response to treatment of the disease.

11.2 Ultrawide field angiography and optical coherence tomography angiography

Ultrawide field (UWF) imaging with a field of view of 110 degrees to 220 degrees allows the visualization of retinal periphery as far as the anterior edge of the ampullae of the vortex veins [79]. They provide not only color fundus photography but also other investigation modalities like fluorescein angiography (FA) and indocyanine green angiography (ICGA). They are non-contact and allow photography without mydriasis. The most significant advantage of these modalities is their ability to assess the retinal periphery, covering about 80% of the retinal area [80]. Assessment of the peripheral retina can help detect lesions that are otherwise missed and help in the prognosis of the disease [81]. Moreover, cohort studies also show that peripheral lesions are independently associated with a greater risk of progression of DR [82]. However, the widespread application of this technology and its role in the classification and prognosis of DR remains to be seen.

Optical coherence tomography angiography (OCTA) is another imaging modality that is increasingly gaining importance in DR assessment and prognostication. OCTA is a non-invasive, non-contact system that provides angiographic information of the retina. Advantages of OCTA include no requirement of invasive dye administration, better visualization of the capillary microvasculature, and depth-resolved segmentation of the superficial, middle and deep capillaries plexuses, which is affected differently in eyes with DR [83, 84]. Since OCTA can provide metric quantification and analysis of retinal vasculature, there is scope for research as to how these metrics can be applied to further prognosticate and give valuable information regarding clinical outcome of DR patients [85].

11.3 Artificial intelligence

Artificial Intelligence (AI) algorithms in ophthalmology, using machine learning algorithms, for automated diagnosis or detection of DR from color fundus photograph (CFP) images have been under development since 2016 [86]. Preliminary studies demonstrated that AI algorithms developed on large datasets reach significantly high levels of diagnostic performance for detection of referable DR and vision-threatening DR [87]. There are now multiple AI-based systems for DR screening that have been approved for clinical use. IDx-DR (IDx LLC, Coralville, IA, USA) and EyeArt (Eyenuk, Inc., Woodlands Hills, CA, USA) have both received approval from the USA Food and Drug Administration (FDA) and are already in clinical use [88, 89]. By 2030, it is projected that AI in diabetic retinopathy screening will be in widespread use. However, certain aspects pertaining to image quality and medicolegal issues need to be dealt with before AI gets worldwide acceptance [90].

Apart from fundus photography, AI can be used to incorporate other imaging modalities such as OCT and OCTA, that already have inbuilt segmentation software, which is amenable to machine learning [91]. This can be another area of groundbreaking research.

12. Conclusion

Diagnosing and managing diabetic retinopathy may not be as simple as it sounds. A lot of effort goes into acquiring the skillset required for the treatment of patients suffering from the consequences of diabetic retinopathy. However, with newer innovations and changing times, a lot of things are slowly becoming plausible and easier to imagine. Newer imaging modalities and the incorporation of AI in detection and prognostication will be a gamechanger in the near future. Nevertheless, we still have a long way to go before applying research from these areas into clinical practice. We can only hope that the unmet needs for managing diabetic retinopathy will slowly disappear in the generations to come.

Author details

Nikita Dash
Vitreo-retinal Fellow, Sir Ganga Ram Hospital, New Delhi, India

*Address all correspondence to: ndash18@gmail.com

References

[1] Sun H, Saeedi P, Karuranga S, Pinkepank M, Ogurtsova K, Duncan BB, et al. IDF diabetes atlas: Global, regional and country-level diabetes prevalence estimates for 2021 and projections for 2045. Diabetes Research and Clinical Practice. 2022;**183**:109119. ISSN 0168-8227

[2] Yau JWY, Rogers SL, Kawasaki R, Lamoureux EL, Kowalski JW, Bek T, et al. Global prevalence and major risk factors of diabetic retinopathy. Diabetes Care. 2012;**35**:556-564. DOI: 10.2337/dc11-1909

[3] Teo ZL, Tham Y-C, Yu M, Chee ML, Rim TH, Cheung N, et al. Global prevalence of diabetic retinopathy and projection of burden through 2045: Systematic review and meta-analysis. Ophthalmology. 2021;**128**:1580-1591. DOI: 10.1016/j.ophtha.2021.04.027

[4] Mitka M. Report quantifies diabetes complications. JAMA. 2007;**297**(21):2337-2338

[5] Klein R, Klein BEK, Moss SE, et al. The Wisconsin epidemiologic study of diabetic retinopathy: II. Prevalence and risk of diabetic retinopathy when age at diagnosis is less than 30 years. Archives of Ophthalmology. 1984;**102**:527-532

[6] Klein R, Klein BEK, Moss SE. Relation of glycemic control to diabetic microvascular complications in diabetes mellitus. Annals of Internal Medicine. 1996;**124**:90-96

[7] Diabetes Control and Complications Trial Research Group. The effect of intensive treatment of diabetes on the development and progression of long-term complications in insulin-dependent diabetes mellitus. The New England Journal of Medicine. 1993;**329**:977-986

[8] Diabetes control and complications trial/epidemiology of diabetes interventions and complications research group. Retinopathy and nephropathy in patients with type 1 diabetes four years after a trial of intensive therapy. The New England Journal of Medicine. 2000;**342**:381-389

[9] UK Prospective Diabetes Study (UKPDS) Group. Effect of intensive blood-glucose control with metformin on complications in over-weight patients with type 2 diabetes (UKPDS 34). Lancet. 1998;**352**:854-865. erratum 1998;352:1557

[10] UK Prospective Diabetes Study Group. Intensive blood-glucose control with sulphonylureas or insulin compared with conventional treatment and risk of complications in patients with type 2 diabetes (UKPDS 33). Lancet. 1998;**352**:837-853. erratum 1999;354:602

[11] UK Prospective Diabetes Study Group. Efficacy of atenolol and captopril in reducing risk of macrovascular and microvascular complications in type 2 diabetes: UKPDS 39. BMJ. 1998;**317**:713-720

[12] UK Prospective Diabetes Study Group. Tight blood pressure control and risk of macrovascular and microvascular complications in type 2 diabetes: UKPDS 38. BMJ. 1998;**317**:703-713. erratum 1999;38:29

[13] Diabetic Retinopathy Study Research Group. Preliminary report on effects of photocoagulation therapy. American Journal of Ophthalmology. 1976;**81**:383-396. DOI: 10.1016/0002-9394(76)90292-0

[14] Diabetic Retinopathy Study Research Group. Photocoagulation treatment of

proliferative diabetic retinopathy: The second report of diabetic retinopathy study findings. Ophthalmology. 1978;**85**:82-106. DOI: 10.1016/S0161-6420(78)35693-1

[15] Early Treatment Diabetic Retinopathy Study Research Group. Early treatment diabetic retinopathy study design and baseline patient characteristics; ETDRS report number 7. Ophthalmology. 1991;**98**:741-756. DOI: 10.1016/S0161-6420(13)38009-9

[16] Early Treatment Diabetic Retinopathy Study Research Group. Fundus photographic risk factors for progression of diabetic retinopathy. ETDRS report number 12. Ophthalmology. 1991;**98**:823-833. DOI: 10.1016/S0161-6420(13)38014-2

[17] Early Treatment Diabetic Retinopathy Study Research Group. Early photocoagulation for diabetic retinopathy. ETDRS report number 9. Ophthalmology. 1991;**98**:766-785. DOI: 10.1016/S0161-6420(13)38011-7

[18] Available from: https://www.public.jaeb.org/drcrnet [Accessed: January 02, 2024]

[19] Yang KB, Feng H, Zhang H. Effects of the COVID-19 pandemic on anti-vascular endothelial growth factor treatment in China. Frontiers in Medicine (Lausanne). 2020;7:576275

[20] DA Paulus YM. A conversation with Dr. Paulus, MD, FACS, on endpoint management™ during COVID. Retina Today. 2020;**15**(7)

[21] Everett LA, Paulus YM. Laser therapy in the treatment of diabetic retinopathy and diabetic macular Edema. Current Diabetes Reports. 2021;**21**(9):35. DOI: 10.1007/s11892-021-01403-6

[22] Fogli S, Del Re M, Rofi E, Posarelli C, Figus M, Danesi R. Clinical pharmacology of intravitreal anti-VEGF drugs. Eye. 2018;**32**:1010-1020

[23] Grisanti S, Ziemssen F. Bevacizumab: Off-label use in ophthalmology. Indian Journal of Ophthalmology. 2007;**55**(6):417-420. DOI: 10.4103/0301-4738.36474

[24] Carmeliet P. Mechanisms of angiogenesis and arteriogenesis. Nature Medicine. 2000;**6**(4):389-395. DOI: 10.1038/74651

[25] Miller JW, Adamis AP, Shima DT, et al. Vascular endothelial growth factor/vascular permeability factor is temporally and spatially correlated with ocular angiogenesis in a primate model. The American Journal of Pathology. 1994;**145**(3):574-584. DOI: 10.1097/00006982-199515020-00021

[26] Nguyen QD, Brown DM, Marcus DM, et al. Ranibizumab for diabetic macular edema: Results from 2 phase III randomized trials: RISE and RIDE. Ophthalmology. 2012;**119**(4):789-801. DOI: 10.1016/j.ophtha.2011.12.039

[27] Heier JS, Korobelnik J-F, Brown DM, et al. Intravitreal aflibercept for diabetic macular edema: 148-week results from the VISTA and VIVID studies. Ophthalmology. 2016;**123**(11):2376-2385. DOI: 10.1016/j.ophtha.2016.07.032

[28] Papadopoulos N, Martin J, Ruan Q, et al. Binding and neutralization of vascular endothelial growth factor (VEGF) and related ligands by VEGF trap, ranibizumab and bevacizumab. Angiogenesis. 2012;**15**(2):171-185. DOI: 10.1007/s10456-011-9249-6

[29] Writing Committee for the Diabetic Retinopathy Clinical Research Network,

Gross JG, Glassman AR, Jampol LM, et al. Panretinal photocoagulation vs intravitreous ranibizumab for proliferative diabetic retinopathy: A randomized clinical trial. Journal of the American Medical Association. 2015;**314**(20):2137-2146. DOI: 10.1001/jama.2015.15217

[30] Bhavsar AR, Torres K, Beck RW, et al. Randomized clinical trial evaluating intravitreal ranibizumab or saline for vitreous hemorrhage from proliferative diabetic retinopathy. JAMA Ophthalmology. 2013;**131**(3):283-293. DOI: 10.1001/jamaophthalmol.2013.2015

[31] Falavarjani KG, Nguyen QD. Adverse events and complications associated with intravitreal injection of anti-VEGF agents: A review of literature. Eye. 2013;**27**:787-794

[32] Shah SM, Khanna CL, Yamanuha J, Bakri SJ. "Glaucomatous fields" after monthly intravitreal injections: Normal tension glaucoma or a mimicker. American Journal of Ophthalmology Case Reports. 2020;**20**:100904

[33] Scappaticci FA, Skillings JR, Holden SN, et al. Arterial thromboembolic events in patients with metastatic carcinoma treated with chemotherapy and bevacizumab. Journal of the National Cancer Institute. 2007;**99**(16):1232-1239. DOI: 10.1093/jnci/djm086

[34] Avery RL, Gordon GM. Systemic safety of prolonged monthly anti-vascular endothelial growth factor therapy for diabetic macular edema: A systematic review and meta-analysis. JAMA Ophthalmology. 2016;**134**(1):21-29. DOI: 10.1001/jamaophthalmol.2015.4070

[35] Jiao C, Eliott D, Spee C, et al. Apoptosis and angiofibrosis in diabetic tractional membranes after vascular endothelial growth factor inhibition: Results of a prospective trial. Report No. 2. Retina. Feb 2019;**39**(2):265-273. DOI: 10.1097/IAE.0000000000001952

[36] Kuiper EJ, Van Nieuwenhoven FA, de Smet MD, et al. The angio-fibrotic switch of VEGF and CTGF in proliferative diabetic retinopathy. PLoS One. 2008;**3**(7):e2675. DOI: 10.1371/journal.pone.0002675

[37] Arevalo JF, Sanchez JG, Saldarriaga L, et al. Pan American collaborative retina study group. Retinal detachment after bevacizumab. Ophthalmology. 2011;**118**(11):2304.e3-2304.e7. DOI: 10.1016/j.ophtha.2011.05.015

[38] Zhang X, Zeng H, Bao S, Wang N, Gillies MC. Diabetic macular edema: New concepts in patho-physiology and treatment. Cell & Bioscience. 2014;**4**:27

[39] Wells JA, Glassman AR, Ayala AR, Jampol LM, Bressler NM, Bressler SB, et al. Aflibercept, bevacizumab, or ranibizumab for diabetic macular edema: Two-year results from a comparative effectiveness randomized clinical trial. Ophthalmology. 2016;**123**:1351-1359

[40] Jonas JB, Söfker A. Intraocular injection of crystalline cortisone as adjunctive treatment of diabetic macular edema. American Journal of Ophthalmology. 2001;**132**:425-427

[41] Boyer DS, Yoon YH, Belfort R Jr, Bandello F, Maturi RK, Augustin AJ, et al. Three-year, randomized, sham-controlled trial of dexamethasone intravitreal implant in patients with diabetic macular edema. Ophthalmology. 2014;**121**:1904-1914

[42] Mathew R, Pearce E, Muniraju R, Abdel-Hay A, Sivaprasad S. Monthly

OCT monitoring of Ozurdex for macular oedema related to retinal vascular diseases: Re-treatment strategy (OCTOME report 1). Eye (London, England). 2014;**28**:318-326

[43] Campochiaro PA, Hafiz G, Shah SM, Bloom S, Brown DM, Busquets M, et al. Sustained ocular delivery of fluocinolone acetonide by an intravitreal insert. Ophthalmology. 2010;**117**:1393-19e3

[44] Campochiaro PA, Brown DM, Pearson A, Chen S, Boyer D, Ruiz-Moreno J, et al. Sustained delivery fluocinolone acetonide vitreous inserts provide benefit for at least 3 years in patients with diabetic macular edema. Ophthalmology. 2012;**119**:2125-2132

[45] Eaton A, Koh SS, Jimenez J, Riemann CD. The USER study: A chart review of patients receiving a 0.2 μg/day fluocinolone acetonide implant for diabetic macular edema. Ophthalmology and Therapy. 2019;**8**:51-62

[46] Pochopien M, Beiderbeck A, McEwan P, Zur R, Toumi M, Aballéa S, et al. Cost-effectiveness of fluocinolone acetonide implant (ILUVIEN®) in UK patients with chronic diabetic macular oedema considered insufficiently responsive to available therapies. BMC Health Services Research. 2019;**19**:22

[47] Callanan DG, Loewenstein A, Patel SS, Massin P, Corcóstegui B, Li XY, et al. A multicenter, 12-month randomized study comparing dexamethasone intravitreal implant with ranibizumab in patients with diabetic macular edema. Graefe's Archive for Clinical and Experimental Ophthalmology. 2017;**255**:463-473

[48] Gillies MC, Lim LL, Campain A, Quin GJ, Salem W, Li J, et al. A randomized clinical trial of intravitreal bevacizumab versus intravitreal dexamethasone for diabetic macular edema: The BEVORDEX study. Ophthalmology. 2014;**121**:2473-2481

[49] Raman R, Bhende M. Diabetic macular edema. Scientific Journal of Medical & Vision Research Foundations. 2015;**XXXIII**:50-56

[50] Elman MJ, Aiello LP, Beck RW, Bressler NM, Bressler SB, Edwards AR. Randomized trial evaluating ranibizumab plus prompt or deferred laser or triamcinolone plus prompt laser for diabetic macular edema. Ophthalmology. 2010;**117**:1064-1077

[51] Aiello LP, Beck RW, Bressler NM, Browning DJ, Chalam KV, Davis M. Rationale for the diabetic retinopathy clinical research network treatment protocol for center-involved diabetic macular edema. Ophthalmology. 2011;**118**:e5-e14

[52] Cekiç O, Bardak Y, Tiğ US, Yildizoğlu U, Bardak H. Quantitative evaluation of reduction of plaque-like hard exudates in diabetic macular edema after intravitreal triamcinolone injection. International Ophthalmology. 2008;**28**(2):95-99. DOI: 10.1007/s10792-007-9120-3

[53] Wenick AS, Bressler NM. Diabetic macular edema: Current and emerging therapies. Middle East African Journal of Ophthalmology. 2012;**19**:4-12

[54] Payne JF, Wykoff CC, Clark WL, Bruce BB, Boyer DS, Brown DM. Randomized trial of treat and extend ranibizumab with and without navigated laser versus monthly dosing for diabetic macular edema: TREX-DME 2-year outcomes. American Journal of Ophthalmology. 2019;**202**:91-99

[55] Karim R, Tang B. Use of antivascular endothelial growth factor for diabetic

macular edema. Clinical Ophthalmology. 2010;**4**:493-517

[56] Regillo CD, Callanan DG, Do DV, Fine HF, Holekamp NM, Kuppermann BD. Use of corticosteroids in the treatment of patients with diabetic macular edema who have a suboptimal response to anti-VEGF: Recommendations of an expert panel. Ophthalmic Surgery, Lasers & Imaging Retina. 2017;**48**:291-301

[57] Mukkamala L, Bhagat N, Zarbin MA. Practical lessons from protocol I for the management of diabetic macular edema. Developments in Ophthalmology. 2017;**60**:91-108

[58] Amoaku WM, Ghanchi F, Bailey C, Banerjee S, Banerjee S, Downey L. Diabetic retinopathy and diabetic macular oedema pathways and management: UK consensus working group. Eye. 2020;**34**:1-51

[59] Australian Government, Department of Health, Therapeutic Goods Administration. Product information for AusPAR: Lucentis, ranibizumab, Novartis pharmaceuticals Australia, PM-2013-00985-1-5. 2014

[60] Chen Y-Y, Chen P-Y, Chen F-T, Chen YJ, Wang JK. Comparison of efficacy of intravitreal ranibizumab between non-vitrectomized and vitrectomized eyes with diabetic macular edema. International Ophthalmology. 2018;**38**:293-299

[61] Papastefanou VP, Dooley I, Zambarakji H. Management of macular edema in vitrectomized patients with diabetes. Expert Review of Ophthalmology. 2018;**13**:87-103

[62] Machemer R, Buettner H, Norton RWD, Parel JM. Vitrectomy in the management of severe diabetic retinopathies. Trans Am Acad Ophthalmol Otolayngol. 1971;**75**(4):813-820

[63] Early vitrectomy for severe vitreous hemorrhage in diabetic retinopathy. Two-year results of a randomized trial. Diabetic retinopathy vitrectomy study report 2. The diabetic retinopathy vitrectomy study research group. Archives of Ophthalmology. 1985;**103**:1644-1652

[64] Tan Y, Fukutomi A, Sun MT, Durkin S, Gilhotra J, Chan WO. Anti-VEGF crunch syndrome in proliferative diabetic retinopathy: A review. Survey of Ophthalmology. 2021;**66**(6):926-932

[65] Thompson JT, Bustrop S, Michels RG, Rice TA. Results and prognostic factors in vitrectomy for diabetic traction retinal detachment of macula. Archives of Ophthalmology. 1987;**105**:497-502

[66] Yang CM, Su PY, Yeh PT, Chen MS. Combined rhegmatogenous and traction retinal detachment in proliferative diabetic retinopathy: Clinical manifestations and surgical outcome. Canadian Journal of Ophthalmology. 2008;**43**:192-198

[67] Gupta V, Arevalo JF. Surgical management of diabetic retinopathy. Middle East African Journal of Ophthalmology. 2013;**20**(4):283-292

[68] Fathy C, Patel S, Sternberg P Jr, Kohanim S. Disparities in adherence to screening guidelines for diabetic retinopathy in the United States: A comprehensive review and guide for future directions. Seminars in Ophthalmology. 2016;**31**(4):364-377

[69] Orji A, Rani PK, Narayanan R, Sahoo NK, Das T. The economic burden of diabetic retinopathy care

at a tertiary eye care center in South India. Indian Journal of Ophthalmology. 2021;**69**(3):666-670. DOI: 10.4103/ijo.IJO_1538_20

[70] Ranade SV, Wieland MR, Tam T, Rea JC, Horvath J, Hieb AR, et al. The port delivery system with ranibizumab: A new paradigm for long-acting retinal drug delivery. Drug Delivery. 2022;**29**(1):1326-1334

[71] Lim JI, Fung AE, Wieland M, Hung D, Wong V. Sustained-release intravitreal liquid drug delivery using triamcinolone acetonide for cystoid macular edema in retinal vein occlusion. Ophthalmology. 2011;**118**(7):1416-1422

[72] Kalogeropoulos D, Kalogeropoulos C, Stefaniotou M, Neofytou M. The role of tele-ophthalmology in diabetic retinopathy screening. Journal of Optometry. 2020;**13**(4):262-268

[73] Padhy SK, Takkar B, Chawla R, Kumar A. Artificial intelligence in diabetic retinopathy: A natural step to the future. Indian Journal of Ophthalmology. 2019;**67**(7):1004-1009

[74] Tan TE, Wong TY. Diabetic retinopathy: Looking forward to 2030. Frontiers in Endocrinology (Lausanne). 2023;**13**:1077669. DOI: 10.3389/fendo.2022.1077669

[75] Sohn EH, Han IC, Abramoff MD. Diabetic retinal neurodegeneration-should we redefine retinopathy from diabetes? JAMA Ophthalmology. 2019;**137**(10):1132-1133. DOI: 10.1001/jamaophthalmol.2019.2536

[76] Chen X, Nie C, Gong Y, Zhang Y, Jin X, Wei S, et al. Peripapillary retinal nerve fiber layer changes in preclinical diabetic retinopathy: A meta-analysis. PLoS One. 2015;**10**:e0125919. DOI: 10.1371/journal.pone.0125919

[77] Aschauer J, Pollreisz A, Karst S, Hülsmann M, Hajdu D, Datlinger F, et al. Longitudinal analysis of microvascular perfusion and neurodegenerative changes in early type 2 diabetic retinal disease. The British Journal of Ophthalmology. 2022;**106**(4):528-533. DOI: 10.1136/bjophthalmol-2020-317322

[78] Obara EA, Hannibal J, Heegaard S, Fahrenkrug J. Loss of melanopsin-expressing retinal ganglion cells in patients with diabetic retinopathy. Investigative Ophthalmology & Visual Science. 2017;**58**:2187-2192. DOI: 10.1167/iovs.16-21168

[79] Choudhry N, Duker JS, Freund KB, Kiss S, Querques G, Rosen R, et al. Classification and guidelines for widefield imaging: Recommendations from the international widefield imaging study group. Ophthalmology Retina. 2019;**3**:843-849. DOI: 10.1016/j.oret.2019.05.007

[80] Byberg S, Vistisen D, Diaz L, Charles MH, Hajari JN, Valerius M, et al. Optos wide-field imaging versus conventional camera imaging in Danish patients with type 2 diabetes. Acta Ophthalmologica. 2019;**97**:815-820. DOI: 10.1111/aos.14118

[81] Silva PS, El-Rami H, Barham R, Gupta A, Fleming A, van Hemert J, et al. Hemorrhage and/or microaneurysm severity and count in ultrawide field images and early treatment diabetic retinopathy study photography. Ophthalmology. 2017;**124**:970-976. DOI: 10.1016/j.ophtha.2017.02.012

[82] Sadda SR, Nittala MG, Taweebanjongsin W, Verma A, Velaga SB, Alagorie AR, et al. Quantitative assessment of the severity of diabetic retinopathy. American Journal of Ophthalmology. 2020;**218**:342-352. DOI: 10.1016/j.ajo.2020.05.021

[83] Sun Z, Yang D, Tang Z, Ng DS, Cheung CY. Optical coherence tomography angiography in diabetic retinopathy: An updated review. Eye (London, England). 2021;**35**(1):149-161. DOI: 10.1038/s41433-020-01233-y

[84] Nesper PL, Roberts PK, Onishi AC, Chai H, Liu L, Jampol LM, et al. Quantifying microvascular abnormalities with increasing severity of diabetic retinopathy using optical coherence tomography angiography. Investigative Ophthalmology & Visual Science. 2017;**58**:BIO307-BIO315. DOI: 10.1167/iovs.17-21787

[85] Tsai ASH, Jordan-Yu JM, Gan ATL, Teo KYC, Tan GSW, Lee SY, et al. Diabetic macular ischemia: Influence of optical coherence tomography angiography parameters on changes in functional outcomes over one year. Investigative Ophthalmology & Visual Science. 2021;**62**:9. DOI: 10.1167/iovs.62.1.9

[86] Ting DSW, Pasquale LR, Peng L, Campbell JP, Lee AY, Raman R, et al. Artificial intelligence and deep learning in ophthalmology. The British Journal of Ophthalmology. 2019;**103**:167-175. DOI: 10.1136/bjophthalmol-2018-313173

[87] Gulshan V, Peng L, Coram M, Stumpe MC, Wu D, Narayanaswamy A, et al. Development and validation of a deep learning algorithm for detection of diabetic retinopathy in retinal fundus photographs. JAMA. 2016;**316**:2402-2410. DOI: 10.1001/jama.2016.17216

[88] Abràmoff MD, Lavin PT, Birch M, Shah N, Folk JC. Pivotal trial of an autonomous AI-based diagnostic system for detection of diabetic retinopathy in primary care offices. npj Digital Medicine. 2018;**1**:39. DOI: 10.1038/s41746-018-0040-6

[89] Bhaskaranand M, Ramachandra C, Bhat S, Cuadros J, Nittala MG, Sadda SR, et al. The value of automated diabetic retinopathy screening with the EyeArt system: A study of more than 100,000 consecutive encounters from people with diabetes. Diabetes Technology & Therapeutics. 2019;**21**:635-643. DOI: 10.1089/dia.2019.0164

[90] Xie Y, Nguyen QD, Hamzah H, Lim G, Bellemo V, Gunasekeran DV, et al. Artificial intelligence for teleophthalmology-based diabetic retinopathy screening in a national programme: An economic analysis modelling study. The Lancet Digital Health. 2020;**2**:e240-e249. DOI: 10.1016/S2589-7500(20)30060-1

[91] Schlegl T, Waldstein SM, Bogunovic H, Endstraßer F, Sadeghipour A, Philip A-M, et al. Fully automated detection and quantification of macular fluid in OCT using deep learning. Ophthalmology. 2018;**125**:549-558. DOI: 10.1016/j.ophtha.2017.10.031